...tional Physical ...tion Standards

FOURTH EDITION

...APE AMERICA –
...LTH AND PHYSICAL EDUCATORS

Na...
Educa...

SOCIETY O...

National Physical Education Standards

FOURTH EDITION

SHAPE AMERICA – SOCIETY OF HEALTH AND PHYSICAL EDUCATORS

PRINCIPAL WRITERS

Cory Dixon, PhD

Suzanna Dillon, PhD, CAPE

Fran Cleland, PED

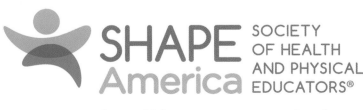

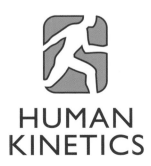

Library of Congress Cataloging-in-Publication Data

Names: SHAPE America (Organization), author.
Title: National physical education standards / SHAPE America - Society of
  Health and Physical Educators ; principal writers Cory Dixon, Suzanna
  Dillon, Fran Cleland.
Other titles: National standards & grade-level outcomes for K-12 physical
  education
Description: Fourth edition. | Champaign, IL : Human Kinetics, 2025. |
  Revised edition of: National standards & grade-level outcomes for K-12
  physical education. 2014. | Includes bibliographical references.
Identifiers: LCCN 2024004266 (print) | LCCN 2024004267 (ebook) | ISBN
  9781718230835 (paperback) | ISBN 9781718230842 (epub) | ISBN
  9781718230859 (pdf)
Subjects: LCSH: Physical education and training--Standards--United States.
  | BISAC: EDUCATION / Teaching/Subjects/Physical Education
Classification: LCC GV365 .A48 2025 (print) | LCC GV365 (ebook) | DDC
  613.7/071--dc23/eng/20240213
LC record available at https://lccn.loc.gov/2024004266
LC ebook record available at https://lccn.loc.gov/2024004267

ISBN: 978-1-7182-3083-5 (print)

Acquisitions Editor: Mark Manross; **Managing Editor:** Anna Lan Seaman; **Copyeditor:** Marissa Wold Uhrina; **Permissions Managers:** Adam Pomerantz and Laurel Mitchell; **Senior Graphic Designers:** Nancy Rasmus and Sean Roosevelt; **Cover Designer:** Keri Evans, **Cover Design Specialist:** Susan Rothermel Allen; **Photograph (cover):** FatCamera/E+/Getty Images; SolStock/E+/ Getty Images; © Human Kinetics; **Photo Asset Manager:** Laura Fitch; **Photo Production Manager:** Jason Allen, **Senior Art Manager:** Kelly Hendren; **Illustrations:** © Human Kinetics, unless otherwise noted; **Printer:** Walsworth

Printed in the United States of America   10 9 8 7 6 5 4 3 2 1

The paper in this book was manufactured using responsible forestry methods.

Human Kinetics
1607 N. Market Street
Champaign, IL 61820
USA

United States and International
Website: **US.HumanKinetics.com**
Email: info@hkusa.com
Phone: 1-800-747-4457

Canada
Website: **Canada.HumanKinetics.com**
Email: info@hkcanada.com

SHAPE America – Society of Health and Physical Educators
PO Box 225
Annapolis Junction, MD 20701
Website: **www.shapeamerica.org**
Phone: 1-800-213-7193

E9565

CONTENTS

STATEMENT OF SUPPORT FROM THE AMERICAN FEDERATION OF TEACHERS

Students enter school with a vast array of social, emotional, physical, and academic needs. SHAPE America's effort to update the National Health Education Standards and the National Physical Education Standards is a crucial part of the work to address these needs and improve children's well-being. The new standards bolster students' learning by doing; skills-based health education best equips students to lead active and healthy lifelong wellness journeys.

Educators across the nation face deprofessionalization and demoralization—we see it and fight it daily. The AFT applauds SHAPE America for understanding that educators today need a culture of collaboration, proper teaching and learning conditions, and real voice and agency. Inclusive task forces worked deliberately and thoughtfully to develop the updated National HE Standards and National PE Standards through admirably open and iterative engagement. As a result, the new standards reflect educators' commitment to real solutions for children's well-being.

Randi Weingarten
President, American Federation of Teachers

ACKNOWLEDGMENTS

SHAPE America wishes to acknowledge the following members of the taskforce who worked diligently for three years to revise the 2024 SHAPE America National Physical Education Standards.

Brad Brummel, MEd, Cochair
Coordinator of Physical Education, Health, and
Engagement Activities
Springfield Public Schools, Missouri

Sally Jones, PhD, Cochair
Physical Education Adapted Physical Education
Consultant
Asheville, NC

Amanda Amtmanis, MEd
Physical Education Teacher
Middletown Public Schools, Connecticut

Langston Clark, PhD
Associate Professor
University of Texas at San Antonio

Fran Cleland, PED
Professor Emeritus
West Chester University, Pennsylvania

Kelly Cornett, MS
Health Scientist
Centers for Disease Control and Prevention

Dan DeJager, MS, NBCT
Physical Education Teacher
San Juan Unified School District, California

Suzanna Dillon, PhD, CAPE
Associate Professor
Texas Woman's University

Cory Dixon, PhD
Assistant Professor
Rowan University, New Jersey

Jonathan Jones, MS
Physical Education Resource Teacher
Prince George's County Public Schools, Maryland

Paulo Ribeiro, PhD
Physical Education Teacher
Parkway School District, Missouri

Clancy Seymour, EdD
Associate Professor
Canisius University, New York

CHAPTER 1

Introduction

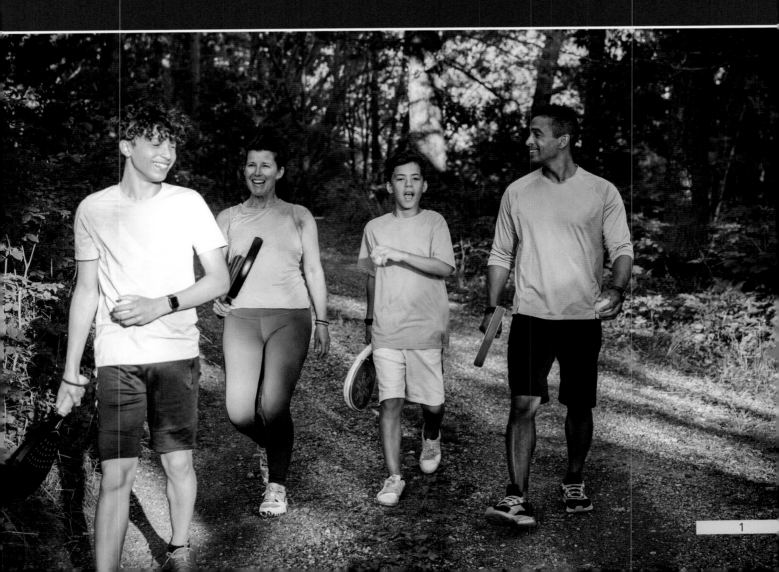

This book introduces physical educators and other key constituents to the revised *National Physical Education Standards*. First, it documents the revision process, including selected empirical evidence for restructuring the *National Standards and Grade-Level Outcomes for K-12 Physical Education*, published in 2014. Second, the book clarifies the framework that is the national standards in preK-12 physical education including support for physical educators on how to use the standards to guide their practice. Third, it clarifies the essential content for preK-12 physical education for key constituents (e.g., students, parents, curriculum directors, administrators, boards of education, and policy makers). Fourth, the appendixes provide critical elements of movement skills, a movement framework used to create Learning Progressions, scope and sequence, and a curriculum map and planning guide. As in the previous editions, to assist readers' understanding, key concepts are presented in **bold**, and corresponding definitions appear in the glossary.

The Standards Revision Process

The 2024 edition of the National Physical Education Standards, which includes Grade-Span Learning Indicators, has been drafted using a range of diverse revision techniques. Those techniques included a willingness to engage with and adapt to a philosophical paradigm shift informed by (1) collaboration with many of the leading researchers and practitioners in the field; (2) an investigation into the content standards of our colleagues internationally; (3) consultation with our field's top diversity, equity, and inclusion (DEI) experts; (4) sifting through evidence-based empirical research; and (5) the analyses of multiple rounds of qualitative and quantitative data in the form of public review and feedback. This section of the chapter highlights the main changes since the third edition (SHAPE America, 2014).

The past, present, and future of physical education and the field's overall contribution to the physical literacy and general well-being of students were considered while amending the previous standards and outcomes. For example, the SHAPE America National Physical Education Standards Task Force created a document outlining guiding principles that detail pedagogical practices teachers observe and implement to ensure proper and equitable access to physical education and assist teachers in helping students find movement more meaningful. These research-based guiding principles helped to shape the early stages of the revision process. They assisted the task force with clarifying pedagogical practices that enhance students' learning of physical education content.

Of notable mention is the expansion of the term *physical literacy*. The previous edition of the national standards textbook defined physical literacy as "the ability to move with competence and confidence in a wide variety of physical activities in multiple environments that benefit the healthy development of the whole person" (SHAPE America, 2014, p. 4), and it identified physical literacy as a primary goal of physical education. Physical literacy, however, is commonly conceptualized as a fixed state to be achieved in the future by a student who has successfully matriculated from the physical education curriculum. As presented in the previous standards documents, physical literacy does not fully capture the essence of the developmental journey students undergo throughout their time as physical education students.

For this reason, in this book, the term *physical literacy* is replaced by the **physical literacy journey**. The revised national standards focus on the well-being of the whole person *and* their physical literacy journey. These national standards consider the psychomotor, cognitive, social, and affective learning domains essential to facilitating the physical literacy journey of preK-12 learners. The physical literacy journey involves the ongoing acquisition and application of knowledge, skills, and dispositions necessary for engagement in a lifetime of healthful and meaningful physical activity. These revised national standards are responsive to the developmental stages of preK-12 learners, which are discussed in chapters 3 through 6, and are designed to help everyone strive to reach their full potential within each grade span.

The physical literacy journey is inclusive; it is for *all individuals* regardless of their ability, age, class, gender, or race. It is based on the premise that everyone can acquire and apply knowledge and skills to move more confidently in physical activities that are motivating and enjoyable to the individual. That said, facilitating the physical literacy journey of preK-12 learners is dependent on quality instruction and opportunities to become more skilled, knowledgeable, and confident movers. These national standards have been designed so that teachers can build relevant and developmentally appropriate learning experiences that engage all preK-12 learners in their own meaningful physical literacy journey.

Another key change is that the fourth iteration of the national standards for preK-12 physical education has moved from five standards to four. The 2014

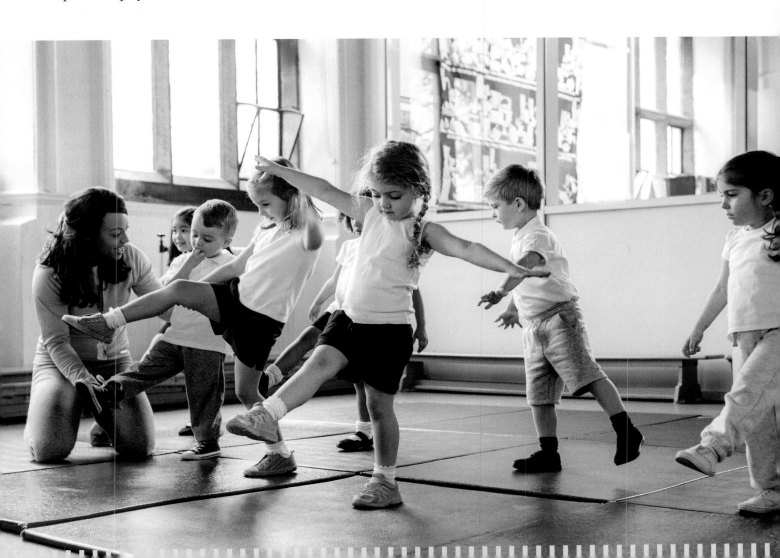

Standard 3 (The physically literate individual demonstrates the knowledge and skills to achieve and maintain a health-enhancing level of physical activity and fitness.) has been integrated into the Learning Indicators addressing the revised Standard 1 (Develops a variety of motor skills.) and Standard 2 (Applies knowledge related to movement and fitness concepts.). The task force decided that a stand-alone fitness standard led to many physical education programs focusing solely on physical fitness, thus not providing a balanced curriculum that meets the needs and interests of all students. Other changes include acknowledging the social domain as a domain of learning in Standard 3 (Develops social skills through movement.). Standard 4 (Develops personal skills, identifies personal benefits of movement, and chooses to engage in physical activity.) addresses the affective domain.

Another key change is the move from Grade-Level Outcomes to Grade-Span Learning Indicators (i.e., preK-2, grades 3-5, grades 6-8, and grades 9-12) with associated Learning Progressions. The **Grade-Span Learning Indicators** articulate the content areas while the **Learning Progressions** provide sample sequential tasks that address a range of skill abilities from pre-kindergarten through high school. The change from Grade-Level Outcomes to Grade-Span Learning Indicators is based on motor development research and is discussed in more depth in this chapter as well as in chapters 3, 4, 5, and 6. The Grade-Span Learning Indicators and associated Learning Progressions are written in a manner that is observable and measurable in order to facilitate appropriate assessment and tracking of student progress within their own physical literacy journey. Additionally, the Grade-Span Learning Indicators and Learning Progressions provide a scope and sequence that leads to progress toward the standards and ultimately prepare the individual to continue their physical literacy journey through adulthood. It should be noted that while considerable research has been completed in the field of physical education since the publication of the *National Standards and Grade-Level Outcomes for K-12 Physical Education* (2014), research in motor development is highlighted within this chapter due to its importance in the restructuring of the standards and Grade-Span Learning Indicators.

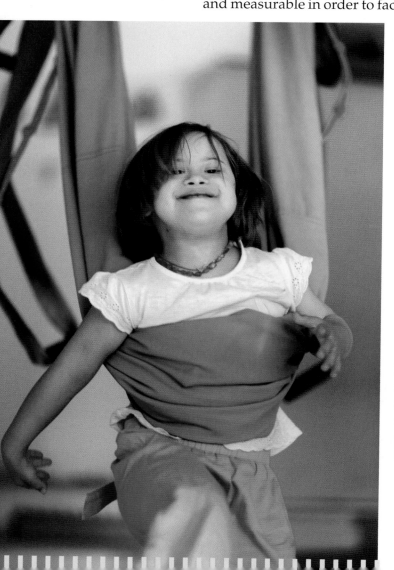

Research in Motor Development Affecting Revisions

Research in motor development provides the foundation for the restructuring of the national standards and Grade-Span Learning Indicators for preK-12 physical education. Developmental principles, including the principle that development is **age-related, not age-dependent**, support the adoption of grade spans. Skill development is not dependent on one's age but on opportunities for practice, instruction, and encouragement. Thus, it would not be expected to have all children in a second-grade class at the same stage of motor skill development.

The **Hourglass Model** is a helpful heuristic for conceptualizing, describing, and explaining the process of motor development (see figure 1.1). The two sources of sand include the environment and heredity, both of which influence the process of motor development. Hereditary factors are more prominent in the first two phases of motor development, whereas instruction, practice, encouragement, and ecology of the environment play a significant role within the fundamental and specialized movement phases of motor development. Each phase of motor development also includes specific stages that describe the characteristics of skill development during that stage. Detailed information about the phases and stages of motor development will be explained in chapters 3, 4, 5, and 6. Understanding the phases and stages of motor development is critical to the design of developmentally appropriate instructional experiences for preK-12 students.

The preK-2 Grade-Span Learning Indicators and associated Learning Progressions reflect children's development within the **fundamental movement phase** (see chapter 3). Similarly, the Grade-Span Learning Indicators and associated Learning Progressions for grades 3-5 reflect children's development within the fundamental movement phase and subsequent **specialized movement phase** (see chapter 4). Finally, the Grade-Span Learning Indicators and associated Learning Progressions for grades 6-8 and 9-12 reflect adolescents' development within the specialized movement phase (see chapters 5 and 6).

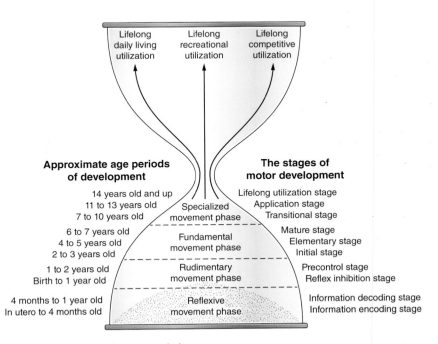

FIGURE 1.1   The Hourglass Model.

Reprinted by permission from J.D. Goodway, J.C. Ozmun, and D.L. Gallahue, *Understanding Motor Development: Infants, Children, Adolescents, and Adults*, 8th ed. (Burlington, MA: Jones & Barlett Learning, 2020), 49.

Use of the Standards in Developing Physical Education Curricula

SHAPE America is committed to advocating for and supporting high-quality physical education programs that provide equitable physical education experiences for all preK-12 students. As a part of that commitment, SHAPE America provides the *National Physical Education Standards* to support states in meeting federal expectations. The United States mandates that states establish standards for every subject and grade level (e.g., Improving America's Schools Act of 1994, Every Student Succeeds Act of 2015). The resources produced by SHAPE America specific to the national standards provide physical educators with guidance on the development of (1) clear and measurable learning goals, (2) instruction, and (3) the assessment of student learning. Whether states choose to adopt the *National Physical Education Standards* directly or choose to use the national standards as a framework to develop physical education content standards that reflect state-level interests, needs, and resources, content standards are essential to the development of standards-based curricula and educational success for our preK-12 learners.

SHAPE America also posits that quality physical education programs facilitate the physical literacy journey of preK-12 learners by providing developmentally appropriate learning experiences across the psychomotor, cognitive, social, and affective learning domains (Bailey et al., 2009; Dettmer, 2005). The revised standards reflect the interdependent nature of learning across all four learning domains in physical education. To that end, these standards are not presented in order of importance. The expectation is that physical education programs should provide preK-12 learners with opportunities to practice, construct, apply, and evaluate their learning across *all* four domains.

Conclusion

The national standards offer physical educators a framework for teaching and learning and provide a trajectory for learning from preK through 12th grade, but they do not prescribe a particular curriculum, teaching methods, or learning activities. The standards articulate what our preK-12 learners are expected to know and be able to do, while the local physical education curriculum describes how physical educators will support students in meeting the standards and progressing in their physical literacy journey.

CHAPTER 2

Reading the National Standards, Grade-Span Learning Indicators, and Learning Progressions

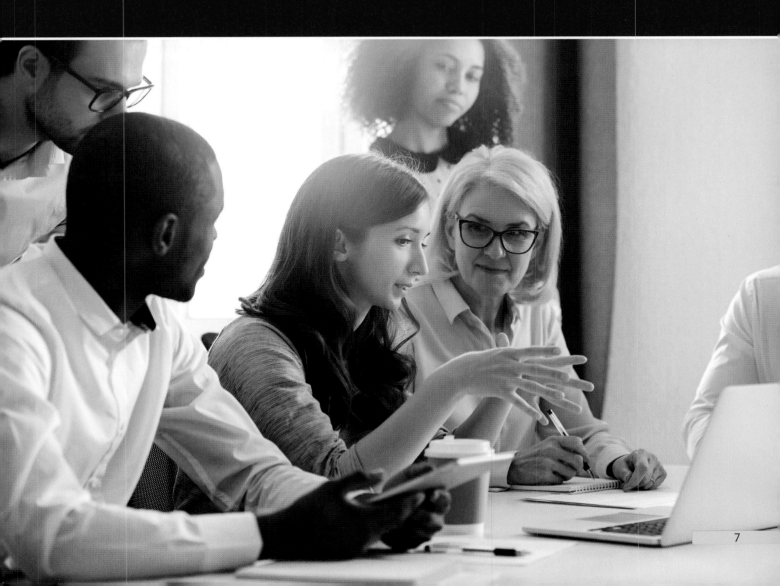

For the past 50 years, content area standards have been used by states and local education agencies as a framework for teaching and learning within content areas, including in physical education (Kober & Rentner, 2020). The 2024 SHAPE America National Physical Education Standards, Grade-Span Learning Indicators and Learning Progressions address learning across the psychomotor, cognitive, affective, and social learning domains, which is essential to supporting preK-12 learners as they progress along their own meaningful physical literacy journey. While the National Physical Education Standards, Grade-Span Learning Indicators, and Learning Progressions articulate the knowledge and skills students are expected to learn across grades preK-12 and provide a general trajectory for that learning, physical literacy is not about mastery but rather is an ongoing process (Castelli et al., 2015). These National PE Standards, along with the corresponding Grade-Span Learning Indicators and Learning Progressions, can be used to create relevant and developmentally appropriate learning experiences that engage all preK-12 learners on a physical literacy journey of holistic competence, to include opportunities to develop the skills, knowledge, confidence, appreciation, and motivation to live an active life—across and beyond their preK-12 years (see figure 2.1).

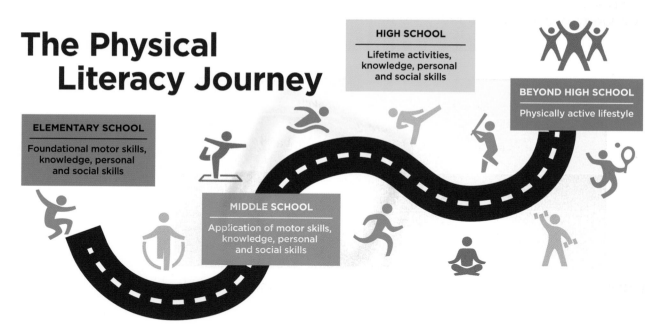

FIGURE 2.1   The process of supporting preK-12 learners on their physical literacy journey through learning experiences in physical education.

The National PE Standards, Grade-Span Learning Indicators, and Learning Progressions presented within this book were developed with the understanding that the goal of high-quality physical education is to support preK-12 students in their physical literacy journey (i.e., the ongoing acquisition and application of knowledge, skills, and dispositions necessary for engagement in a lifetime of healthful and meaningful physical activity) so they have the "ability, confidence, and desire to be physically active for life" (Farrey & Isard, 2015). The current National PE Standards were designed to be responsive to the developmental stages of preK-12 learners and to support physical educators with developing more inclusive, engaging, and meaningful physical education curricula. Through quality instruction and learning experiences in physical education, the National PE Standards, Grade-Span Learning Indicators, and Learning Progressions are designed to ensure that each preK-12 learner accomplishes the following:

■ Develops a variety of motor skills.
■ Applies knowledge related to movement and fitness concepts.
■ Develops social skills through movement.
■ Develops personal skills, identifies personal benefits of movement, and chooses to engage in physical activity.

Please note that the National PE Standards, as presented, are not hierarchical or prioritized in a particular order (see figure 2.2).

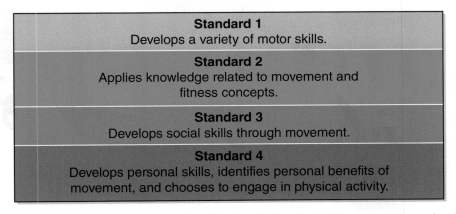

Standard 1
Develops a variety of motor skills.

Standard 2
Applies knowledge related to movement and fitness concepts.

Standard 3
Develops social skills through movement.

Standard 4
Develops personal skills, identifies personal benefits of movement, and chooses to engage in physical activity.

FIGURE 2.2   2024 SHAPE America National Physical Education Standards.

Reading the Grade-Span Learning Indicators

Unlike previous editions, this edition has no Grade-Level Outcomes. Rather, each standard has Grade-Span Learning Indicators with associated Learning Progressions. For each standard, the Grade-Span Learning Indicators are grouped by preK-2, 3-5, 6-8, and 9-12, with the highest grade indicated within the coding structure. Each Grade-Span Learning Indicator is assigned a number, which is not reflective of any hierarchical or prioritized order. This information is combined to create a coding system that identifies each of the standards' Grade-Span Learning Indicators. The coding system allows physical educators to easily locate and use the National PE Standards and their corresponding Grade-Span Learning Indicators. The coding system is structured as follows:

The standard (1, 2, 3, or 4)

The grade span (2, 5, 8, 12)

The Learning Indicator (1, 2, 3, 4, and so on)

Figures 2.3 and 2.4 are examples of the coding system.

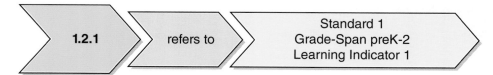

FIGURE 2.3   1.2.1 Demonstrates a variety of locomotor skills with the concepts of space, effort, and relationship awareness.

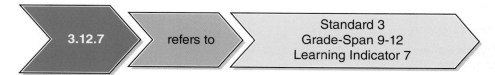

FIGURE 2.4   3.12.7 Thinks critically and solves problems in physical activity settings, both as an individual and in groups.

Within Standard 1 and Standard 2, the Grade-Span Learning Indicators are also grouped by categories, which assists the physical educator with identifying similar Grade-Span Learning Indicators. Table 2.1 presents the categories used for Standard 1 (Develops a variety of motor skills.) by grade span, and table 2.2 presents the categories used for Standard 2 (Applies knowledge related to movement and fitness concepts.) by grade span.

Where appropriate, Learning Progressions for the Grade-Span Learning Indicators provide physical educators with examples of sequential tasks that address a range of skill abilities. The examples of Learning Progressions were designed to assist physical educators with planning and delivering instruction that addresses the varying performance levels that preK-12 students may display and to promote mastery of the Grade-Span Learning Indicators.

As an example, the Learning Progressions for the Grade-Span Learning Indicators for grades 3-5, specific to kicking, are provided in figure 2.5. Across their grades 3-5 experience, students can work toward the Grade-Span Learning Indicator within any of the Learning Progression tasks.

TABLE 2.1 Standard 1 Content Categories Presented by Grade Span

Grades preK-2	Grades 3-5	Grades 6-8	Grades 9-12
Locomotor	Locomotor	Outdoor pursuits	Lifetime activities
Non-locomotor	Dance and rhythms	Dance and rhythms	Dance and rhythms
Bouncing	Non-locomotor	Fitness activities	Fitness activities
Rolling	Target	Target games	Aquatics
Catching and throwing	Striking and fielding	Striking and fielding games	
Kicking and dribbling with feet	Net and wall	Net and wall games	
Striking with hands	Invasion	Invasion games	
Striking with implements	Aquatics	Aquatics	
Dance and rhythms			
Aquatics			

TABLE 2.2 Standard 2 Content Categories Presented by Grade Span

Grades preK-2	Grades 3-5	Grades 6-8	Grades 9-12
Tactics and strategies	Tactics and strategies	Tactics and strategies	Tactics and strategies
Dance and rhythms	Dance and rhythms	Dance and rhythms	Dance and rhythms
Fitness concepts	Fitness concepts	Fitness concepts	Fitness concepts
Physical activity knowledge	Physical activity knowledge	Physical activity knowledge	Physical activity knowledge
Aquatics	Aquatics	Outdoor pursuits	Aquatics
		Aquatics	

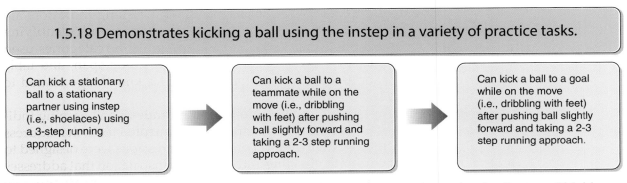

1.5.18 Demonstrates kicking a ball using the instep in a variety of practice tasks.

Can kick a stationary ball to a stationary partner using instep (i.e., shoelaces) using a 3-step running approach. → Can kick a ball to a teammate while on the move (i.e., dribbling with feet) after pushing ball slightly forward and taking a 2-3 step running approach. → Can kick a ball to a goal while on the move (i.e., dribbling with feet) after pushing ball slightly forward and taking a 2-3 step running approach.

FIGURE 2.5 Sample Learning Progression for the Grade-Span Learning Indicator of kicking for grades 3-5.

This flexibility when implementing the standards allows for students in the same class to work at different points along the Learning Progression while still working toward the same Standard and Grade-Span Learning Indicator. While this flexibility supports the use of universal design for learning (CAST, 2018) and differentiated instruction, it does not preclude the need for **adapted physical education** services for students with identified needs in physical education.

If a physical educator suspects that a student may need adapted physical education services to have their needs met in physical education, the educator should follow the special education process that evaluates the student's performance and leads to the development of an **individualized education program (IEP)**. The IEP process is necessary for identifying the **present level of academic achievement and functional performance (PLAAFP)**, the development of individualized goals, and appropriate adapted physical education services, which must all be documented in the IEP. Related to the IEP process, it should be noted that the sample Learning Progressions were not intended to be used as IEP goals, nor should they be considered an exhaustive progression that addresses the learning needs of all students.

As previously mentioned, the change from Grade-Level Outcomes to Grade-Span Learning Indicators is based on motor development research, which will be discussed more fully in chapters 3 through 6. The Grade-Span Learning Indicators and corresponding Learning Progressions also provide physical educators with a scope and sequence to support learners in making progress toward the standards and advancing on their physical literacy journey.

Implications for Teaching Using the Standards

Effective teaching using the standards includes physical educators planning instruction and assessment that is aligned with the standards while also considering the needs and interests of students so that learning experiences are meaningful. Physical educators can use the standards to backward design the local curriculum and corresponding lessons, beginning with identifying the goals of the physical education program (i.e., intended learning outcomes) aligned with the standards and corresponding Grade-Span Learning Indicators. Once the intended learning outcomes (i.e., what the students should know and be able to do as the result of physical education instruction) have been identified, assessment measures can be developed to determine whether student performance meets those goals (i.e., intended learning outcomes). Assessment is critical because it provides evidence of student learning of the skills, knowledge, and behaviors aligned to the standards. Once assessments aligned with the standards have been created, meaningful physical education (MPE) experiences (i.e., learning tasks) can be developed to facilitate learning of the physical education content. See figure 2.6, which explains the backward design process.

As a result of the backward design process, physical educators can (1) clearly establish standards-based learning goals; (2) teach skills, knowledge, and behav-

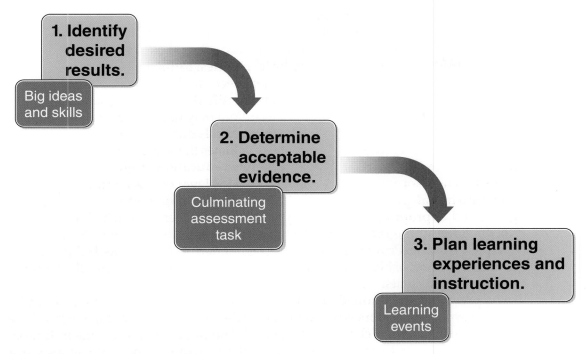

FIGURE 2.6   Understanding by design: the backward design process for curriculum development.

Adapted by permission from G.P. Wiggins and J. McTighe, *Understanding by Design, Expanded 2nd ed.* (Arlington, VA: ASCD. © 2005 by ASCD). All rights reserved.

iors aligned to the standards; (3) formatively assess student learning; (4) provide timely feedback to students to support their achievement of learning goals; and (5) provide opportunities for students to engage with the physical education content and practice the skills and behaviors with an awareness of their individual performance. When physical educators use frequent formative assessments and provide **growth-oriented feedback** focused on individual improvement, students may be more engaged in their learning process and find it more personally relevant.

Meaningful Physical Education

In implementing the standards, physical educators should be mindful that students' desire to be physically active may also be influenced by the "meaningfulness" that they derive from engaging in physical education activities. That is, physical educators should prioritize **meaningful physical education (MPE)** experiences, with their pedagogical decision-making focused on delivering quality and personally relevant experiences for their students that are aligned with the standards and major aims of physical education (Fletcher et al., 2021).

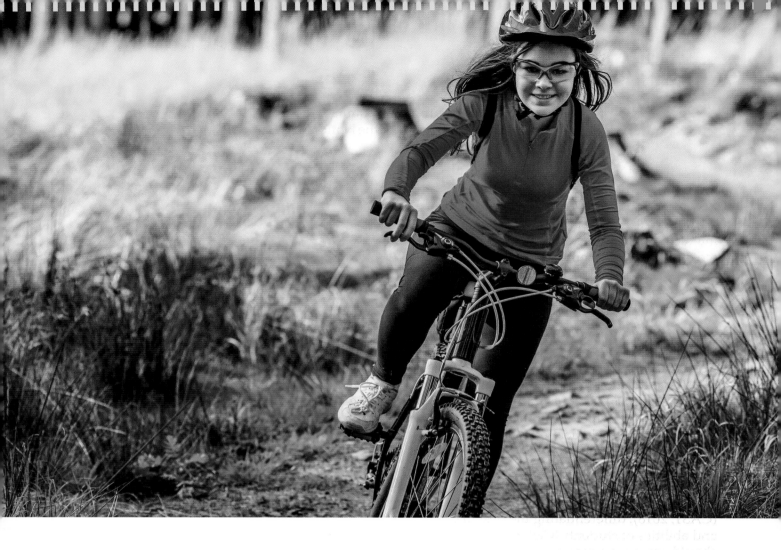

Given that students are more likely to commit to participation in physical activity because of intrinsic motivational factors such as pleasure, joy, and satisfaction (e.g., Cleland Donnelly, 2021; Teixeira et al., 2012), Ennis suggests that physical educators "assist students in their search to find meaningful experiences in which they seek to engage and affiliate with others in an enjoyable physical activity environment" (2017, p. 248). The provision of these MPE experiences to our preK-12 learners reflects best practice.

Gleddie and Harding-Kuriger (2021) suggest that MPE begins with physical educators getting to know their students and better understanding their physical education and movement experiences. They propose that it is worth the time to create opportunities for students to express what make them excited about movement and even find out what kind of movement experiences might create fear or anxiety (2021). For MPE, designing lessons that provide social interaction, challenge, fun, motor competence, personally relevant learning, and delight requires teachers to know not only their content but also their students' developmental needs and interests. Students' reflection on their movement experiences is also essential for understanding if the learning tasks designed are indeed meaningful. The features of a physical education lesson that can contribute to meaningful physical education for children (i.e., social interaction, challenge, fun, motor competence, personally relevant learning, and delight) have been identified by researchers (e.g., Cleland Donnelly, 2021; Fletcher et al., 2021; Walseth et al., 2018) and are discussed in the following section. These features focus on the quality of the learning experiences and how this influences the likelihood of students seeking or avoiding such experiences in the future. It is recommended that physical educators consider these factors when implementing the National PE Standards.

Social Interaction

When physical educators consider how opportunities for social interactions are "organized and structured based on students' needs and desires" (Fletcher et al., 2021, p. 7.), they can cultivate positive student-to-student and student-to-teacher interactions. Fostering the development of personal and social responsibility promotes a sense of community in the physical education classroom and supports children being responsible to each other in making their learning experiences more meaningful (e.g., passing the ball to everyone before scoring or making sure everyone is involved; Azzarito & Ennis, 2003; Lyngstad et al., 2020).

Challenge

Researchers have identified that optimal challenges are critical to students' finding physical education more meaningful (e.g., Dismore & Bailey, 2011; Dyson, 1995; Kretchmar, 2006). The use of student-centered pedagogies fosters inclusivity, encourages the achievement of process-oriented goals, and allows students to adjust their own challenge level—increasing or decreasing challenge to meet individual needs. For example, the use of Mosston and Ashworth's (2008) inclusion style of teaching accommodates individual differences by providing tasks with multiple levels of performance within the same task. The inclusion style of teaching is also consistent with the intent of universal design for learning (CAST, 2018), differentiating the design of instructional tasks to meet the needs and abilities of students (Cleland Donnelly et al., 2017). Physical educators also should consider a measured approach to competition, with the importance of winning and losing being balanced against the achievement of personal bests. Students who perceived themselves as less skilled reported that limiting competition (e.g., keeping team score) while also providing opportunities for "spirited competition" (e.g., keeping class score) led to more meaningful physical education (Beni et al., 2019).

Fun

While the reasons why physical education is fun vary across the preK-12 grades, fun has been clearly identified by students as the primary reason they continue to participate in physical education (Ladwig et al., 2018). Social interaction and challenge were perceived as fun and contributing to MPE by providing opportunities to work with others and be successful in completing hard work with support from others (e.g., Hopple, 2018). In addition, physical educators and students have reported that pairing motor competence with an appropriate level of challenge was perceived as fun, with one student stating, "Now you can have more fun because you know how to play it and you have the right level of challenge" (Beni et al., 2019, p. 615). Physical educators are encouraged to consider creating different levels of challenge by modifying the environment (e.g., performer scaling equipment conditions of size, length, weight, texture) and performer scaling conditions (e.g., space—distance, direction, trajectory, pathway; temporal—speed, rhythm, timing, relationships—alone, partner, small group) as described by Cleland Donnelly and colleagues (2017). When physical educators use these variables to modify instruction and adjust levels of difficulty, they can enhance children's motor competence and contribute to MPE.

Motor Competence

Researchers have reported that physical education is more meaningful when students perceive they are developing motor skill competence (e.g., Beni et al., 2019; Estevan et al., 2021). Though motor competence is an established feature of MPE, caution should be taken in overemphasizing it within physical education because it can contribute to feelings of exclusion or isolation in students who perceive themselves to be less skilled (Fletcher et al., 2021).

Personally Relevant Learning

Physical educators should design learning tasks that help students understand what they are learning, why this learning in physical education is important, and how this learning applies to their lives inside and outside of physical education (Fletcher et al., 2021). The physical education learning tasks should not only increase students' understanding but they also should be perceived as personally and culturally relevant to the students (Braga et al., 2015). This can lead to more buy-in from the students. Decision-making autonomy and choice about their participation also make learning more personally relevant for students (Enright & O'Sullivan, 2010). For example, physical educators can be responsive to students' needs and interests by including students in making decisions and seeking their input on unit and lesson design. When students are provided with opportunities to create or direct their own activities and to take ownership in achieving their goals, they report that physical education is more meaningful (e.g., Dyson, 1995; Houser & Kriellaars, 2023).

Delight

Delight can be developed when physical education experiences lead to students' feeling a genuine sense of accomplishment and fulfillment. These experiences typically take time to develop as students establish and work toward personal goals. While delight may be difficult for some students to articulate, it can be gleaned from students' reflections on their experiences, such as "When you knew what you were doing and working towards something, it meant more" (Chróinín et al., 2023, p. 46) and "I felt so accomplished when I finished the mile. A sense of accomplishment always makes an activity better" (Lynch & Sargent, 2020, p. 636). Goal setting and reflection on progress toward one's goal can facilitate this sense of achievement as well as provide motivation to continue goal setting in the future. The significant investment of effort over time results in meaningful, and perhaps delightful, experiences for the students.

Application of these aforementioned features of a physical education lesson that contributes to meaningful physical education for children is summarized in table 2.3.

TABLE 2.3   Application of Features of Meaningful Physical Education Within Instruction

Feature	Application examples
Social interaction	• Provide students with opportunities to engage individually, with a partner, in a small group, or as a part of a large group. • During gameplay, have students pass to all teammates before taking a shot on the goal. • Provide students with opportunities to engage with the content as a player or participant and in an alternative or peripheral role (e.g., referee, scorekeeper, spotter).
Fun	• Provide students with choice within participation (e.g., use of inclusion-style teaching). • Provide students with opportunities to participate in novel physical activities (e.g., new games or physical activities, social dances) and creative movement experiences (e.g., creating dance routines). • Structure learning tasks so that interpersonal competition is minimized.
Challenge	• Provide opportunities for challenge by choice where students decide to take on a challenge without external pressure from others. • Provide opportunities for goal setting and reflection on goal setting so that students can determine an appropriate level of challenge.
Movement competence	• Provide opportunities for self-evaluation of skill and comfort in performing the skill. • Provide differentiated levels of participation as well as differentiated levels of student support (e.g., visual supports or physical assistance from a teacher or peer). • Emphasize that it is "okay to be a beginner" (Rink, 2004, p.31) when learning a new skill, and honor approximations of the skill as students try new skills and activities.
Personally relevant learning	• Provide opportunities for reflection or discussion of how social and motor skills learned in physical education can be applied outside of physical education. • Ensure learning tasks include information about why a skill is being learned. • Provide opportunities for movement that are culturally relevant to the students and accessible to them within their community.

The Importance of Practice, Critical Elements, Feedback, and Demonstration

In addition to considering the ecology of the physical education environment and the meaningfulness of the learning experiences, physical educators should also understand the role of practice, critical elements, feedback, and demonstration. Physical educators must plan for the use of practice, critical elements, feedback, and demonstration because they are critical to the development of effective learning experiences for students with and without disabilities.

Physical practice involves repetition of movements to learn or improve motor skill performance. **Constant practice** is repeating a skill using the same movement characteristics (i.e., spatial, temporal, and relationship variables). Two examples of constant practice are repetitively performing an underhand toss to a target from the same distance and direction and repetitively performing a sequence of dance steps to the same tempo and rhythm. Constant practice is used when learners have not yet progressed to the mature stage of motor skill development and are acquiring the critical elements (stable features) of a motor skill. The repetition of motor skills through constant practice enhances the rhythmic coordination of

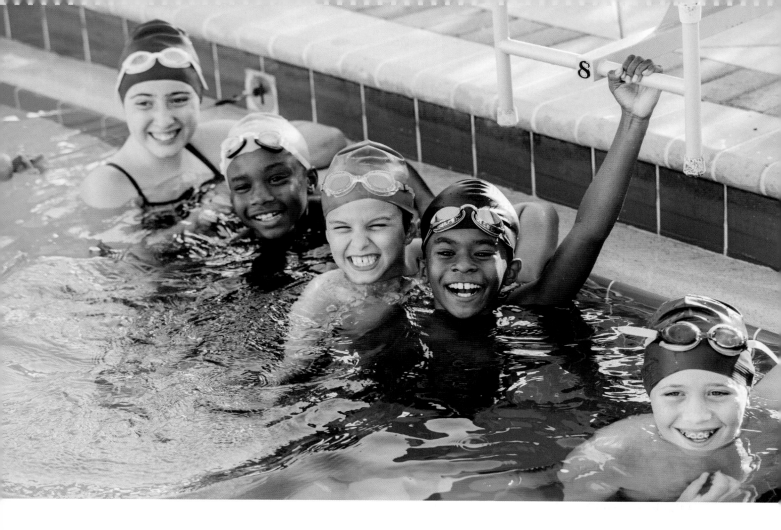

movements. Most often, constant practice is used only for as long as it takes the learner to demonstrate adequate timing and execution of the critical elements of the skill.

Variable practice is practice that includes variations of the skill itself or the context of the skill in variable order such as varying an underhand toss to targets at different levels, distances, or directions (Beach et al., 2024, p. 391). Whereas constant practice contributes to the learner's gaining the critical elements (stable features) of a generalized motor program, variable practice helps the learner gain the characteristics (flexible features) that vary skill execution from one performance to the next. The flexible features involve performing skills using different parameters such as level, direction, distance, speed, trajectory, or in relationship to a partner.

Practicing a skill using many different movement parameters expands the learner's **generalized motor program**. This leads to the learner's attaining a greater variety of ways to perform **closed skills** (i.e., skills that take place in a stable, predictable environment in which objects or events are stationary). For instance, dancers could vary turns by the number of revolutions or the position of nonsupporting body parts. Volleyball serves could be varied by placement in different locations. For **open skills** (i.e., in an environment in which objects, people, and events are changing or unpredictable), a generalized motor program with many flexible features leads to a faster, more accurate response to an unpredictable environment. When structuring variable practice for open skills, teachers need to design progressions that start with more predictable environments and transition to less predictable environments.

The critical elements of the fundamental movement skills within Standard 1 Grade-Span Learning Indicators are provided in appendix A. Within these skills, manipulative skills include preparation, execution (or force phase), and follow-through; locomotor and non-locomotor skills include preparation, execution, and recovery. As children progress to the mature stage of motor skill development, they are capable of consistently performing the critical elements of the fundamental movement skills.

Practice, when accompanied by feedback, influences the rate of learning and level of performance achieved (Coker, 2004; Young et. al., 2000). Feedback is information performers receive about their movement responses. Just as in practice, for optimum performance results, physical educators need to match the types and amounts of feedback to the learner, task, and environment.

Intrinsic feedback is when the information comes from the performer's senses (e.g., they see the ball, feel it in their hands, and adjust their balance to prepare to throw). **Augmented feedback** is when the information comes from a source other than the performer (e.g., teacher, heart rate monitor, time-delayed video feedback). Augmented feedback is used to guide, motivate, and reinforce the learner. Feedback used to guide performance should point out errors and ways to correct them. Ultimately, the goal is to enable learners to become more capable of detecting and correcting their own errors—a skill that is critical to their physical literacy journey beyond their preK-12 experience. Feedback is motivating when it informs learners about their progress toward a predetermined goal. Physical educators may tell learners, "Keep trying; you're almost there," to encourage them to keep working on their performance goals. When physical educators describe the specific movements while reinforcing correct performance, it is more likely that the learner will perform the movements similarly under like circumstances in the future. Examples of specific reinforcing feedback include "Nice job; by moving quickly you were able to intercept the ball" and "Way to go; that tight tuck made your roll smooth." One way to classify feedback is by whether the goal of the skill is process- or outcome-oriented. **Process goals** address the pattern of the movement and focus on biomechanical efficiency of the critical elements of the skill. **Outcome goals** address the product of the movement and focus on end results such as how high, how far, how accurate, or how fast.

Knowledge of performance (KP) is augmented feedback about the process or movement characteristics of the performance and includes information about the location, speed, direction, or coordination of body actions. Since the purpose of KP is to reinforce or change the way the performer moves, physical educators must be knowledgeable about the critical elements and biomechanical principles that determine correct performance. Examples of such feedback include, "Step forward with the other foot," "Keep your knees closer to your chest," and "Keep your head still and eyes on the ball." These KP feedback statements are all **prescriptive feedback** because they focus on what performers specifically need to do to correct their movements. Specific, prescriptive KP feedback is especially important for learners whose goal is to minimize errors and develop the correct movements of a new skill. Teachers should also employ **descriptive feedback**. When giving descriptive feedback, physical educators verbally describe what students did correctly (e.g., "Great job; you stepped with your opposite foot during your throw"). Descriptive feedback is also important because it can serve as a motivational factor, thus encouraging continued practice.

Knowledge of results (KR) is either intrinsic or augmented feedback about the outcome or end results of the movement performance. Information about goal attainment is critical for acquiring and performing movement skills (Young et al., 2000). Most often KR is intrinsically known to performers because they see the ball, hit a target, feel themselves going off balance, or hear the ball hit the sweet spot of the bat. Physical educators can provide augmented KR that is unknown or less obvious to the learner to aid in goal attainment, such as "You finished the dash in 10 seconds," "Your foot was out of bounds," or "You successfully fielded 40 percent of the ground balls." These KR feedback statements are all descriptive because they simply describe what happened in the performance. For preK-2 students who are within the fundamental movement phase of motor development and progressing from the emerging elementary to mature stage of motor skill development, KP is more important than KR to assist them in demonstrating the critical elements of movement skills.

Another feature of best practices in delivering instruction is demonstration. Physical educators can provide their students with correct demonstrations in multiple ways, including the use of technology. Many physical educators project an image or video of a motor skill during practice so that students can reference the correct performance of the skill. Demonstrations should adhere to the following basic guidelines (e.g., Chen et al., 2016; Goodway et al., 2003; Zittel & Houston-Wilson, 2000): Demonstrations should be visible for all students to observe and be repeated with and without verbal cues, multiple times. When teaching complex skills, the skills can be demonstrated as a whole and then in parts. Additionally, students should be allowed to shadow the teacher during demonstrations.

Conclusion

As physical educators begin to plan and implement a curriculum based on the new standards and Grade-Span Learning Indicators, it is essential that they connect with and identify the needs of their students and consider the supports necessary to facilitate their physical literacy journey. As shared in this chapter, teachers should make concerted efforts to plan physical education learning tasks that facilitate social interaction between students and between the teacher and students, provide opportunities for challenge and fun, support the development of motor competence, and engage the students in personally relevant learning. Physical education learning tasks should also be designed to provide ample practice; across differentiated levels; supported with the use of critical elements, feedback, and demonstration.

CHAPTER 3

Grades PreK-2 National Physical Education Standards, Grade-Span Learning Indicators, and Learning Progressions

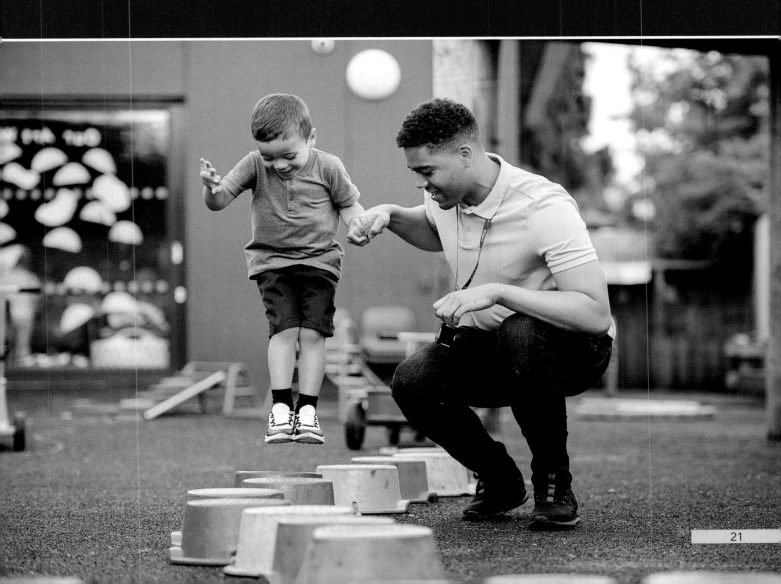

Understanding the Learner

The preschool and early elementary years have been recognized as critical in the development of fundamental movement skills. Goodway and colleagues (2021) remind us that fundamental movement skills are not determined maturationally; rather, they are influenced by "opportunities for practice, encouragement and instruction and the ecology (context) of the environment with conditions of the learning environment playing important roles in the degree to which the fundamental movement skills develop" (p. 51). Additionally, links exist between fundamental movement skills and later engagement in physical activity (Logan et al., 2015). Skill acquisition is essential for continued participation in physical activity in adolescence and beyond (Lubans et al., 2010; Goodway et al., 2021; Stodden et al., 2009).

Children do not naturally develop fundamental movement skills; rather, carefully designed instruction is necessary for young children to achieve fundamental movement competence. The Grade-Span Learning Indicators described in this chapter inform teachers about what preK-2 children should know and be able to do and guide teachers in designing meaningful learning experiences. Teachers must take the time to review and be familiar with the developmental characteristics of preK-2 children because it will aid them in understanding the Grade-Span Learning Indicators and associated Learning Progressions.

Developmental Characteristics Within the Psychomotor Domain of Learning

Children two to three years of age are typically in the initial stage of motor skill development (see chapter 1). During the initial stage, children make their first observable and purposeful attempts at performing fundamental motor skills. Children in preK-2 are in the fundamental movement phase of motor development. PreK (ages four to five) students are progressing through the **emerging elementary stage** of fundamental motor skill development. The emerging elementary stage of fundamental movement skill development is typical of the performance of three- to five-year-old children; however, these age ranges are not absolute. Development through the elementary stage and into the mature stage is partly dependent on growth and maturation and largely dependent on opportunities for practice, encouragement, quality instruction, and the ecology of the environment. During the transitional period between the initial and mature stages, the increases in strength with growth and gradual lengthening of the trunk and limbs allow moderate ranges of flexion, extension, and rotation, although short, stubby fingers still hamper object handling. Emerging elementary–stage performers gain greater control of their movements but still appear somewhat awkward and lacking in fluidity.

By ages six or seven years (i.e., grades 1 and 2), children's slow and steady growth in height, weight, and strength supports their developmental potential to be at the **mature stage** in most fundamental movement skills. The mature stage is characterized by progress in gaining a well-coordinated and biomechanically efficient movement performance. By six years of age, children can move through full ranges of flexion, extension, and rotation because their body proportions are more similar to adults. Through growth, they have become stronger, and their fingers have lengthened, making object manipulation easier. Within this stage, performance has the potential to improve rapidly. Children can throw farther, run faster, and jump higher. It is important to note that even though children have the potential to attain the mature stage in most fundamental skills by age six or seven years, they get there at varying rates. Opportunities for practice and encouragement, the quality of instruction, and the ecology of the environment may limit or enhance the attainment of motor skill proficiency. Thus, few opportunities for practice with little to no encouragement or instruction in an environment with regulation equipment might delay achievement of the mature stage, whereas developmentally appropriate equipment, practice, encouragement, and instruction could lead to a more rapid achievement of the mature stage. Meeting the needs of all children requires considering the ecology of the environment (i.e., equipment and condition variables; see figures 3.1 through 3.3). By adjusting the equipment, spatial, temporal, and relationship variables, teachers can differentiate instruction. Teachers of elementary physical education control these variables within their instruction and thus are key players in the development of fundamental motor skills. The core of the physical education

Equipment Variables							
Affordance	Size	Width	Length	Weight	Height	Texture	Motion
Easy	Large Small	Wide	Short	Light	Low	Soft	Stationary
↓	↓ ↓	↓	↓	↓	↓	↓	↓
Difficult	Small Large	Narrow	Long	Heavy	High	Solid	Moving

FIGURE 3.1 Performer scaling conditions: equipment.

Reprinted by permission from F. Cleland-Donnelly, S.S. Mueller, and D. Gallahue, *Developmental Physical Education for All Children*, 5th ed. (Champaign, IL: Human Kinetics, 2017).

Condition Variables							
Affordance	Spatial					Temporal	
	Distance	Direction	Pathway	Level	Trajectory	Speed	Rhythm	Timing
Easy	Near	Front	Straight	Low	Horizontal	Slow Moderate	Even	Predictable
		Sides	Curved		Vertical	Slow		
↓	↓	↓	↓	↓	↓	↓ ↓	↓	↓
Difficult	Far	Back	Zigzag	High	Arc	Fast Fast	Uneven	Unpredictable

FIGURE 3.2 Performer scaling conditions: spatial and temporal.

Reprinted by permission from F. Cleland-Donnelly, S.S. Mueller, and D. Gallahue, *Developmental Physical Education for All Children*, 5th ed. (Champaign, IL: Human Kinetics, 2017).

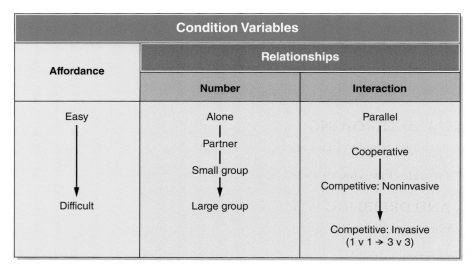

Condition Variables		
Affordance	**Relationships**	
	Number	**Interaction**
Easy ↓ Difficult	Alone | Partner | Small group ↓ Large group	Parallel | Cooperative | Competitive: Noninvasive ↓ Competitive: Invasive (1 v 1 → 3 v 3)

FIGURE 3.3 Performer scaling conditions: relationships.

Reprinted by permission from F. Cleland-Donnelly, S.S. Mueller, and D. Gallahue, *Developmental Physical Education for All Children*, 5th ed. (Champaign, IL: Human Kinetics, 2017).

program for preK-2 students is developmentally appropriate movement goals and skill development using **body-scaled** equipment and performance contexts to support children becoming mature movers by refining, varying, and combining a wide variety of fundamental movement skills.

Based on the developmental characteristics of preK-2 children within the **psychomotor domain**, preK-2 Standard 1 Grade-Span Learning Indicators and Learning Progressions are provided. The range of practice tasks provided in the Learning Progressions support **differentiated instruction** in physical education with the goal of meeting the needs of all children.

Standard 1: Develops a variety of motor skills.

Rationale. Through learning experiences in physical education, the student develops motor skills across a variety of environments. Motor skills are a foundational part of child development and support the movements of everyday life. The development of motor skills contributes to an individual's physical literacy journey.

Learning Indicators

LOCOMOTOR

1.2.1 Demonstrates a variety of locomotor skills with the concepts of space, effort, and relationship awareness.

1.2.2 Demonstrates jumping and landing in a non-dynamic environment.

1.2.3 Demonstrates transferring weight on multiple body parts.

NON-LOCOMOTOR

1.2.4 Demonstrates non-locomotor skills with the concepts of space, effort, and relationship awareness.

1.2.5 Demonstrates balancing on different body parts in a non-dynamic environment.

BOUNCING

1.2.6 Demonstrates bouncing a ball in a variety of non-dynamic practice tasks.

ROLLING

1.2.7 Demonstrates rolling a ball in a variety of non-dynamic practice tasks.

CATCHING AND THROWING

1.2.8 Demonstrates catching in a variety of non-dynamic practice tasks.

1.2.9 Demonstrates throwing in a variety of non-dynamic practice tasks.

KICKING AND DRIBBLING WITH FEET

1.2.10 Demonstrates kicking a ball in a variety of non-dynamic practice tasks.

1.2.11 Demonstrates dribbling with feet in a variety of non-dynamic practice tasks.

STRIKING WITH HANDS

1.2.12 Demonstrates striking with hands in a variety of non-dynamic practice tasks.

STRIKING WITH IMPLEMENTS

1.2.13 Demonstrates striking with a short-handled implement in a variety of non-dynamic practice tasks.

1.2.14 Demonstrates striking with a long-handled implement in a variety of non-dynamic practice tasks.

DANCE AND RHYTHMS

1.2.15 Demonstrates locomotor, non-locomotor, and manipulative movements based on a variety of dance forms.

1.2.16 Demonstrates jumping rope in a non-dynamic environment.

AQUATICS

1.2.17 Demonstrates water safety skills. If a pool facility is available, demonstrates water safety and basic swimming skills.

Developmental Characteristics Within the Cognitive Domain of Learning

Understanding preK-2 children's cognitive development is integral to the design of developmentally appropriate learning experiences in physical education. The **pre-operational stage** describes the intellectual capabilities of preK-2 children ages two to seven. During this early childhood period, "the child uses elementary logic and reasoning as they learn to use past experiences and the beginning use of symbols to represent objects in their environment. This process leads the way to oral communication" (Nichols, 1994, p. 23).

In social situations the child is often **egocentric** in their thinking. According to Beach and colleagues (2024), "This does not imply selfishness, but rather, that children are unable to view the world from a perspective other than their own. Thus, it makes little sense for the child to spread out on a playing field in the hope that someone will pass him the ball, or even to wait his turn on a playground" (p. 289).

Preschoolers' vivid imaginations make it possible for them to jump from "great heights," climb "high mountains," leap over "raging rivers," and run "faster" than an assorted variety of "wild beasts." Children of preschool age are rapidly expanding their horizons, asserting their individuality, developing their abilities, and testing their limits.

Kindergarten is a readiness time in which children begin making the gradual transition from an egocentric, home-centered play world to the group-oriented world of adult concepts and logic. In first grade, the first formal demands for cognitive understanding are made. The major cognitive milestone of the first and second grader is learning how to read at a reasonable level. The child is involved in developing the first real understanding of time and money, the concepts of movement (e.g., personal and general space; fast, medium, and slow speeds; following and leading), and numerous other concrete cognitive concepts. By second grade, children should be well on their way to meeting and surmounting a broadening array of cognitive, affective, and motor tasks. Table 3.1 provides an overview of preK-2 children's cognitive development with relevant teaching implications. Standard 2 (Applies knowledge related to movement and fitness concepts) reflects preK-2 children's stage of cognitive development.

Based on the developmental characteristics of preK-2 children within the **cognitive domain**, preK-2 Standard 2 Grade-Span Learning Indicators and Learning Progressions are provided here.

TABLE 3.1 Developmental Characteristics of Learners in the Cognitive Domain

	PreK	Grades K-2
Stage of cognitive development and learner characteristics	Pre-operational stage during which children are egocentric and unable to view the world from another's perspective. Children are curious and imaginative and enjoy exploring their environment and testing their limits.	Pre-operational stage during which children use elementary logic; reasoning reflects past experiences. Children use symbols to represent objects in their environment (learning to read).
Teaching implications	Teachers can implement the following strategies: simple instructions and task cards with pictures; activities of short duration; variety of tasks; moving into activity quickly; brief (3-5 minutes) use of whole-class format, with small bits of information provided at one time; station format, each with a single focus; activities that stimulate imagination and creativity.	Teachers can implement the following strategies: simple instructions; task cards with few words and pictures; increasingly longer periods of whole-class format; station format, each with a single focus; activities that stimulate imagination and creativity. Elementary logic enables children to look for one movement cue when observing a peer. They can correct their own performance based on feedback and can design or vary a short movement combination and follow simple rules. Children begin to develop a movement vocabulary.

Reprinted by permission from F. Cleland-Donnelly, S.S. Mueller, and D. Gallahue, *Developmental Physical Education for All Children*, 5th ed. (Champaign, IL: Human Kinetics, 2017).

Standard 2: Applies knowledge related to movement and fitness concepts.

Rationale. Through learning experiences in physical education, the student uses their knowledge of movement concepts, tactics, and strategies across a variety of environments. This knowledge helps the student become a more versatile and efficient mover. Additionally, the student applies knowledge of health-related and skill-related fitness to enhance their overall well-being. The application of knowledge related to various forms of movement contributes to an individual's physical literacy journey.

Learning Indicators

TACTICS AND STRATEGIES

2.2.1 Recognizes personal space and where to move in general space.

2.2.2 Identifies simple strategies in chasing and fleeing activities.

2.2.3 Identifies movement concepts related to locomotor, non-locomotor, and manipulative skills.

2.2.4 Demonstrates knowledge of locomotor, non-locomotor, and manipulative skills in movement settings.

DANCE AND RHYTHMS

2.2.5 Demonstrates knowledge of locomotor, non-locomotor, and movement concepts used in dance and rhythms.

FITNESS CONCEPTS

2.2.6 Identifies physical activities that contribute to fitness.

2.2.7 Recognizes the importance of stretching before and after physical activity.

2.2.8 Identifies the heart as a muscle that gets stronger with physical activity.

PHYSICAL ACTIVITY KNOWLEDGE

2.2.9 Recognizes that regular physical activity is good for their health.

2.2.10 Recognizes physiological changes in their body during physical activities.

2.2.11 Recognizes food and hydration choices that provide energy for physical activity.

AQUATICS

2.2.12 Demonstrates knowledge of water safety skills. Demonstrates knowledge of basic swimming skills.

Developmental Characteristics Within the Social Domain of Learning

The work of leading psychology and education scholars, such as Erikson (1980), has informed our understanding of psychosocial development. According to Erikson (1980), **industry versus inferiority** is the stage of psychosocial development attributed to children ages 6 to 12 years. During this stage of development, children are learning to relate to others. Through social interactions, children begin to develop a sense of pride in their accomplishments and abilities. Given that children spend much of their day in school, teachers and peers become important social agents; thus the child must conform to a set of social expectations beyond the realm of family. According to Beach and colleagues (2024), "The need to produce mobilizes children beyond play and to acquire cognitive skills such as reading and writing, as well as social skills appropriate to the culture. They learn to cooperate with others to achieve shared goals" (p. 308). Teachers facilitate industry by helping children establish and attain realistic criterion-referenced goals using evidence from personal data and refrain from exclusively using social comparisons that could lead to feelings of inferiority.

Physical education classes are rich in opportunities for developing **social competence**, which involves both social awareness and relationship awareness. **Social awareness** refers to the ability to understand the perspectives of and empathize with others, including those from diverse backgrounds, cultures, and contexts (CASEL, 2023). Examples of such behaviors for preK-2 students may include but are not limited to (1) recognizing strengths in others, (2) showing concern for the

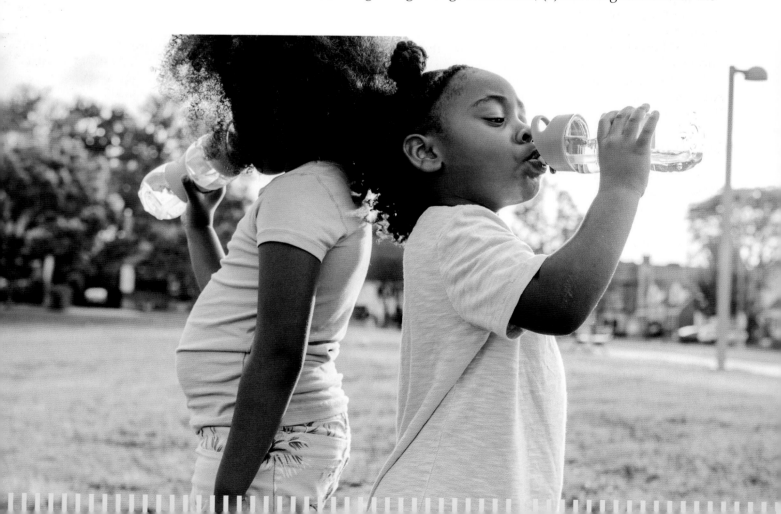

feelings of others, and (3) understanding and expressing gratitude. **Relationship awareness** refers to the ability to establish and maintain healthy and supportive relationships and to effectively navigate settings with diverse individuals and groups (CASEL, 2023). Examples of such behaviors for preK-2 students may include but are not limited to (1) seeking or offering support and help when needed, (2) communicating effectively, (3) developing positive relationships, and (4) resolving conflicts.

In a school physical education setting children are always participating in relation to one another. Sharing space while practicing a motor skill next to a classmate, cooperating to solve a movement problem, or competing against others in a small-sided game requires children to demonstrate social competence. Teachers need to plan a sequence of learning experiences that lead children to understand and positively respond to others and gain the social skills to positively interact. Responding positively to others is based on feelings of empathy: "Empathy is the identification with and understanding of another's situation, feelings and motives" (Mercier & Hutchinson, 2003, p. 274). Learning social and relationship skills provides the vehicle for children to interact with others, solve conflicts peacefully, and build positive feelings that lead to successful performance in pairs, small groups, and teams.

Communication, cooperation, and conflict resolution are also relationship skills important for children to develop to work productively with others. Communication involves the ability to be courteous, listen, provide feedback, encourage, and compliment others. Cooperation involves being honest, fair, patient, tolerant, and sensitive to others' ideas. Cooperative activities can also facilitate positive interdependence because students take personal responsibility while working with a group toward a common goal. During cooperative challenges, students must monitor their interactions and reflect on how these contributed to the outcome. When students have disagreements, they need to apply communication and problem-solving skills that will lead to a positive resolution.

Based on these developmental characteristics of preK-2 children within the **social domain**, preK-2 Standard 3 Grade-Span Learning Indicators and Learning Progressions are provided.

Standard 3: Develops social skills through movement.

Rationale. Through learning experiences in physical education, students develop the social skills necessary to exhibit empathy and respect for others and foster and maintain relationships. In addition, students develop skills for communication, leadership, cultural awareness, and conflict resolution in a variety of physical activity settings.

Learning Indicators

3.2.1 Recognizes the feelings of others during a variety of physical activities.

3.2.2 Demonstrates ability to encourage others.

3.2.3 Uses communication skills to share space and equipment.

3.2.4 Responds appropriately to directions and feedback from the teacher.

3.2.5 Demonstrates respectful behaviors that contribute to positive social interactions in movement.

3.2.6 Describes why following rules is important for safety and fairness.

3.2.7 Makes safe choices with physical education equipment.

3.2.8 Discusses problems and solutions with teacher support in a physical activity setting.

3.2.9 Makes fair choices as directed by the teacher.

3.2.10 Identifies and participates in physical activities representing different cultures.

Developmental Characteristics Within the Affective Domain of Learning

The affective domain is one of the three domains in Bloom's Taxonomy. It involves feelings, attitudes, and emotions. It includes the ways in which people deal with external and internal phenomena emotionally, such as values, enthusiasms, and motivations. Self-awareness is a component of the affective domain. **Self-awareness** is defined as the ability to understand one's own emotions, thoughts, and values and how they influence behavior across contexts (CASEL, 2023). Developing interests and a sense of purpose is part of self-awareness. As such, when teachers design instruction, they should keep in mind that preK-2 students need to identify the purpose of the lesson. Choosing to engage in physical activity also involves **self-management**, which is defined as the ability to manage one's emotions, thoughts, and behaviors effectively in different situations and to achieve goals and aspirations (CASEL, 2023). Examples of such self-management behaviors for preK-2 students may include but are not limited to (1) showing the courage to take initiative or, in preK-2 vocabulary, "being willing to try something new," and (2) setting personal and collective goals. Students' development of self-management skills contributes to **responsible decision-making**, which is defined as the ability to make caring and constructive choices about one's personal behavior and social interactions across diverse situations (CASEL, 2023). For preK-2 students, part of the decision-making process includes setting goals. These goals are concrete, **short-term goals** that could be accomplished during a physical education class, such as staying on task, sharing a piece of equipment with a classmate, or trying a new motor skill. When students discover why it is beneficial to engage in physical activity, they may subsequently choose to engage in physical activity.

Students' motivation to move and engage in physical activity within and outside of the school environment may also be affected by features or aspects of their self-determination, competence motivation, and self-efficacy. These constructs and their relationship to preK-2 students will be explained.

According to Beach and colleagues (2024), "**Self-determination** theory postulates that humans have basic needs to feel competent, autonomous, and connected with other people (i.e., relatedness)" (p. 313). Young children are known to play for hours for the sheer joy of participating in such activities as hide-and-seek or tag. When children choose to engage in play, their need for autonomy is met. This type of play also suggests children are intrinsically motivated and are engaging in physical activity for the pleasure and satisfaction derived without the need for material rewards or constraints (i.e., rules or guidelines from teachers or parents). Self-determination research suggests that when teachers maintain a learning environment that provides choice, fun (i.e., relevant activities), and developmentally appropriate challenges students are motivated to participate and learn new skills.

Harter's (1999) observations of young children's intrinsic interest in mastery of their world through free play (e.g., playing with blocks) led to his formation of a model of **competence motivation**. Competence motivation represents the fundamental desire of humans to be competent (i.e., successful and skillful). Standard 1 aims to foster students' motor skill development and, in doing so, their competence. Students' desire for competence leads to their participation in the psychomotor domain. This research suggests that physical education teachers should provide developmentally appropriate or optimal challenges so that preK-2 students experience success and develop a feeling of competence and thus are motivated to move.

Self-efficacy also plays an important role in preK-2 students' motivation to move. Bandura (1997) defined perceived self-efficacy as "beliefs in one's capabilities to organize and execute the courses of action required to produce given attainments" (p. 3). Beach and colleagues (2024) further clarified that when self-efficacy is defined as an individual's confidence in their ability to be physically active in a given physical activity situation, "it becomes the most consistently identified psychosocial determinant of physical activity in children, adolescents, and adults" (p. 315). PreK-2 students' self-efficacy is influenced primarily by their caregivers, family members, and teachers. Self-efficacy may be fostered when students experience success in physical education. In addition, verbal persuasion (i.e., when teachers express faith in their students' abilities) may positively affect preK-2 students' self-efficacy.

Based on the developmental characteristics of preK-2 children within the **affective domain**, preK-2 Standard 4 Grade-Span Learning Indicators and Learning Progressions are provided.

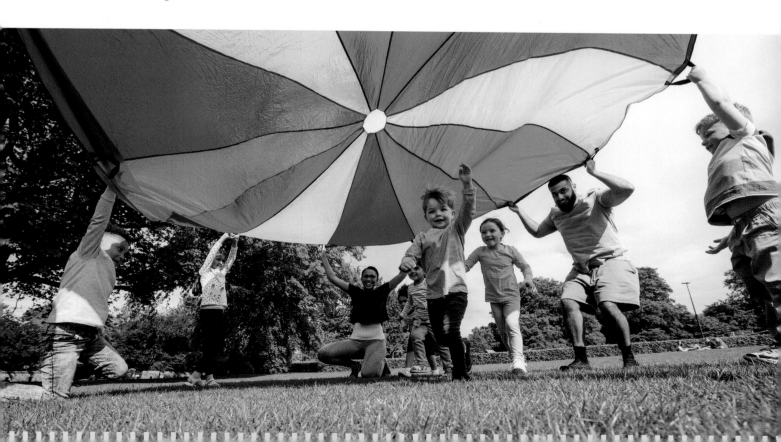

Standard 4: Develops personal skills, identifies personal benefits of movement, and chooses to engage in physical activity.

Rationale. Through learning experiences in physical education, the student develops an understanding of how movement is personally beneficial and subsequently chooses to participate in physical activities that are personally meaningful (e.g., activities that offer social interaction, cultural connection, exploration, choice, self-expression, appropriate levels of challenge, and added health benefits). The student develops personal skills including goal setting, identifying strengths, and reflection to enhance their physical literacy journey.

Learning Indicators

4.2.1 Identifies physical activities that can meet the need for self-expression.

4.2.2 Identifies physical activities that can meet the need for social interaction.

4.2.3 Lists ways that movement positively affects personal health.

4.2.4 Identifies preferred physical activities based on personal interests.

4.2.5 Recognizes individual challenges through movement.

4.2.6 Sets observable short-term goals.

4.2.7 Recognizes movement strengths and the need for practice for individual improvement.

4.2.8 Recognizes the opportunity for physical activity within physical education class.

4.2.9 Demonstrates techniques (e.g., breathing, counting) to assist with managing emotions and behaviors in a physical activity.

4.2.10 Reflects on movement experiences during physical education to develop understanding of how movement is personally meaningful.

Conclusion

Physical educators are encouraged to intentionally design instruction based on Standards 1 through 4 to foster preK-2 children's physical literacy journey. The Learning Indicators and Learning Progressions are provided to help teachers design purposeful and relevant lessons for preK-2 students.

DANCE AND RHYTHMS

2.5.6 Applies movement concepts to different types of dances, gymnastics, rhythms, and individual performance activities.

FITNESS CONCEPTS

2.5.7 Defines and provides examples of movement activities for developing the health-related fitness components.

2.5.8 Establishes goals related to enhancing fitness development.

2.5.9 Defines and explains how to implement the FITT Principle for fitness development.

2.5.10 Defines and provides examples of movement activities for developing the skill-related fitness components.

2.5.11 Identifies the need for warm-up and cool-down relative to various physical activities.

2.5.12 Identifies location of pulse and provides examples of activities that increase heart rate.

PHYSICAL ACTIVITY KNOWLEDGE

2.5.13 Explains the benefits of physical activity.

2.5.14 Recognizes and explains how physical activity influences physiological changes in their body.

2.5.15 Recognizes the critical elements that contribute to proper execution of a skill.

2.5.16 Identifies technology tools that support physical activity goals.

2.5.17 Describes the impact of food and hydration choices on physical activity.

AQUATICS

2.5.18 Demonstrates knowledge of water safety skills. Demonstrates knowledge of basic swimming skills.

Developmental Characteristics Within the Social Domain of Learning

During grades 3-5 children are acquiring a new set of social skills, including but not limited to making friends, becoming part of a group, listening carefully, and responding considerately to others. In addition, in grades 3-5 children begin to accurately recognize nonverbal behavior and verbal qualities such as tone of voice and volume. Developing social competence also involves sharing, cooperating, displaying appropriate levels of assertiveness as well as regulating one's own emotions and behaviors.

As children move toward later childhood, they can differentiate between additional competence domains such as academic, athletic, social, physical appearance, and behavior. With the aid of language and increased cognitive functioning, they are now aware of social comparisons as they interact with others in school and sports environments. They know others have an opinion of them, which influences their self-esteem positively if they know others have positive opinions of them. They understand competence within domains; that is, they can be a good swimmer but a poor baseball player. At this point, children have a more balanced and accurate view of themselves. (Beach et al., 2024, p. 310)

Children in grades 3-5 continue to be within the industry versus inferiority stage of psychosocial development. Teachers should continue to facilitate industry by helping children establish and attain realistic criterion-referenced goals using evidence from personal data and refrain from exclusively using social comparisons that could lead to feelings of inferiority (e.g., using personal fitness data to set a goal for engaging in some type of aerobic activity daily versus comparing themselves to a classmate). Additionally, physical educators can integrate personal and social skills within the context of developmentally appropriate games, dance, and gymnastic lesson content.

As noted in chapter 3, students in grades 3-5 are further developing social competence (i.e., social awareness and relationship awareness). Given that students in grades 3-5 are entering the formal operations stage of cognitive development, they are even more capable of understanding the perspectives of and empathizing with others, including those from diverse backgrounds, cultures, and contexts (CASEL, 2023). The behaviors of students in grades 3-5 are expanding, and in addition to those characteristics of preK-2 children, they may include but are not limited to taking others' perspectives and recognizing strengths in others.

Relationship awareness involves the ability to establish and maintain healthy and supportive relationships and to effectively navigate settings with diverse

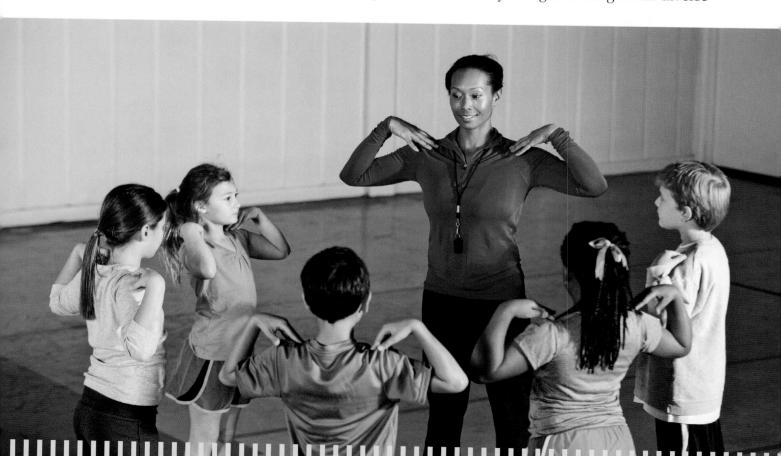

individuals and groups (CASEL, 2023). Examples of such behaviors for students in grades 3-5 may include but are not limited to (1) seeking or offering support and help when needed, (2) communicating effectively, (3) developing positive relationships, and (4) conflict resolution.

Based on these developmental characteristics of children in grades 3-5 within the social domain, Grades 3-5 Standard 3 Grade-Span Learning Indicators and Learning Progressions are provided.

Standard 3: Develops social skills through movement.

Rationale. Through learning experiences in physical education, students develop the social skills necessary to exhibit empathy and respect for others and foster and maintain relationships. In addition, students develop skills for communication, leadership, cultural awareness, and conflict resolution in a variety of physical activity settings.

Learning Indicators

3.5.1 Describes the perspective of others during a variety of activities.

3.5.2 Uses communication skills to negotiate roles and responsibilities in a physical activity setting.

3.5.3 Demonstrates respectful behaviors that contribute to positive social interaction in group activities.

3.5.4 Demonstrates safe behaviors independently with limited reminders.

3.5.5 Solves problems independently, with partners, and in small groups.

3.5.6 Makes choices that are fair according to activity etiquette.

3.5.7 Describes physical activities that represent a variety of cultures around the world.

Developmental Characteristics Within the Affective Domain of Learning

Students in grades 3-5 are developing a keener self-awareness and thus have a greater ability to discern their own emotions, thoughts, and values. They are now entering the formal operations stage of cognitive development, which enables them to think abstractly and contemplate more complex ideas. Understanding the personal benefits of engaging in physical activity and recognizing their strengths and personal challenges encourages them to take personal ownership of managing their level of engagement in physical activity. As noted in chapter 3, choosing to engage in physical activity involves self-management. In addition to managing one's emotions, additional examples of self-management behaviors for students in grades 3-5 may include but are not limited to (1) identifying and using stress management strategies, (2) exhibiting self-discipline and self-motivation, (3) setting personal and collective goals, and (4) showing the courage to take initiative. Students' development of self-management skills contributes to responsible decision-making. For students in grades 3-5, part of the decision-making process includes setting goals. Students in grades 3-5 can now set personal goals (e.g., exercising daily or participating with new classmates during physical education class) and group goals (e.g., everyone touching the ball prior to scoring or everyone offering a solution to an adventure problem-solving initiative).

Students' motivation to move and engage in physical activity within and outside of the school environment may also be affected by features or aspects of their self-determination, competence motivation, and self-efficacy. Both constructs will be explained and the relationship of them to students in grades 3-5 will be highlighted.

Students in grades 3-5 continue to have the basic need of feeling competent as well as having autonomy (i.e., teachers providing them with opportunities to make activity choices) within the physical education setting. Competence motivation, or the fundamental desire of humans to be competent (i.e., successful and skillful), continues to be a characteristic of students in grades 3-5. As with preK-2 students, self-efficacy also plays an important role in the motivation to move for students in grades 3-5. In grades 3-5, students' self-efficacy is not only influenced by family members and teachers but expands to include their peers.

Positive feedback about students' motor skill performance can augment their feeling of competence and enhance their self-efficacy. Additionally, allowing student input about lesson activities and assessment options may in turn provide them with a sense of autonomy.

Based on these developmental characteristics of children in grades 3-5 within the affective domain, Grades 3-5 Standard 4 Grade-Span Learning Indicators and Learning Progressions are provided.

Standard 4: Develops personal skills, identifies personal benefits of movement, and chooses to engage in physical activity.

Rationale. Through learning experiences in physical education, the student develops an understanding of how movement is personally beneficial and subsequently chooses to participate in physical activities that are personally meaningful (e.g., activities that offer social interaction, cultural connection, exploration, choice, self-expression, appropriate levels of challenge, and added health benefits). The student develops personal skills including goal setting, identifying strengths, and reflection to enhance their physical literacy journey.

Learning Indicators

4.5.1 Explains how preferred physical activities meet the need for personal self-expression.

4.5.2 Explains how preferred physical activities meet the need for social interaction.

4.5.3 Describes how movement positively affects personal health.

4.5.4 Explains the rationale for one's choices related to physical activity based on personal interests.

4.5.5 Recognizes group challenges through movement.

4.5.6 Sets observable long-term goals.

4.5.7 Identifies movement strengths and opportunities for practice for individual improvement.

4.5.8 Identifies physical activity opportunities outside of physical education class.

4.5.9 Recognizes personally effective techniques that assist with managing one's emotions and behaviors in a physical activity setting.

4.5.10 Reflects on movement experiences during physical education to develop understanding of how movement is personally meaningful.

Conclusion

Physical educators are encouraged to intentionally design instruction based on Standards 1 through 4 to foster grades 3-5 children's physical literacy journey. The Learning Indicators and Learning Progressions are provided to help teachers design purposeful and relevant lessons for grades 3-5.

CHAPTER 5

Grades 6-8
National Physical Education Standards, Grade-Span Learning Indicators, and Learning Progressions

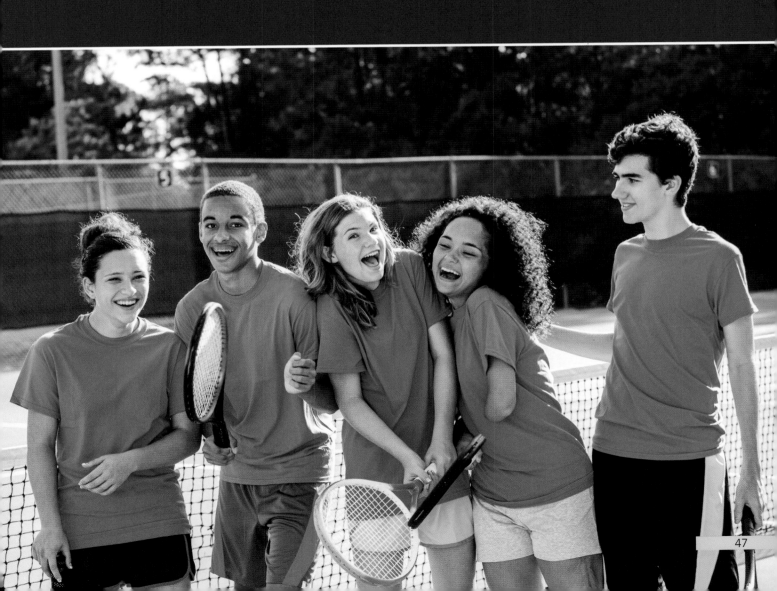

Understanding the Learner

The physical literacy journey for students in grades 6 through 8 reflects the influence of early and emerging adolescence on their psychomotor, cognitive, social, and affective learning. Transitions prompted by changes (e.g., biological, social, emotional, cognitive) during early and emerging adolescence directly affect learning in physical education. During adolescence, students experience rapid development, shape their beliefs and attitudes, adopt physical activity and health habits, and develop social behaviors that serve as the foundation for adulthood (McCarthy et al., 2016).

The Grade-Span Learning Indicators described in this chapter inform teachers about what students in grades 6 to 8 should know and be able to do and guide teachers in designing meaningful learning experiences. Teachers must take the time to review and be familiar with the developmental characteristics of students in grades 6-8 because it will aid them in understanding the Grade-Span Learning Indicators and associated Task Progressions.

Developmental Characteristics Within the Psychomotor Domain of Learning

Physically, students in grades 6 through 8 experience puberty, neural change, and periods of rapid and uneven growth, with most students growing between 2 and 4 inches (5-10 cm) per year and gaining 8 to 10 pounds (4-5 kg) per year (Patton et al., 2016; Snowman & McCown, 2014). It is worth noting that the growth experienced by adolescent students is more rapid than any other period of development except the period from birth to two years of age (Brinegar & Caskey, 2022). These changes in height, weight, and body proportions lead to motor performance and coordination issues as well as growing pains as the result of skeletal growth preceding muscular development. The growth hormones responsible for the physical changes also tend to make female students mature (e.g., hips widen, breasts develop, body weight increases) one to two years earlier than their male counterparts (Wood et al., 2019). Early maturing male students experience limb growth disproportionate to growth in their trunk that results in awkwardness and motor coordination disturbances. Following the growth spurt, these early maturing male students do experience increases in strength and coordination greater than those of their less-mature peers of the same age (Cleland Donnelly et al., 2017). All in total, these noticeable physical changes lead to increased self-awareness among male and female adolescent students (Harrison et al., 2019).

Regarding motor skill development, students in grades 6 through 8 are in the specialized movement phase, which begins around the age of seven years and progresses into adulthood through the transitional stage, application stage, and lifelong utilization stage (Cleland Donnelly et al., 2017). During their middle school years, students are exiting the transitional stage, wherein they refine the performance of fundamental motor skills and develop the mature stage characteristics of fundamental movement skills (see appendix A) with improvements in form, accuracy, and control, and are progressing into the application stage.

As mentioned in chapter 4, development through these stages of the specialized movement phase is largely dependent on the quality of the movement and practice experiences received by the students.

Motor skill development in the application stage is typical for middle school students between the ages of 11 and 13 years. During this stage, students use prior successful experiences, body type, and environmental, emotional, social, and cultural factors in the decision-making process as they decide whether to participate (or not) in physical activities that require more advanced skill levels. This participation in selected or preferred physical activities is often accompanied by an increased desire for competence (Cleland Donnelly et al., 2017). The desire for competence in form, precision, accuracy, and the skills needed for good performance is increasingly important to the learner in the application stage.

During grades 6 through 8, individual differences in growth and maturation rates will require differentiated instruction and developmentally appropriate **accommodations**. As previously mentioned, skill acquisition is greatly dependent on how teachers design programs and engage learners in meaningful practice and culturally relevant movement experiences. When children are provided with developmentally appropriate and culturally relevant physical activities that provide opportunities for social interaction, challenge, fun, motor competence, and personally relevant learning, they are more likely to be successful in the learning tasks and motivated to continue participating. These sustained learning experiences allow students to refine, vary, combine, and apply specialized skills across a variety of culturally relevant physical activities and support progress within their physical literacy journey.

Based on the developmental characteristics of students in grades 6-8 within the psychomotor domain, the Grades 6-8 Standard 1 Grade-Span Learning Indicators and Learning Progressions are provided. The example practice tasks provided in the Learning Progressions support differentiated instruction in physical education and the meeting of physical education needs of all children. It is important to note that some Learning Indicators do not need associated Learning Progressions.

Standard 1: Develops a variety of motor skills.

Rationale. Through learning experiences in physical education, the student develops motor skills across a variety of environments. Motor skills are a foundational part of child development and support the movements of everyday life. The development of motor skills contributes to an individual's physical literacy journey.

Learning Indicators

OUTDOOR PURSUITS

1.8.1 Demonstrates correct technique in a variety of outdoor activities.

DANCE AND RHYTHMS

1.8.2 Demonstrates movement sequences within varied dance forms.

FITNESS ACTIVITIES

1.8.3 Demonstrates appropriate form in a variety of health-related fitness activities.

1.8.4 Demonstrates appropriate form in a variety of skill-related fitness activities.

TARGET GAMES

1.8.5 Demonstrates a striking motion with a long-handled implement.

1.8.6 Demonstrates a correct rolling and throwing (underhand, sidearm, overhand) technique in a variety of practice tasks and modified target games.

STRIKING AND FIELDING GAMES

1.8.7 Demonstrates striking a self-tossed/pitched ball with an implement to open space in a variety of practice tasks and small-sided games.

1.8.8 Demonstrates a proper catch with or without an implement in a variety of practice tasks and small-sided games.

1.8.9 Demonstrates throwing for accuracy, distance, and power in a variety of practice tasks and small-sided games.

NET AND WALL GAMES

1.8.10 Demonstrates a proper underhand and overhand serve using the hand in a variety of practice tasks and modified small-sided games.

1.8.11 Demonstrates a proper underhand and overhand serve using a short- or long-handled implement in a variety of practice tasks and modified small-sided games.

1.8.12 Demonstrates the correct form of a forehand and backhand stroke with a short-handled and long-handled implement in a variety of practice tasks and modified small-sided games.

1.8.13 Demonstrates a volley using a short-handled and long-handled implement in a variety of practice tasks and modified net and wall games.

INVASION GAMES

1.8.14 Demonstrates sending and receiving in combination with locomotor skills in a variety of small-sided games.

1.8.15 Demonstrates a dribbling skill in a variety of practice tasks and small-sided games.

1.8.16 Demonstrates dribbling an object with an implement in a variety of practice tasks and small-sided games.

1.8.17 Demonstrates a shot on goal with and without an implement in a variety of practice tasks and small-sided games.

1.8.18 Demonstrates multiple techniques to create open space during a variety of practice tasks and small-sided games (offense).

1.8.19 Demonstrates a defensive ready position in a variety of practice tasks and small-sided games.

AQUATICS

1.8.20 Demonstrates water safety skills. If a pool facility is available, demonstrates water safety and basic swimming skills.

Developmental Characteristics Within the Cognitive Domain of Learning

Between the ages of 11 and 14, cognitive development for students in grades 6-8 can be as intense and significant as their physical development (Brinegar & Caskey, 2022). These students tend to be curious and engaged in learning about content they find interesting, personally relevant (Bishop et al., 2019), and representative of their intersecting identities (e.g., gender, race, disability, culture, sexuality, class; Harrison et al., 2019). Understanding the cognitive development of adolescents in grades 6-8 is critical to physical educators' designing and implementing developmentally appropriate and meaningful learning experiences for these students in physical education.

Students in grades 6 through 8 are progressing through the concrete operations stage of cognitive development and onto formal operational thought (Piaget, 1952, 1954, 1974; Piaget et al., 1969). Within the concrete operations stage (ages 6 to 12 years), students focus on physical realities and hierarchical classifications. Their thinking is logical but requires learning through situations that are directly experienced, heard, or seen. Through these direct experiences, they also develop the ability to judge the reactions of others, make social comparisons, and consider the feelings of others (Smart, 2019).

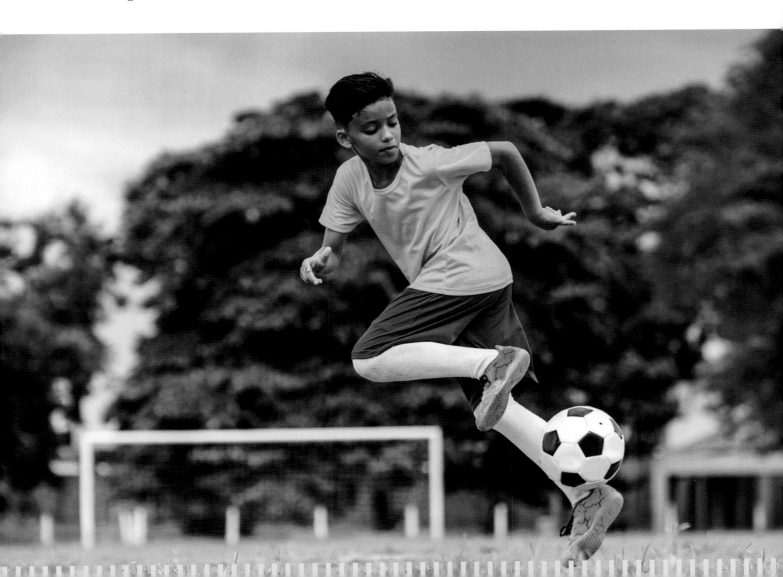

Around the age of 11 or 12 years, students move into the final stage of cognitive development, the formal operations stage, which begins in adolescence and persists through adulthood. Students can think in abstract and symbolic terms, and project themselves in future situations. For example, students can envision themselves in gameplay, anticipate player moves or responses, and determine defensive strategies to address those moves (Beach et al., 2024). In grades 6-8, students begin to develop metacognition skills, which allows them to understand and evaluate the way they perceive, remember, and learn new things. The characteristics of formal operational thinkers (the ability to use logical and abstract reasoning and prediction and planning skills) can be used by students in grades 6-8.

Based on students' cognitive development in grades 6-8, the Grades 6-8 Standard 2 Grade-Span Learning Indicators and Learning Progressions are designed to facilitate their physical literacy journey.

Standard 2: Applies knowledge related to movement and fitness concepts.

Rationale. Through learning experiences in physical education, the student uses their knowledge of movement concepts, tactics, and strategies across a variety of environments. This knowledge helps the student become a more versatile and efficient mover. Additionally, the student applies knowledge of health-related and skill-related fitness to enhance their overall well-being. The application of knowledge related to various forms of movement contributes to an individual's physical literacy journey.

Learning Indicators

TACTICS AND STRATEGIES

2.8.1 Identifies the effective use of movement concepts within multiple dynamic environments.

2.8.2 Demonstrates knowledge of offensive tactics to create space with movement in invasion games.

2.8.3 Demonstrates knowledge of reducing open space with movement and denial in invasion games.

2.8.4 Selects and applies the appropriate shot and technique in net and wall games.

2.8.5 Demonstrates knowledge of offensive tactics in striking and fielding games.

2.8.6 Demonstrates knowledge of defensive positioning tactics in striking and fielding games.

2.8.7 Demonstrates problem-solving skills in a variety of games and activities.

DANCE AND RHYTHMS

2.8.8 Applies knowledge of movement concepts for the purpose of varying different types of dances and rhythmic activities.

FITNESS CONCEPTS

2.8.9 Identifies and compares the components of health and skill-related fitness.

2.8.10 Self-selects and monitors physical activity goals based on a self-selected health-related fitness assessment.

2.8.11 Implements the principles of exercise (progression, overload, and specificity) for different types of physical activity.

2.8.12 Applies knowledge of skill-related fitness to different types of physical activity.

2.8.13 Explains the relationship of aerobic fitness and RPE Scale to physical activity effort.

2.8.14 Applies knowledge of dynamic and static stretching to exercise in warm-up, cool-down, flexibility, endurance, etc. physical activities.

2.8.15 Demonstrates knowledge of heart rate and describes its relationship to aerobic fitness.

PHYSICAL ACTIVITY KNOWLEDGE

2.8.16 Identifies ways to be physically active.

2.8.17 Examines how rest impacts the body's response to physical activity.

2.8.18 Analyzes skill performance by identifying critical elements.

2.8.19 Evaluates usefulness of technology tools to support physical activity and fitness goals.

2.8.20 Explains the relationships among nutrition, physical activity, and health factors.

OUTDOOR PURSUITS

2.8.21 Demonstrates knowledge of safety protocols in teacher-selected outdoor activities.

AQUATICS

2.8.22 Demonstrates knowledge of water safety skills. Demonstrates knowledge of basic swimming skills.

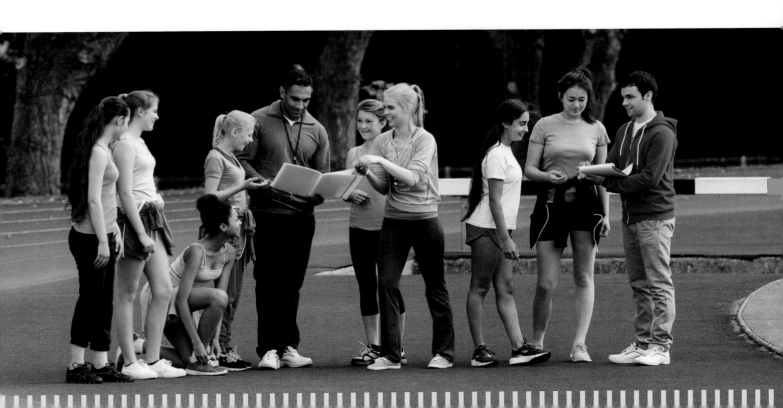

Developmental Characteristics Within the Social Domain of Learning

Physical educators' understanding of the social development of adolescents in grades 6-8 is critical to designing and implementing developmentally appropriate and meaningful learning experiences within physical education in these grades. As noted in previous chapters, students in grades 6-8 continue to develop social competence (i.e., social awareness and relationship awareness) across the middle school years. As defined by CASEL (2023), social awareness is the ability to understand the perspectives of and empathize with others, including those from diverse backgrounds, cultures, and contexts; while relationship awareness is the ability to establish and maintain healthy and supportive relationships and to effectively navigate settings with diverse individuals and groups (CASEL, 2023).

The social development of students in grades 6-8 can be further understood using Erikson's stages of psychosocial development (Erikson, 1963). In the transition from childhood to adulthood, adolescents experience two stages of identity formation: (1) industry versus inferiority and (2) identity versus role confusion (Erikson, 1968). As 10- to 11-year-olds in the industry versus inferiority stage, they develop their sense of self based on the skills and behaviors they perform well. Between the ages of 12 and 15 years, students progress through the **identity versus role confusion** stage, exploring various roles and experiences as they further develop their sense of individuality, uniqueness, and autonomy (Erikson, 1968). Through this ongoing process, adolescents search to find their identity and independence and to answer the question, "Who am I?" According to Scales (2010), as adolescents engage in the ongoing process of integrating prior identifications, self-images, experiences, beliefs, and values to develop a sense of self, they may experience feelings of vulnerability if they discover or sense differences between themselves and their peers. In resolving the social crisis of identity confusion and developing their identity, adolescents identify with others who are socially appealing, accept or reject family or peer values, and begin to accept the individual strengths and weaknesses that make them unique (Beach et al., 2024). Physical educators can assist students with development of their identity and self-concept by providing physical education learning activities that (1) are relevant and related to student interests, (2) build and support relationships between students and between the teacher and students, and (3) celebrate individual accomplishments. When adolescents are not allowed to explore and examine different identities, it may result in role confusion. Role confusion results in students being unsure of themselves and who they are, difficulties with maintaining relationships, and feelings of confusion or disappointment about their place in life. Role confusion also contributes to poor psychological well-being, which in turn affects social-emotional, cognitive, and physical development.

Based on these developmental characteristics of children in grades 6-8 within the social domain, Grades 6-8 Standard 3 Grade-Span Learning Indicators and Learning Progressions are provided.

Standard 3: Develops social skills through movement.

Rationale. Through learning experiences in physical education, students develop the social skills necessary to exhibit empathy and respect for others, and foster and maintain relationships. In addition, students develop skills for communication, leadership, cultural awareness, and conflict resolution in a variety of physical activity settings.

Learning Indicators

3.8.1 Understands and accepts others' differences during a variety of physical activities.

3.8.2 Demonstrates consideration for others and contributes positively to the group or team.

3.8.3 Uses communication skills to negotiate strategies and tactics in a physical activity setting.

3.8.4 Implements and provides constructive feedback to and from others when prompted and supported by the teacher.

3.8.5 Explains the value of a specific physical activity in culture.

3.8.6 Demonstrates the ability to follow game rules in a variety of physical activity situations.

3.8.7 Recognizes and implements safe and appropriate behaviors during physical activity and with exercise equipment.

3.8.8 Solves problems amongst teammates and opponents.

3.8.9 Applies and respects the importance of etiquette in a physical activity setting.

3.8.10 Explains how communication, feedback, cooperation, and etiquette relate to leadership roles.

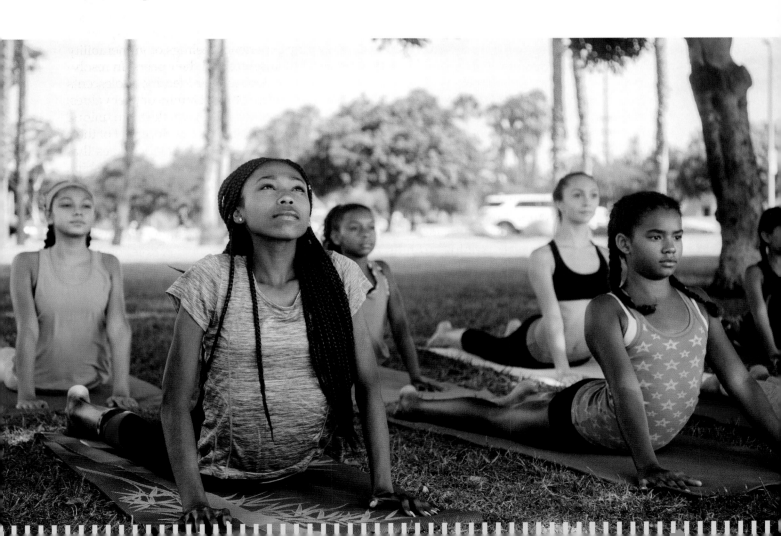

Developmental Characteristics Within the Affective Domain of Learning

As in previous chapters, the framework developed by the Collaborative for Academic, Social and Emotional Learning (CASEL) was used to examine the affective development of adolescents in grades 6-8 (e.g., self-awareness, self-management, and responsible decision-making). The attitudes, values, interests, and appreciation of a learner are several of the main focuses of the affective domain. The skills associated with this domain typically range from general awareness to allowing one's values to affect their behaviors and decisions (i.e., self-management). At this developmental stage in adolescents' lives, their personal beliefs, values, and standards are now more salient and identifiable with their own nature.

Adolescents are in the developmental stage where they are no longer young children but also not yet adults. Development of a strong sense of self-awareness, or the ability to understand emotions, thoughts, and values and how they influence one's behavior (CASEL, 2023), supports adolescents in being personally confident and successful as well as helping others be successful. For students in grades 6-8, physical education learning experiences that help them reflect objectively on their skills and behaviors and develop an awareness of their strengths and character traits will also help them learn how to use those traits to accomplish goals and everyday tasks. These experiences help students be more adept at identifying stressors and motivators, as well as self-management of their emotions, thoughts, and behaviors. Self-management contributes directly to a student's decision to engage in physical activity and progress within their own physical literacy journey.

The development of self-management skills for adolescents is critical to their responsible decision-making (the ability to make caring and constructive choices about one's personal behavior and social interactions across diverse situations; CASEL, 2023). For students in grades 6-8, responsible decision-making could include goal setting for teacher-selected and student-selected activities as well as identifying strategies to overcome barriers to physical activity participation. These physical education learning experiences for students in grades 6-8 also facilitate the development of their self-efficacy (beliefs in one's personal capabilities to achieve a successful outcome), which affects cognitive, motivational, affective, and decisional processes (Bandura, 1997). Development of students' self-efficacy specific to physical activity is central to engagement in physical education learning experiences in class as well as engagement in physical activities outside of physical education, including beyond their preK-12 years.

Based on these developmental characteristics of children in grades 6-8 within the affective domain, the Grades 6-8 Standard 4 Grade-Span Learning Indicators and Learning Progressions are provided.

Standard 4: Develops personal skills, identifies personal benefits of movement, and chooses to engage in physical activity.

Rationale. Through learning experiences in physical education, the student develops an understanding of how movement is personally beneficial and subsequently chooses to participate in physical activities that are personally meaningful (e.g., activities that offer social interaction, cultural connection, exploration, choice, self-expression, appropriate levels of challenge, and added health benefits). The student develops personal skills including goal setting, identifying strengths, and reflection to enhance their physical literacy journey.

Learning Indicators

4.8.1 Describes how self-expression impacts individual engagement in physical activity.

4.8.2 Describes how social interaction impacts individual engagement in physical activity.

4.8.3 Participates in a variety of physical activities that can positively affect personal health.

4.8.4 Connects how choice and personal interests impact individual engagement in physical activity.

4.8.5 Examines individual and group challenges through movement.

4.8.6 Sets goals to participate in physical activities based on examining individual ability.

4.8.7 Examines opportunities and barriers to participating in physical activity outside of physical education class.

4.8.8 Utilizes a variety of techniques to manage one's emotions and behaviors in a physical activity setting.

4.8.9 Reflects on movement experiences during physical education to develop understanding of how movement is personally meaningful.

Conclusion

Physical educators are encouraged to use the Standards and Grade-Span Learning Indicators for grades 6-8 to intentionally design instruction that supports the physical literacy journey of students in grades 6-8. The Grade-Span Learning Indicators and Learning Progressions are provided as examples to assist teachers with designing purposeful and relevant lessons for grades 6-8.

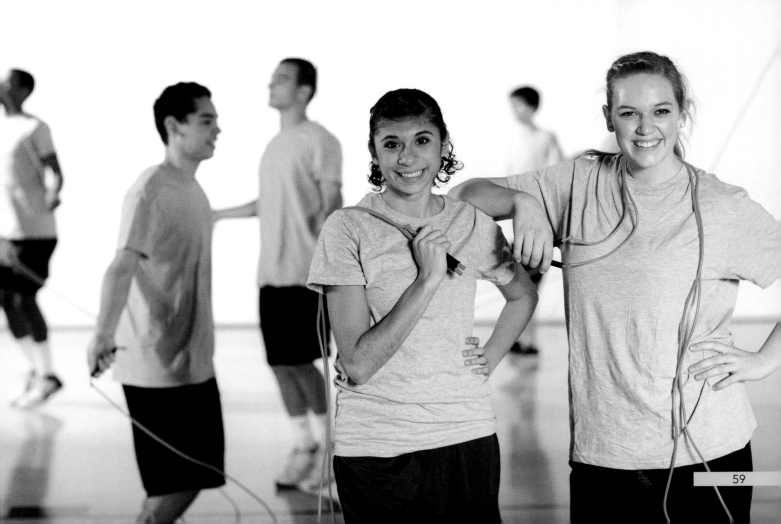

CHAPTER 6

Grades 9-12
National Physical Education
Standards, Grade-Span
Learning Indicators, and
Learning Progressions

Understanding the Learner

The development of an adolescent's physical literacy journey in grades 9-12 is significant because the student exists in a transitional stage between childhood and early adulthood. As students enter grades 9-12, they receive their (often final) structured pedagogical exposure to instruction related to physical activity before entering early adulthood. The knowledge, skills, and dispositions acquired by students prior to and during this pivotal time frame will shape their ability and likeliness to maintain a health-enhancing and physically active lifestyle through adulthood. Building on a growing proficiency with fundamental movement skills, students will be acquiring and refining their performance of specialized movement skills.

The Grade-Span Learning Indicators described in this chapter inform teachers about what grade 9-12 adolescents should know and be able to do and guide teachers in designing meaningful learning experiences. Teachers must take the time to review and be familiar with the developmental characteristics of grades 9-12 adolescents because it will aid them in understanding the Grade-Span Learning Indicators and associated Learning Progressions.

Developmental Characteristics Within the Psychomotor Domain of Learning

Adolescents in grades 9-12 are entering the final stage of the specialized movement phase of motor development. As discussed in previous chapters, during preK-8 years, these individuals have progressed through stages of the fundamental movement phase and, more recently, through the first two stages of the specialized movement phase. Essentially, at this point in an adolescent's development, they have progressed through the transitional and application stages of the specialized movement phase. In those two stages, adolescents have learned to combine and apply fundamental movement skills for sport and recreational performance in addition to refining more complex skills to be used in the narrower scope of lifetime physical activities (e.g., individual and team sports, outdoor pursuits, and other various activities) based on improved cognitive ability and increased movement experiences.

Thus, after progressing through the transitional and application stages of the specialized movement phase, adolescents now enter the third and final stage: lifelong utilization. The lifelong utilization stage, in a sense, is comprehensive and an application of an adolescent's motor development process and physical literacy journey. Additionally, this stage is marked by the choices, experiences, and refined complex skills acquired by adolescents in previous years that are now being applied to day-to-day, organized, and unorganized activities or movement experiences.

The lifelong utilization stage, as its name implies, is not intended to end at the completion of grades 9-12 but rather continue through one's life span. Therefore, at this stage, lifetime activities, dance and rhythms, and fitness activities are vital in the education of adolescents because they need to learn how to select, enjoy, and participate in movement experiences. For adolescents in this age group, success is dependent on proficiency in the fundamental movement phase.

Extensive developmentally appropriate opportunities, high-quality instruction, and encouragement are needed for appropriate development to continue in and beyond grade 12.

Based on the developmental characteristics of adolescents in grades 9-12 within the psychomotor domain, Grades 9-12 Standard 1 Grade-Span Learning Indicators are provided. Though the Grades 9-12 Learning Indicators are brief, when thoroughly unpacked, they are quite complex. These Learning Indicators, as written, allow for curricular flexibility so teachers and students can make choices that meet the diverse needs of all students.

Standard 1: Develops a variety of motor skills.

Rationale. Through learning experiences in physical education, the student develops motor skills across a variety of environments. Motor skills are a foundational part of child development and support the movements of everyday life. The development of motor skills contributes to an individual's physical literacy journey.

Learning Indicators

LIFETIME ACTIVITIES

1.12.1 Demonstrates activity-specific movement skills in a variety of lifetime sports and activities.

1.12.2 Demonstrates activity-specific movement skills in a variety of recreational and backyard games.

1.12.3 Demonstrates activity-specific movement skills in a variety of outdoor pursuits.

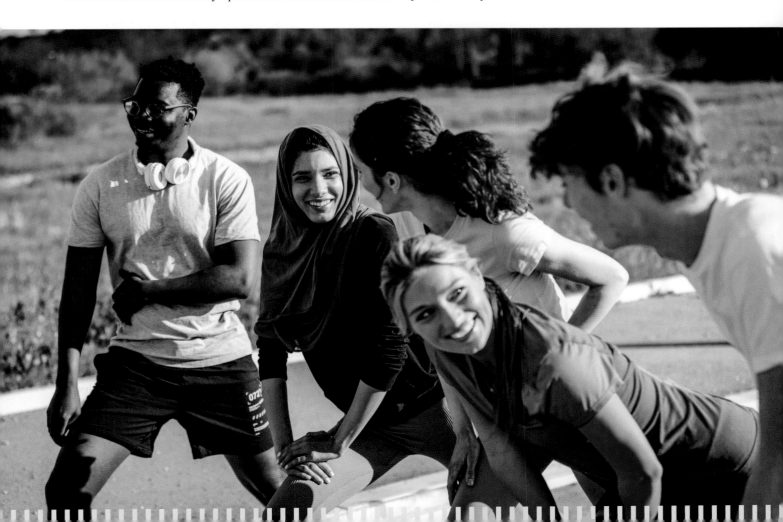

DANCE AND RHYTHMS
1.12.4 Demonstrates and creates movement sequences based on one or more forms of dance.

FITNESS ACTIVITIES
1.12.5 Demonstrates appropriate technique in cardiovascular training.

1.12.6 Demonstrates appropriate technique in muscular strength and endurance training.

1.12.7 Demonstrates appropriate technique in flexibility training.

1.12.8 Demonstrates appropriate technique in skill-related fitness training.

1.12.9 Demonstrates water safety skills. If a pool facility is available, demonstrates water safety and basic swimming skills.

Developmental Characteristics Within the Cognitive Domain of Learning

Understanding the cognitive development of grades 9-12 adolescents is vital in any effort to design and deliver developmentally appropriate learning experiences within physical education. Psychologist Jean Piaget has provided a theoretical approach to understanding human development as it relates to cognition. The **developmental milestone theory** (Piaget, 1952, 1954, 1974; Piaget et al., 1969) gives us a valuable conceptual framework that provides insight into the developmental characteristics of adolescents in grades 9-12 within the cognitive domain.

Adolescents in grades 9-12 engage in Piaget's process of **adaptation**. This includes both **accommodation** (adapting responses to new information) and **assimilation** (interpreting new information within present cognitive structures) and takes place in four stages. Starting in early adolescence, students are in the third stage: concrete operations. In that stage, adolescents' mental actions are still tied to concrete objects; however, they also begin to **conserve**. This describes the ability of one to focus on multiple variables in a given environment (e.g., solving tactical problems in an invasion game).

By high school, though, adolescents should be several years into cognitive adaptation and entering the fourth and final phase: formal operations. This phase (similar to the lifelong utilization phase mentioned in the previous section) persists into and through adulthood. Adolescents in the formal operational stage can reason logically but now are able to do so without concrete objects or events experienced personally. They can cognitively manage games, activities, and movement experiences that are more complex. Within the context of physical education, adolescents in the formal operational phase can now understand and apply tactics and strategies, compare and contrast various movement experiences, analyze factors that would affect participation in activity beyond high school, and create plans that support an active and healthy lifestyle. These are but a few markers of developmental appropriateness in this phase.

Based on the developmental characteristics of adolescents in grades 9-12 within the cognitive domain, Grades 9-12 Standard 2 Grade-Span Learning Indicators and Learning Progressions are provided.

Standard 2: Applies knowledge related to movement and fitness concepts.

Rationale. Through learning experiences in physical education, the student uses their knowledge of movement concepts, tactics, and strategies across a variety of environments. This knowledge helps the student become a more versatile and efficient mover. Additionally, the student applies knowledge of health-related and skill-related fitness to enhance their overall well-being. The application of knowledge related to various forms of movement contributes to an individual's physical literacy journey.

Learning Indicators

TACTICS AND STRATEGIES

2.12.1 Demonstrates knowledge of tactics and strategies within lifetime sports and activities.

2.12.2 Demonstrates knowledge of tactics and strategies within recreational and backyard games.

2.12.3 Demonstrates knowledge of tactics and strategies within outdoor pursuits.

DANCE AND RHYTHMS

2.12.4 Applies knowledge of movement sequences to create or participate in one or more forms of dance.

FITNESS CONCEPTS

2.12.5 Analyzes how health and fitness will impact quality of life after high school.

2.12.6 Establishes a goal and creates a practice plan to improve performance for a self-selected skill.

2.12.7 Applies the principles of exercise in a variety of self-selected lifetime physical activities.

2.12.8 Designs and implements a plan that applies knowledge of aerobic, strength and endurance, and flexibility training exercises.

2.12.9 Evaluates perceived exertion during physical activity and adjusts effort.

2.12.10 Applies heart rate concepts to ensure safety and maximize health-related fitness outcomes.

PHYSICAL ACTIVITY KNOWLEDGE

2.12.11 Discusses the benefits of a physically active lifestyle as it relates to young adulthood.

2.12.12 Applies knowledge of rest when planning regular physical activity.

2.12.13 Applies movement concepts and principles (e.g., force, motion, rotation) to analyze and improve performance of self and/or others in a selected skill (e.g., overhand throw, back squat, archery).

2.12.14 Identifies and discusses the historical and cultural roles of games, sports and dance in a society.

2.12.15 Analyzes and applies technology as tools to support a healthy, active lifestyle.

2.12.16 Identifies snacks and food choices that help and hinder performance, recovery, and enjoyment during physical activity.

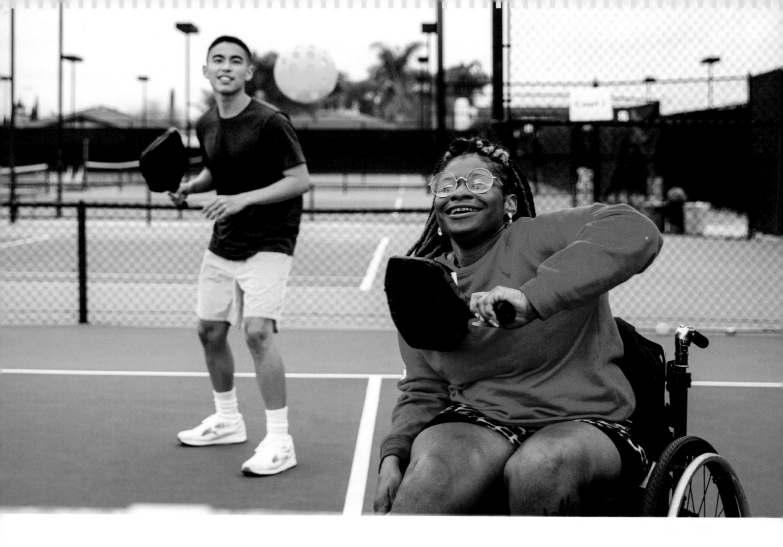

AQUATICS

2.12.17 Demonstrates knowledge of water safety skills. Demonstrates knowledge of basic swimming skills.

Developmental Characteristics Within the Social Domain of Learning

Understanding the social development of grades 9-12 adolescents is essential for pedagogical attempts to plan and present developmentally appropriate learning experiences within physical education. As noted in previous chapters, students in grades 9-12 are further developing social competence (i.e., social awareness and relationship awareness). Social awareness involves the ability to understand the perspectives of and empathize with others, including those from diverse backgrounds, cultures, and contexts (CASEL, 2023). Additionally, relationship awareness involves the ability to establish and maintain healthy and supportive relationships and to effectively navigate settings with diverse individuals and groups (CASEL, 2023).

Psychoanalyst Erik Erikson has provided a theoretical approach to understanding human psychosocial development. The phase-stage theory (Erikson, 1963, 1980) gives us an indispensable conceptual framework that provides insight into the developmental characteristics of adolescents in grades 9-12 within the social domain. Young people who are transitioning from early adolescence to late adolescence are mainly entering and exiting two of Erikson's stages of psychosocial development: identity versus role confusion and intimacy versus isolation. During the identity versus role confusion stage, younger adolescents begin to develop more masculine or feminine identities as they experience rapid changes in physical and sexual maturation. Additionally, perceived peer acceptance and rejection start to take significant precedence. When the values and perspectives that begin to arise conflict with what a student is experiencing in relationships and society, there is a risk for role confusion. As adolescents begin (and continue) to be immersed in society, identity formation becomes vital and they make decisions regarding who they will be and what they will do in life. In this phase, adolescents often gain a sense of identity from having opportunities to solve the regulated social challenges that arise from movement-related learning experiences curated by physical education teachers. Role confusion, again, becomes a risk without exposure to occasions for competence and success in these experiences.

Furthermore, as adolescents enter the **intimacy versus isolation stage**, healthy and intimate relationships begin to outweigh or supersede other social factors. This stage is marked by one's ability to accept the identity established in the previous stages of development and begin to accept and synthesize the identities formed by others with their own. Adolescents in this stage are able to foster a sense of belonging and intimacy with peers through participation in various movement experiences. Through cooperation, teamwork, etiquette, communication, respect, cultural awareness, leadership, and critical thinking opportunities during movement, relational intimacy can develop among adolescent peers. Unfortunately, failure to develop the requisite knowledge, skills, and dispositions necessary for participation in physical activity can lead students to a deep sense of isolation from social groups.

Based on the developmental characteristics of adolescents in grades 9-12 within the social domain, Grades 9-12 Standard 3 Grade-Span Learning Indicators and Learning Progressions are provided.

Standard 3: Develops social skills through movement.

Rationale. Through learning experiences in physical education, students develop the social skills necessary to exhibit empathy and respect for others, and foster and maintain relationships. In addition, students develop skills for communication, leadership, cultural awareness, and conflict resolution in a variety of physical activity settings.

Learning Indicators

3.12.1 Demonstrates awareness of other people's emotions and perspectives in a physical activity setting.

3.12.2 Exhibits proper etiquette, respect for others, and teamwork while engaging in physical activity.

3.12.3 Encourages and supports others through their interactions in a physical activity setting.

3.12.4 Implements and provides feedback to improve performance without prompting from the teacher.

3.12.5 Analyzes the value of a specific physical activity in a variety of cultures.

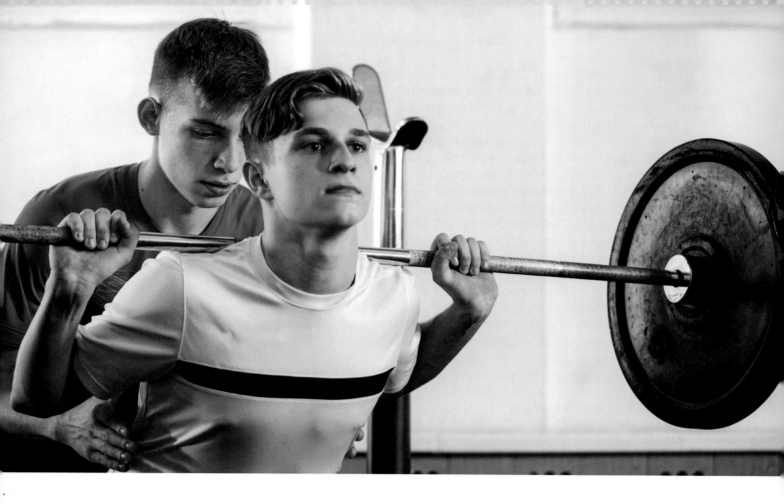

3.12.6 Applies best practices for participating safely in physical activity (e.g., injury prevention, spacing, hydration, use of equipment, implementation of rules, sun protection).

3.12.7 Thinks critically and solves problems in physical activity settings, both as an individual and in groups.

3.12.8 Evaluates the effectiveness of leadership skills when participating in a variety of settings.

Developmental Characteristics Within the Affective Domain of Learning

As in previous chapters, the concepts of self-awareness, self-management, and responsible decision-making (CASEL, 2023) provide a valuable framework with which to view the affective developmental characteristics of grades 9-12 adolescents. The attitudes, values, interests, and appreciation of a learner are several of the main focuses of the affective domain. The skills associated with this domain typically range from general awareness to allowing one's values to affect their behaviors and decisions (i.e., self-management). At this developmental stage in adolescents' lives, their personal beliefs, values, and standards are now more salient and identifiable with their own nature.

Essentially, self-awareness begins to become more clearly internally driven rather than driven by parents, coaches, teachers, or peers. For students in grades 9-12, their perceived competence likely will affect their decision-making as it relates to physical activity. While it is debatable if perceived competence increases simply with age, high perceptions of competence in physical skills can lead to positive emotional connections with activity and thus increase participation (Beach et al., 2024).

Additionally, as adolescents in grades 9-12 become more self-determined (Ryan & Deci, 2000), their need to feel competent and autonomous has an even greater impact on their intrinsic and extrinsic motivation (or lack thereof) to move. Not meeting these needs negatively influences the affective experience of students. As students in grades 9-12 rely less and less on parent and teacher beliefs and values, they must start to identify and act on intrinsic desires to be physically active (e.g., personal meaningfulness or improved health).

Providing adolescents with choices, occasions to set goals, positive feedback, and an emphasis on personal improvement can help to facilitate more responsible decision-making. Relatedly, a student's self-efficacy (Bandura, 1997) can be improved with those same strategies. Self-efficacy is vital for anyone's likelihood of continuing to participate in physical activity beyond high school.

Based on the developmental characteristics of adolescents in grades 9-12 within the affective domain, Grades 9-12 Standard 4 Grade-Span Learning Indicators and Learning Progressions are provided.

Standard 4: Develops personal skills, identifies personal benefits of movement, and chooses to engage in physical activity.

Rationale. Through learning experiences in physical education, the student develops an understanding of how movement is personally beneficial and subsequently chooses to participate in physical activities that are personally meaningful (e.g., activities that offer social interaction, cultural connection, exploration, choice, self-expression, appropriate levels of challenge, and added health benefits). The student develops personal skills including goal setting, identifying strengths, and reflection to enhance their physical literacy journey.

Learning Indicators

4.12.1 Selects and participates in physical activities (e.g., dance, yoga, aerobics) that meet the need for self-expression.

4.12.2 Selects and participates in physical activities that meet the need for social interaction.

4.12.3 Identifies and participates in physical activity that positively affects health.

4.12.4 Chooses and participates in physical activity based on personal interests.

4.12.5 Chooses and successfully participates in self-selected physical activity at a level that is appropriately challenging.

4.12.6 Sets and develops movement goals related to personal interests.

4.12.7 Analyzes factors on regular participation in physical activity after high school (e.g., life choices, economics, motivation, accessibility).

4.12.8 Analyzes and applies self-selected techniques to manage one's emotions in a physical activity setting.

4.12.9 Reflects on movement experiences during physical education to develop understanding of how movement is personally meaningful.

Conclusion

Physical educators are encouraged to intentionally design instruction based on Standards 1 through 4 to foster grades 9-12 adolescents' physical literacy journey. The Learning Indicators and Learning Progressions are provided to help teachers design purposeful and relevant lessons for grades 9-12 students.

CHAPTER 7

The National Physical Education Standards, Grade-Span Learning Indicators, and Learning Progressions

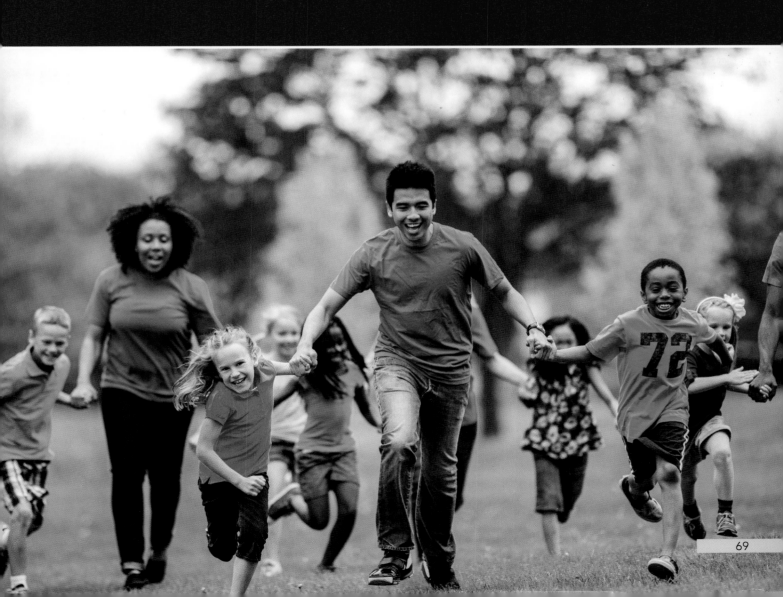

The 2024 SHAPE America National Physical Education Standards, Grade-Span Learning Indicators, and Learning Progressions provide a framework for ensuring consistency and quality in physical education programs and address the holistic development of students across the nation. In chapters 3 through 6, the Grade-Span Learning Indicators were presented in isolation by grade span. In this chapter, the National Physical Education Standards and Grade-Span Learning Indicators are presented with their associated Learning Progressions.

For each standard, the Grade-Span Learning Indicators for grades preK-12 will be listed first in an Indicators at a Glance table. This table is a list of all the indicators for a standard and is not designed to show alignment across grade spans. On the subsequent pages, Grade-Span Learning Indicators are organized by grade span: preK-2, grades 3-5, grades 6-8, and grades 9-12. Each Grade-Span Learning Indicator is then listed with its associated Learning Progressions.

Learning Progressions provide examples of qualitative descriptors to guide teachers in unpacking the Grade-Span Learning Indicators. Learning Progressions should not be viewed as the only way teachers can break down Grade-Span Learning Indicators but as one of many ways teachers can break them down. They are designed to be measurable, observable, and of use to teachers as they develop assessments and learning experiences for their students.

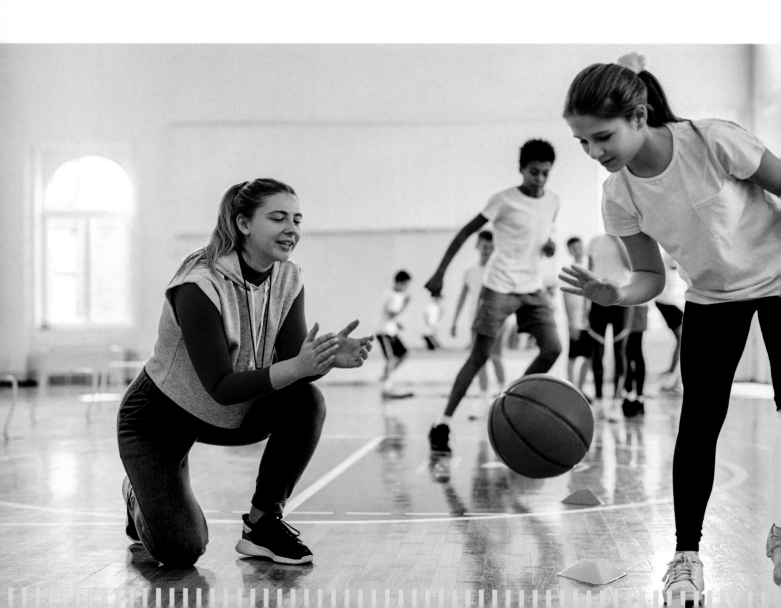

INDICATORS AT A GLANCE

Note: *This chart is intended to list the Grade-Span Learning Indicators for grades preK-12. This chart is not intended to show alignment across Grade-Span Learning Indicators. However, some indicators may align across grade spans and some may not due to the content and skills being taught within a specific grade span.*

STANDARD 1	Develops a variety of motor skills.
RATIONALE	Through learning experiences in physical education, the student develops motor skills across a variety of environments. Motor skills are a foundational part of child development and support the movements of everyday life. The development of motor skills contributes to an individual's physical literacy journey.

Grades preK-2 Learning Indicators	Grades 3-5 Learning Indicators	Grades 6-8 Learning Indicators	Grades 9-12 Learning Indicators
1.2.1 Demonstrates a variety of locomotor skills with the concepts of space, effort, and relationship awareness.	1.5.1 Combines varied locomotor skills in a variety of practice tasks.	1.8.1 Demonstrates correct technique in a variety of outdoor activities.	1.12.1 Demonstrates activity-specific movement skills in a variety of lifetime sports and activities.
1.2.2 Demonstrates jumping and landing in a non-dynamic environment.	1.5.2 Demonstrates transferring weight from feet to hands and hands to feet in a non-dynamic environment.	1.8.2 Demonstrates movement sequences within varied dance forms.	1.12.2 Demonstrates activity-specific movement skills in a variety of recreational and backyard games.
1.2.3 Demonstrates transferring weight on multiple body parts.	1.5.3 Demonstrates rolling with the body in a non-dynamic environment.	1.8.3 Demonstrates appropriate form in a variety of health-related fitness activities.	1.12.3 Demonstrates activity-specific movement skills in a variety of outdoor pursuits.
1.2.4 Demonstrates non-locomotor skills with the concepts of space, effort, and relationship awareness.	1.5.4 Combines jumping and landing, rolling, balancing and transfer of weight from feet to hands in a non-dynamic environment.	1.8.4 Demonstrates appropriate form in a variety of skill-related fitness activities.	1.12.4 Demonstrates and creates movement sequences based on one or more forms of dance.
1.2.5 Demonstrates balancing on different body parts in a non-dynamic environment.	1.5.5 Combines locomotor, non-locomotor, and manipulative movements based on a variety of dance forms.	1.8.5 Demonstrates a striking motion with a long-handled implement.	1.12.5 Demonstrates appropriate technique in cardiovascular training.
1.2.6 Demonstrates bouncing a ball in a variety of non-dynamic practice tasks.	1.5.6 Demonstrates jumping rope in a variety of practice tasks.	1.8.6 Demonstrates a correct rolling and throwing (underhand, sidearm, overhand) technique in a variety of practice tasks and modified target games.	1.12.6 Demonstrates appropriate technique in muscular strength and endurance training.
1.2.7 Demonstrates rolling a ball in a variety of non-dynamic practice tasks.	1.5.7 Demonstrates jumping and landing in a non-dynamic environment.	1.8.7 Demonstrates striking a self-tossed/pitched ball with an implement to open space in a variety of practice tasks and small-sided games.	1.12.7 Demonstrates appropriate technique in flexibility training.

>continued

STANDARD 1   >continued

Grades preK-2 Learning Indicators	Grades 3-5 Learning Indicators	Grades 6-8 Learning Indicators	Grades 9-12 Learning Indicators
1.2.8 Demonstrates catching in a variety of non-dynamic practice tasks.	1.5.8 Demonstrates balancing on different body parts in a non-dynamic environment.	1.8.8 Demonstrates a proper catch with or without an implement in a variety of practice tasks and small-sided games.	1.12.8 Demonstrates appropriate technique in skill-related fitness training.
1.2.9 Demonstrates throwing in a variety of non-dynamic practice tasks.	1.5.9 Demonstrates rolling a ball in a non-dynamic environment.	1.8.9 Demonstrates throwing for accuracy, distance, and power in a variety of practice tasks and small-sided games.	1.12.9 Demonstrates water safety skills. If a pool facility is available, demonstrates water safety and basic swimming skills.
1.2.10 Demonstrates kicking a ball in a variety of non-dynamic practice tasks.	1.5.10 Demonstrates throwing in a variety of practice tasks.	1.8.10 Demonstrates a proper underhand and overhand serve using the hand in a variety of practice tasks and modified small-sided games.	
1.2.11 Demonstrates dribbling with feet in a variety of non-dynamic practice tasks.	1.5.11 Demonstrates striking with a long-handled implement in a variety of practice tasks.	1.8.11 Demonstrates a proper underhand and overhand serve using a short- or long-handled implement in a variety of practice tasks and modified small-sided games.	
1.2.12 Demonstrates striking with hands in a variety of non-dynamic practice tasks.	1.5.12 Demonstrates catching in a variety of practice tasks.	1.8.12 Demonstrates the correct form of a forehand and backhand stroke with a short-handled and long-handled implement in a variety of practice tasks and modified small-sided games.	
1.2.13 Demonstrates striking with a short-handled implement in a variety of non-dynamic practice tasks.	1.5.13 Demonstrates striking with hands above waist in a variety of practice tasks.	1.8.13 Demonstrates a volley using a short-handled and long-handled implement in a variety of practice tasks and modified net and wall games.	
1.2.14 Demonstrates striking with a long-handled implement in a variety of non-dynamic practice tasks.	1.5.14 Demonstrates striking with hands below waist in a variety of practice tasks.	1.8.14 Demonstrates sending and receiving in combination with locomotor skills in a variety of small-sided games.	

Grades preK-2 Learning Indicators	Grades 3-5 Learning Indicators	Grades 6-8 Learning Indicators	Grades 9-12 Learning Indicators
1.2.15 Demonstrates locomotor, non-locomotor, and manipulative movements based on a variety of dance forms.	**1.5.15** Demonstrates serving an object in a non-dynamic environment.	**1.8.15** Demonstrates a dribbling skill in a variety of practice tasks and small-sided games.	
1.2.16 Demonstrates jumping rope in a non-dynamic environment.	**1.5.16** Demonstrates striking an object with a short-handled implement in a variety of practice tasks.	**1.8.16** Demonstrates dribbling an object with an implement in a variety of practice tasks and small-sided games.	
1.2.17 Demonstrates water safety skills. If a pool facility is available, demonstrates water safety and basic swimming skills.	**1.5.17** Demonstrates sending and receiving an object in a variety of practice tasks.	**1.8.17** Demonstrates a shot on goal with and without an implement in a variety of practice tasks and small-sided games.	
	1.5.18 Demonstrates kicking a ball using the instep in a variety of practice tasks.	**1.8.18** Demonstrates multiple techniques to create open space during a variety of practice tasks and small-sided games (offense).	
	1.5.19 Demonstrates dribbling with hands in a variety of practice tasks.	**1.8.19** Demonstrates a defensive ready position in a variety of practice tasks and small-sided games.	
	1.5.20 Demonstrates dribbling with feet in a variety of practice tasks.	**1.8.20** Demonstrates water safety skills. If a pool facility is available, demonstrates water safety and basic swimming skills.	
	1.5.21 Combines manipulative skills and traveling for execution to a target in a variety of practice tasks.		
	1.5.22 Demonstrates water safety skills. If a pool facility is available, demonstrates water safety and basic swimming skills.		

STANDARD 1	Develops a variety of motor skills.			
Grades preK-2	**PROGRESSIONS**			
	LOCOMOTOR			

INDICATORS					
1.2.1 Demonstrates a variety of locomotor skills with the concepts of space, effort, and relationship awareness.	**Horizontal jump**	Demonstrates jumping horizontally across space. Inconsistent push-off and landing from both feet, limited knee flexion, and no arm swing.	• Demonstrates jumping horizontally across space achieving small to moderate distance. • Exhibits some knee flexion and arm swing from back to front to generate force and achieve a flight phase.	Demonstrates jumping horizontally across space achieving greater distance.	
	Galloping	Gallops consecutively forward but back foot passes beyond heel of lead foot; limited arm swing and no flight phase.	Gallops consecutively forward but back foot trails lead foot; limited arm swing and no flight phase; moderate arm action and flight phase.	Gallops consecutively forward but back foot trails lead foot; limited arm swing and no flight phase; full arm swing and flight phase.	
	Sliding sideways	Leads sliding action with side, but during slide stomach leads action; limited flight phase during main action.	Leads sliding action with side; arms stay extended out to side; moderate flight phase created by step-together-step action.	Leads sliding action with side; arms stay extended out to side; complete flight phase created by step-together-step action.	
	Hopping	Performs 1 hop; limited arm and non-hopping leg action.	Performs 3 consecutive hops; limited arm and non-hopping leg action.	Performs 3 consecutive hops with moderate arm and non-hopping leg.	
	Skipping	Performs skipping forward; arms do not alternate; knees not waist high.	Performs skipping forward with limited alternating arm action; knees waist high.	Performs skipping forward along varied pathways with full range of motion.	
	Leaping	Demonstrates transferring weight from one foot to the opposite foot over a low lying object placed on the floor. Legs are not straight and there is little flight phase. Leap resembles a running step.	Demonstrates a brief run and transfer of weight from one foot to the opposite foot over a low lying object placed on the floor. There is a greater flight phase and more distance is achieved during the leap. Legs are not straight.	• Demonstrates a run and transfer of weight from one foot to the opposite foot over a low lying object placed on the floor. • There is a greater flight phase and more distance is achieved during the leap. Legs are almost straight during the flight phase.	
1.2.2 Demonstrates jumping and landing in a non-dynamic environment.	• Jumps off a low object onto the floor. • Does not consistently take off of both feet and land on both feet. Little arm action, knee flexion and extension.	Jumps off a low object onto the floor consistently taking off two feet and landing on two feet. Little arm action, knee flexion.	Jumps off a low object onto the floor consistently taking off two feet and landing on two feet. Arms swing from back to front and there is some knee flexion and extension to produce force.	Jumps over a low object (rope on floor, polyspot, foam noodle) onto the floor consistently taking off two feet and landing on two feet. Arms swing from back to front and there is some knee flexion and extension to produce force.	

Gallops along varied pathways.	Gallops in general space in response to designated beats/rhythms.		
Can slide leading with right side and then turn and perform with left side leading the slide; complete flight phase.	Can slide to an external beat through general space.		
Performs consecutive hops along varied pathways	Performs consecutive hops to an external beat.		
Performs skipping forward to an external beat.	Performs skipping and turning forward through general space.		
Can run and jump over a low object (rope on floor, polyspot, foam noodle) onto the floor consistently taking off two feet and landing on two feet or one to two feet.			

>continued

STANDARD 1   >continued

STANDARD 1	Develops a variety of motor skills.			
Grades preK-2	PROGRESSIONS			

LOCOMOTOR

1.2.3 Demonstrates transferring weight on multiple body parts.	Transfers weight on one or more body parts to another (e.g., animal walks).	Rolls using different body positions from side to side on a flat surface.	Rolls forward using a round body position.	

NON-LOCOMOTOR

1.2.4 Demonstrates non-locomotor skills with the concepts of space, effort, and relationship awareness.	Performs curling, stretching, twisting, and bending in self-space.	Performs curling, stretching, twisting, and bending in self-space to an external rhythm in self-space.		
1.2.5 Demonstrates balancing on different body parts in a non-dynamic environment.	Maintains momentary stillness on different bases of support.	Maintains stillness on different bases of support with different body shapes.	Balances on different bases of support, combining levels and shapes.	Balances in an inverted position with one foot above head while maintaining stillness.

BOUNCING

1.2.6 Demonstrates bouncing a ball in a variety of non-dynamic practice tasks.	Drops ball and catches it on the rebound while stationary.	Pushes down (applies force) on ball with both hands and catches it on rebound while stationary.	Pushes down (applies force) on ball with both hands repetitively while stationary.	Pushes down (applies force) on ball with both hands repetitively while moving slowly.

ROLLING

1.2.7 Demonstrates rolling a ball in a variety of non-dynamic practice tasks.	Rolls a small ball (hand size) toward the wall or large target. Minimal arm swing alongside of body. Feet side by side and no step in opposition.	Rolls a small ball (hand size) toward the wall or large target. Larger arms swing during preparation. Forward/backward stance, steps with opposition while rolling.	Rolls a playground ball using full range of arm motion and leg actions toward a stationary target.	Rolls a playground ball using full range of arm motion and greater force for the purpose of hitting/reaching a target.

CATCHING AND THROWING

1.2.8 Demonstrates catching in a variety of non-dynamic practice tasks.	Can reach up with two hands to catch a suspended balloon.	Tosses to self just above head and catches in front of chest with two hands.	While stationary catches an oncoming large ball from a short distance and slow speed using forearms to "hug" or "scoop" ball into chest.	While stationary catches an oncoming large ball from a short distance and slow speed using two hands.

INDICATORS

Pushes down (applies force) on ball with preferred hand repetitively while stationary.	Pushes down (applies force) on ball with preferred hand repetitively while moving through open space.	Bounces with preferred hand while moving and avoiding obstacles.	Pushes down (applies force) on ball with preferred hand repetitively while following a partner who is also bouncing through general space.
Rolls a playground ball using full range of arm and legs to a stationary partner 15 feet (5 m) away.	Rolls a playground ball using full range of arm and legs to a moving partner 15 feet (5 m) away.		
While stationary catches an oncoming large ball from a medium distance and medium speed using two hands.	• Can move a short distance to get behind the oncoming ball from a horizontal trajectory, medium speed and medium distance. • Catches with two hands only.		

>continued

STANDARD 1   >continued

STANDARD 1	Develops a variety of motor skills.			
Grades preK-2	**PROGRESSIONS**			

CATCHING AND THROWING

| 1.2.9 Demonstrates throwing in a variety of non-dynamic practice tasks. | Throws a small object (fits in one's hand) using any arm motion (underhand, sidearm, overhand) in a non-dynamic practice task. | Refines underhand throwing technique using greater arm motion (i.e., preparation and execution or force phase) in a non-dynamic practice task. | Refines underhand throwing technique adding forward/ backward stance for the purpose of shifting weight during the execution of the throw in a non-dynamic practice task. | Refines underhand throwing technique by increasing range of motion of arm action and also starts with feet together and steps with opposition during the execution of the throw in a non-dynamic practice task. |

KICKING AND DRIBBLING WITH FEET

| 1.2.10 Demonstrates kicking a ball in a variety of non-dynamic practice tasks. | Kicks a stationary ball from a stationary position into general space with limited range of motion and force. | Kicks a stationary ball from a stationary position toward a stationary target with medium force and distance. | Kicks a stationary ball with a two-step approach into general space. | Kicks a stationary ball with a two-step approach toward a stationary object. |
| 1.2.11 Demonstrates dribbling with feet in a variety of non-dynamic practice tasks. | Dribbles a ball with the inside of either foot at a slow speed through general space. | Dribbles a ball with the inside of either foot at a slow speed around stationary objects in general space. | Dribbles a ball with the inside of either foot around stationary objects while changing speeds. | Dribbles a ball with the inside of either foot around stationary objects changing speeds and directions upon command. |

STRIKING WITH HANDS

| 1.2.12 Demonstrates striking with hands in a variety of non-dynamic practice tasks. | Strikes with one or both hands a lightweight object (balloon), sending it upward while in personal space. | Strikes with one or both hands a lightweight object, sending it upward with consecutive hits. | Strikes with both hands a lightweight object, sending it upward with consecutive hits. | Strikes a lightweight object over a horizontal rope (4-5 ft [1-2 m] high) tossed to them at a medium trajectory and distance of 5-10 feet (2-3 m). |

STRIKING WITH IMPLEMENTS

| 1.2.13 Demonstrates striking with a short-handled implement in a variety of non-dynamic practice tasks. | Using a short-handled racquet strikes a suspended ball. | Using a short-handled racquet strikes a balloon using a sidearm striking motion (low to high). | Using a short-handled racquet strikes a balloon using a sidearm striking motion (low to high) toward a partner. | Using a short-handled racquet strikes a self-bounced foam tennis ball toward the wall using a sidearm motion. |
| 1.2.14 Demonstrates striking with a long-handled implement in a variety of non-dynamic practice tasks. | Using a bat (appropriate size for student) strikes a suspended object. | Using a bat (appropriate size for student) strikes an object off of a tee toward open space or a large stationary target. | Using a bat (appropriate size for student) strikes an object off of a tee toward open space or a large stationary target. | Using a bat (appropriate size for student) strikes a soft object tossed underhand to them from a distance of 5 feet (2 m). |

INDICATORS

Demonstrates overhand throw to large stationary targets at different levels and distances without full range of motion.	Demonstrates the overhand throw using full range of motion in a non-dynamic practice task.		
Kicks a moving ball (e.g., from a partner roll) with a two-step approach into open space.	Kicks a moving ball (e.g., from a partner roll) with a two-step approach toward a large stationary target.		
Using a bat (appropriate size for student) strikes a soft object tossed underhand to them from a distance of 10 feet (3 m).			

>continued

STANDARD 1   >continued

STANDARD 1	Develops a variety of motor skills.				
Grades preK-2	**PROGRESSIONS**				
	DANCE AND RHYTHMS				
1.2.15 Demonstrates locomotor, non-locomotor, and manipulative movements based on a variety of dance forms.	Demonstrates lyric-directed dances using simple steps (e.g., step-touch to right/left; slide to right/left, walk forward 4 counts and back 4 counts) with simple upper body movements (e.g., clapping hands; hand actions).	Demonstrates locomotor skills while traveling in a circle to a rhythmic beat.	Performs simple locomotor and non-locomotor skills while manipulating a scarf, ribbon or small prop.	Combines locomotor and non-locomotor movements to a rhythmic beat along varied pathways and in different directions.	
1.2.16 Demonstrates jumping rope in a non-dynamic environment.	Jumps in and out of a rope positioned in a shape on the floor.	Executes a single jump with a self-turned rope.	Executes multiple jumps forward with a self-turned rope.	Executes a single jump backward with a self-turned rope.	
	AQUATICS				
1.2.17 Demonstrates water safety skills. If a pool facility is available, demonstrates water safety and basic swimming skills.	Demonstrates safety rules strategies.	Demonstrates floating skills.	Demonstrates glide to kick.	Demonstrates swimming stroke.	

INDICATORS

Executes multiple jumps backward with a self-turned rope.	Jumps a long rope with teacher-assisted turning.	Can enter a long jump rope with teacher-assisted turning and jump 1-2 times.	Can enter a long jump rope with teacher-assisted turning and jump multiple times.

STANDARD 1	Develops a variety of motor skills.				
Grades 3-5	PROGRESSIONS				

LOCOMOTOR

INDICATORS						
1.5.1 Combines varied locomotor skills in a variety of practice tasks.	Demonstrates a movement sequence of three different locomotor skills across general space with full range of movement (e.g., skip, run and leap, slide sideways or gallop, skip, run and leap).	Demonstrates a movement sequence of three different locomotor skills across general space with full range of movement (e.g., skip, run and leap, slide sideways or gallop, skip, run and leap).	Demonstrates a movement sequence of three different locomotor skills across general space with full range of movement (e.g., skip, run and leap, slide sideways or gallop, skip, run and leap).	Demonstrates a movement sequence of three different locomotor skills across general space with full range of movement (e.g., skip, run and leap, slide sideways or gallop, skip, run and leap).	
1.5.2 Demonstrates transferring weight from feet to hands and hands to feet in a non-dynamic environment.	Can perform a modified cartwheel (i.e., hand, hand, foot, foot) with hands on a 12-18 inches (30-46 cm) foam shape and kicking legs over the shape.	Can perform a cartwheel on a mat; legs are not fully extended; arms not fully extended above head in recovery.	Can perform a cartwheel covering space, legs fully extended and recovering with arms above head.	Can sequence 2 or more cartwheels with body control.	Modified tuck vault: Can walk up to spring board, transfer weight from 1 to 2 feet (30-61 cm) off of a spring board, place hands on top of foam vault and tuck knees up on to the foam shape.
1.5.3 Demonstrates rolling with the body in a non-dynamic environment.	Can perform a rocker on a mat surface, keeping knees tucked to chest, chin to chest with hands flat on the mat, thumbs next to ears.	Safety roll on a mat: Roll forward over one shoulder on the diagonal and land with one foot in front of the other.	Safety roll forward after jumping off of a foam shape.	Can perform a backward shoulder roll to right or left side of body.	Can perform a forward roll from a "down-dog" position on a mat recovering on both feet with arms extended forward.
1.5.4 Combines jumping and landing, rolling, balancing and transfer of weight from feet to hands in a non-dynamic environment.	Can combine three different skills into a movement sequence across general space.	Can combine four different skills into a movement sequence across general space.	Can perform a movement sequence with a partner in unison or meeting and parting.	Can create a movement sequence with a small group connecting jumping and landing, rolling, balancing and transfer of weight skills.	

DANCE AND RHYTHMS

1.5.5 Combines locomotor, non-locomotor, and manipulative movements based on a variety of dance forms.	Replicates simple dance sequences combining 3-4 different movements at a slow to moderate tempo within cultural, social and contemporary (hip-hop) dance forms.	Creates dance sequences based on one or more elements of body, space, effort and relationship awareness (e.g., making different body shapes at different levels).	Replicates dance sequences combining several different movements at a moderate to fast tempo within cultural, social and contemporary (hip-hop) dance forms.		

Modified tuck vault: Can run up to spring board, transfer weight from 1 to 2 feet (30-61 cm) off of a spring board, place hands on top of foam vault and tuck knees to chest, landing on both feet on to the foam shape.	Tuck vault: Can run up to spring board, transfer weight from 1 to 2 feet (30-61 cm) off of a spring board, take off with force and tuck over the foam vault landing on 2 feet.				
Can perform a forward roll down an incline mat.	Can perform a forward roll on a mat.	Can perform a backward roll down an incline mat.	Can perform a backward roll on a mat.	From a standing position can bend over and perform a forward roll.	Can perform a forward roll in a straddle position.

>continued

STANDARD 1   >continued

STANDARD 1	Develops a variety of motor skills.			
Grades 3-5	**PROGRESSIONS**			

DANCE AND RHYTHMS

INDICATORS					
1.5.6 Demonstrates jumping rope in a variety of practice tasks.	**Short rope**	Can perform a spread eagle, rocker, twister, scissor and wounded duck jump with a self-turned short rope.			
	Long rope	Adding a "jumper" but the jumper will not jump. The jumper will stand beside one of the turners and watch the rope for the timing. As it turns the jumper will run through to the other side and around the other turner (in a figure 8 pattern).	The jumper needs to recognize the "front door" direction of the rope being turned. It is easier to jump into the rope from the "front door" side. The jumper will stand beside the turner's shoulder and watch the rope as it comes by their eyes. The rope should come down past the jumper's eyes, hit the floor and then go away from them and up into an arc as it repeats again. This way it gives the jumper a chance to jump into the middle of rope.	Have the jumper stand on the "front door" side of one turner, and when the rope hits the floor and goes away they should take 2-3 steps into the middle and start jumping. Jump 3-4 times and run out of rope to the opposite side of other turner (figure 8 pattern they practiced on the run through).	Once the jumper can consistently jump in the long rope—and turners can consistently turn—jumper can work on adding different footwork in rope. Jumper can add a short rope in the long rope. Turners can add a second rope (double Dutch).

NON-LOCOMOTOR

1.5.7 Demonstrates jumping and landing in a non-dynamic environment.	Can jump from 2 to 2 feet and land with a straight body shape (i.e., pencil jump) pushing off of 2 feet and landing on 2 feet while swinging arms up vertically to create force (for height).	Can jump from 2 to 2 feet and land tucking knees up to chest and extending legs prior to landing.	Can jump from 2 to 2 feet and land making a "letter X" with hands and legs and bringing legs back together before landing.	Can jump from 2 to 2 feet and make a 1/4 turn in the air while maintaining an extended or straight body shape.	Can jump from 2 to 2 feet and make a 1/2 turn in the air while maintaining an extended or straight body shape.
1.5.8 Demonstrates balancing on different body parts in a non-dynamic environment.	Can balance on 3 body parts at any level (e.g., knee scale; side knee scale; one foot and one hand at a low level).	Can balance on one foot with arms extended in a V-position with non-balancing leg extended to the side (i.e., T-scale).	Can perform an arabesque balance.	Can perform an inverted balance with one foot above the head.	Can perform a modified headstand (i.e., head and hands in a triangle shape on mat; bottom up high; feet on floor).

	Can jump from 2 to 2 feet and make a full turn in the air while maintaining an extended or straight body shape.	Jumping off an object from 2 to 2 feet and make varied shapes in the air prior to landing.	Can run through space and take off from 1 foot and land on 2 feet (i.e., jump for distance).		
	Can perform a modified headstand (i.e., head and hands in a triangle shape on mat; knees on elbows as in a tripod).	Can perform a lead-up to a handstand (i.e., hands begin on floor; scissor kick legs).	Can perform a modified handstand (i.e., begin standing and perform a scissor kick action).		

>continued

STANDARD 1   >continued

STANDARD 1	Develops a variety of motor skills.				
Grades 3-5	**PROGRESSIONS**				
	TARGET				
1.5.9 Demonstrates rolling a ball in a non-dynamic environment.	Can roll a lightweight bowling ball with a one-step approach to a target from a distance of 15 feet (5 m), demonstrating moderate range of motion in preparation, execution and follow-through.	Can roll a lightweight bowling ball with a two-step approach to a target from a distance of 15-20 feet (5-6 m), demonstrating full range of motion in preparation, execution and follow-through.	Can roll a lightweight bowling ball with a three-step approach to a target from a distance of 15-20 feet (5-6 m), demonstrating full range of motion in preparation, execution and follow-through.		
	STRIKING AND FIELDING				
1.5.10 Demonstrates throwing in a variety of practice tasks.	While stationary receives an oncoming ball and performs an overhand throw to a stationary partner positioned at a medium distance.	While on the move and in a small-sided practice task catches an oncoming ball and throws it overhand to another player positioned at a medium distance.	While on the move in a small-sided practice task catches an oncoming ball and throws it to appropriate base.		
1.5.11 Demonstrates striking with a long-handled implement in a variety of practice tasks.	Using two-hand grip, can strike an object into general space while demonstrating proper grip, stance, body orientation, swing plane, and follow-through.	Using two-hand grip, can strike an object to a specific area while demonstrating proper grip, stance, body orientation, swing plane, and follow-through.	Using two-hand grip, can strike an object from a distance or to a greater distance while demonstrating proper grip, stance, body orientation, swing plane, and follow-through.		
1.5.12 Demonstrates catching in a variety of practice tasks.	While on the move and in a small-sided practice task (1 v 2 or 2 v 2) catches an oncoming object at a fast speed from any trajectory (angled, high, low) and absorbs force by giving in with elbows. Positions body to get behind oncoming object.	While on the move and in a small-sided practice task (3 v 3) catches an oncoming object at a fast speed from any trajectory (angled, high, low) and absorbs force by giving in with elbows. Positions body to get behind oncoming object.	Combines catching with immediately touching a base and throwing.	Combines catching and throwing to a base.	

>continued

STANDARD 1   >continued

STANDARD 1	Develops a variety of motor skills.				
Grades 3-5	PROGRESSIONS				
	NET AND WALL				
1.5.13 Demonstrates striking with hands above waist in a variety of practice tasks.	Demonstrates striking overhead with two hands (i.e., set) a tossed ball from 10 feet (3 m) distance, high trajectory back to tosser.	Demonstrates striking overhead with two hands (i.e., set) a tossed ball from 10 feet (3 m) distance, high trajectory back and forth with a partner.	Demonstrates overhead set within a modified volleyball game.		
1.5.14 Demonstrates striking with hands below waist in a variety of practice tasks.	Demonstrates striking with both forearms (i.e., making a flat platform) a tossed ball from 10 feet (3 m) distance, high trajectory back to tosser with proper grip, bending/ extending knees to get under and lift the ball and extending arms below shoulders.	Demonstrates striking with forearms (i.e., making a flat platform) a tossed ball from 10 feet (3 m) distance, high trajectory back and forth to a partner bending/ extending knees to get under and lift the ball and extending arms below shoulders.	Demonstrates striking with both forearms within a modified volleyball game.		
1.5.15 Demonstrates serving an object in a non-dynamic environment.	Can hit a trainer volleyball over a lowered volleyball net from modified shorter distance out of one's hand to an open court space.	Can hit a trainer volleyball over a lowered volleyball net from a modified shorter distance out of one's hand to specific court areas.			
1.5.16 Demonstrates striking a an object with a short-handled implement in a variety of practice tasks.	Can strike a self-bounced ball or self-tossed shuttlecock toward a wall from a distance of 10-15 feet (3-5 m) and repeat striking the ball off of the wall.	Can strike a ball tossed underhand by a partner (partner has their back to a wall) from a distance of 10 feet (3 m) toward the wall.	Can strike a ball tossed underhand by a partner over a rope suspended on tall cones.	With a partner, can hit a ball or shuttlecock back and forth over a low rope or tennis net from a 10-15 foot (3-5 m) distance.	With a partner, can hit a ball or shuttlecock back and forth over a low rope, tennis net or badminton net.
	INVASION				
1.5.17 Demonstrates sending and receiving an object in a variety of practice tasks.	Sends object in varied pathways from a stationary position to a stationary partner.	Moves the object in a 3 v 1 practice task in a grid-like space.	Maintains possession of object while moving around cold or warm defenders and using jab step to avoid defender.	Maintains possession and sends object to a teammate within a 2 v 2 keep-away practice task.	Maintains possession and sends object to teammate within a 3 v 3 or 4 v 4 small-sided game.

INDICATORS

>continued

STANDARD 1   >continued

STANDARD 1	Develops a variety of motor skills.				
Grades 3-5	PROGRESSIONS				
	INVASION				
1.5.18 **Demonstrates kicking a ball using the instep in a variety of practice tasks.**	Can kick a stationary ball to a stationary partner using instep (i.e., shoelaces) using a 3-step running approach.	Can kick a ball to a teammate while on the move (i.e., dribbling with feet) after pushing ball slightly forward and taking a 2- to 3-step running approach.	Can kick a ball to a goal while on the move (i.e., dribbling with feet) after pushing ball slightly forward and taking a 2- to 3-step running approach.		
1.5.19 **Demonstrates dribbling with hands in a variety of practice tasks.**	Demonstrates dribbling a ball with preferred hand through general space at a moderate speed.	Demonstrates dribbling a ball with preferred hand through general space while avoiding others.	Demonstrates dribbling a ball with preferred hand through general space along varied pathways and while changing speeds.	Demonstrates dribbling a ball with either hand through general space along varied pathways and while changing speeds.	Demonstrates dribbling a ball with either hand through general space along varied pathways, while changing speeds and avoiding a "cold" defender.
1.5.20 **Demonstrates dribbling with feet in a variety of practice tasks.**	Dribbles with inside of feet at a slow or medium speed while moving around stationary objects in general space.	Dribbles with inside of feet at a medium or fast speed while moving around stationary objects in general space.	Dribbles with inside of feet at a slow or medium speed while moving around others who are also dribbling in general space.	Dribbles with inside and outside of feet at a slow speed while moving around stationary objects in general space.	Dribbles with inside and outside of feet at a medium or fast speed while moving around stationary objects in general space.
1.5.21 **Combines manipulative skills and traveling for execution to a target in a variety of practice tasks.**	Demonstrates moving a game object through general space when alone and scoring on goal.	Demonstrates passing and receiving a game object with a partner and then scoring on goal.	Demonstrates passing and receiving a game object in a small-sided practice task and then scoring on goal.		
	AQUATICS				
1.5.22 **Demonstrates water safety skills. If a pool facility is available, demonstrates water safety and basic swimming skills.**	Demonstrates safety rules strategies.	Demonstrates floating skills.	Demonstrates glide to kick.	Demonstrates swimming stroke.	

INDICATORS

	Demonstrates dribbling a ball with either hand while moving around a "cold" defender with a spin dribble or crossover dribble.				
	Dribbles with inside and outside of feet at a slow or medium speed while moving around others who are also dribbling in general space.	Dribbles with inside and outside of feet changing directions and speeds in a 3 v 3 small-sided practice task.			

STANDARD 1	Develops a variety of motor skills.			
Grades 6-8	**PROGRESSIONS**			
	OUTDOOR PURSUITS			
1.8.1 Demonstrates correct technique in a variety of outdoor activities.	Demonstrates correct technique for skills in a variety of cooperative or practice tasks.	Demonstrates correct technique for skills in 1 self-selected outdoor activity.	Demonstrates correct technique for skills in at least 2 self-selected outdoor activities.	
	DANCE AND RHYTHMS			
1.8.2 Demonstrates movement sequences within varied dance forms.	Coordinates 3-4 upper and lower body movements (i.e., repeating or creating a movement sequence or pattern) to a slow or moderate tempo while maintaining correct rhythm. Above can be performed individually, with a partner or in a group.	Individually, with a partner or in groups, coordinates 5-6 upper and lower body movements (i.e., repeating or creating a movement sequence or pattern), with one direction change to a moderate tempo while maintaining correct rhythm.	Individually, with a partner or in groups, coordinates 5-6 upper and lower body movements (i.e., repeating or creating a movement sequence or pattern), with 2-3 direction changes and a level change (e.g., pivots, turns) to a moderate tempo while maintaining correct rhythm.	
	FITNESS ACTIVITIES			
1.8.3 Demonstrates appropriate form in a variety of health-related fitness activities.	Cardiovascular endurance	Demonstrates cardiovascular exercises that focus on lower intensity and shorter duration.	Demonstrates cardiovascular exercises that focus on higher intensity and longer duration.	
	Muscular strength and endurance	Demonstrates muscular strength and endurance exercises that focus on body weight and functional movements.	Demonstrates muscular strength and endurance exercises that focus on using resistance (e.g., machines, bands, balls).	
	Flexibility	Demonstrates appropriate flexibility exercises (static and dynamic) for warm-up and cool-down.	Demonstrates appropriate flexibility exercises (static and dynamic) to target a specific muscle group or to prepare for a specific movement/activity.	
1.8.4 Demonstrates appropriate form in a variety of skill-related fitness activities.	Demonstrates activities that target a specific skill-related fitness component in a closed environment.	Demonstrates activities that target a specific skill-related fitness component in an open environment.		
	TARGET GAMES			
1.8.5 Demonstrates a striking motion with a long-handled implement.	Performs the striking motion with an implement in activities such as croquet, shuffleboard, or golf.	Strikes a stationary object with an implement using correct form in activities such as croquet, shuffleboard, or golf.	Strikes, with an implement, a stationary object for distance/power in activities such as croquet, shuffleboard, or golf.	

INDICATORS

Demonstrates correct technique for skills in 3 or more self-selected outdoor activities.			
Individually, with a partner or in groups, coordinates multiple upper and lower body movements (i.e., repeating or creating a movement sequence or pattern), with two direction changes, a level change and add accents to a fast tempo while maintaining correct rhythm.	Create simple dance sequence based on the elements of the movement framework (i.e., body, space, effort and relationship awareness) alone, with a partner and in small group.		
Demonstrates muscular strength and endurance exercises that focus on using free weights.			
Strikes, with an implement, a stationary object for distance/power and accuracy in activities such as croquet, shuffleboard, or golf.			

>continued

STANDARD 1   >continued

STANDARD 1	Develops a variety of motor skills.		
Grades 6-8	**PROGRESSIONS**		
	TARGET GAMES		
1.8.6 Demonstrates a correct rolling and throwing (underhand, sidearm, overhand) technique in a variety of practice tasks and modified target games.	Demonstrates correct rolling or throwing technique to produce force and achieve distance and accuracy in modified target games.		
	STRIKING AND FIELDING GAMES		
1.8.7 Demonstrates striking a self-tossed/pitched ball with an implement to open space in a variety of practice tasks and small-sided games.	Strikes a self-tossed ball with an implement with force in a variety of practice tasks.	Strikes a pitched ball with an implement with force in a variety of practice tasks.	Strikes a pitched ball with an implement for power to open space in a variety of small-sided games.
1.8.8 Demonstrates a proper catch with or without an implement in a variety of practice tasks and small-sided games.	Catches, with correct form, using a variety of objects in a variety of practice tasks.	Catches, with correct form, from different trajectories using a variety of objects in a variety of practice tasks.	Catches, with correct form, from different trajectories in combination with locomotor skills using different objects in a variety of practice tasks.
1.8.9 Demonstrates throwing for accuracy, distance, and power in a variety of practice tasks and small-sided games.	Performs a correct throw for distance and power appropriate to a variety of practice tasks.	Performs a correct throw for distance and power appropriate to a variety of practice tasks in a dynamic environment.	Throw for distance and power in combination with locomotor skills appropriate to a variety of practice tasks in a dynamic environment.
	NET AND WALL GAMES		
1.8.10 Demonstrates a proper underhand and overhand serve using the hand in a variety of practice tasks and modified small-sided games.	Performs a proper underhand serve using the hand in a variety of practice tasks.	Performs a proper underhand serve using the hand in modified net and wall games.	Performs a proper overhand serve using the hand in a variety of practice tasks.
1.8.11 Demonstrates a proper underhand and overhand serve using a short- or long-handled implement in a variety of practice tasks and modified small-sided games.	Performs a proper underhand serve using a short-handled implement in a variety of practice tasks.	Performs a proper underhand serve using a short-handled implement in modified net and wall games.	Performs a proper overhand serve using a short-handled implement in a variety of practice tasks.
1.8.12 Demonstrates the correct form of a forehand and backhand stroke with a short-handled and long-handled implement in a variety of practice tasks and modified small-sided games.	Performs correct form of the forehand stroke with a short-handled implement in a variety of practice tasks.	Performs the correct form of the backhand stroke with a short-handled implement in a variety of practice tasks.	Performs the correct form of the forehand and backhand stroke with a short-handled implement in modified net and wall games.
1.8.13 Demonstrates a volley using a short-handled and long-handled implement in a variety of practice tasks and modified net and wall games.	Forehand volleys with correct form and control using a short-handled implement in a variety of practice tasks.	Forehand volleys with correct form and control using a short-handled implement in a modified net and wall game.	Backhand volleys with correct form and control using a short-handled implement in a variety of practice tasks.

INDICATORS

Passes and receives a leading pass (using hands, feet, or implement) in combination with locomotor patterns of running and change of direction and speed with competency in modified activities such as basketball, flag football, speedball, team handball, soccer, lacrosse or hockey (floor, field, ice).	Passes and receives (using hands, feet, or implement) a lead pass to a moving partner off a dribble or pass in modified activities such as basketball, flag football, speedball, team handball, soccer, lacrosse or hockey (floor, field, ice).		
Executes a dribbling skill with dominant and non-dominant hand, foot, or both using a change of speed and direction in small-sided game play.			
Executes dribbling an object with an implement using a change of speed and direction in small-sided game play.			
Shoots on goal in combination with locomotor patterns with and without an implement for power and accuracy in modified small-sided invasion games.			
Executes the following offensive skills during modified or small-sided game play: pivot, give and go, and fakes.			
Executes drop-steps or quick turns in the direction of the pass during player-to-player in modified or small-sided invasion games.			
Demonstrates swimming skills over greater distances and speeds.			

STANDARD 1	Develops a variety of motor skills.		
Grades 9-12	**PROGRESSIONS**		
	LIFETIME ACTIVITIES		
1.12.1 Demonstrates activity-specific movement skills in a variety of lifetime sports and activities.	Demonstrates activity-specific movement skills solo, with a partner, or in a small group within a non-dynamic/stationary environment.	Demonstrates activity-specific movement skills solo, with a partner, or in a small group within a structured dynamic environment.	
1.12.2 Demonstrates activity-specific movement skills in a variety of recreational and backyard games.	Demonstrates activity-specific movement skills solo, with a partner, or in a small group within a non-dynamic/stationary environment.	Demonstrates activity-specific movement skills solo, with a partner, or in a small group within a structured dynamic environment.	
1.12.3 Demonstrates activity-specific movement skills in a variety of outdoor pursuits.	Demonstrates activity-specific movement skills solo, with a partner, or in a small group within a non-dynamic/stationary environment.	Demonstrates activity-specific movement skills solo, with a partner, or in a small group within a structured dynamic environment.	
	DANCE AND RHYTHMS		
1.12.4 Demonstrates and creates movement sequences based on one or more forms of dance.	Structured dance	• Demonstrates dances with slow to moderate tempo, 3-4 different steps and few changes of directions. • Dance steps can be done alone, with a partner, or with a group.	
	Creative dance	Demonstrates dance sequences based on elements of the movement framework (body, space, effort, and relationship awareness, etc.). *See appendix A.*	
	FITNESS ACTIVITIES		
1.12.5 Demonstrates appropriate technique in cardiovascular training.	Demonstrates cardiovascular exercises that focus on lower intensity and shorter duration.	Demonstrates cardiovascular exercises that focus on higher intensity and longer duration.	
1.12.6 Demonstrates appropriate technique in muscular strength and endurance training.	Demonstrates muscular strength and endurance exercises that focus on body weight and functional movements.	Demonstrates muscular strength and endurance exercises that focus on using resistance (e.g., machines, bands, balls).	
1.12.7 Demonstrates appropriate technique in flexibility training.	Demonstrates appropriate flexibility exercises (static and dynamic) for warm-up and cool-down.	Demonstrates appropriate flexibility exercises (static and dynamic) to target a specific muscle group or to prepare for a specific movement/activity.	
1.12.8 Demonstrates appropriate technique in skill-related fitness training.	Demonstrates activities that target a specific skill-related fitness component in a closed environment.	Demonstrates activities that target a specific skill-related fitness component in an open environment.	
	AQUATICS		
1.12.9 Demonstrates water safety skills. If a pool facility is available, demonstrates water safety and basic swimming skills.	Demonstrates safety rules and life saving techniques.	Demonstrates basic swimming skills. Land and water skills.	

INDICATORS

Demonstrates activity-specific movement skills solo, with a partner, or in a small group within a dynamic and game-like environment.	
Demonstrates activity-specific movement skills solo, with a partner, or in a small group within a dynamic and game-like environment.	
Demonstrates activity-specific movement skills solo, with a partner, or in a small group within a dynamic and real-world environment.	
Demonstrates dances with moderate to faster tempo, increasing number of steps and changes of directions. Dance steps can be done alone, with a partner, or with a group.	
Demonstrates a dance sequence using a prop.	Demonstrates a dance sequence based on a theme or idea.
Demonstrates muscular strength and endurance exercises that focus on using free weights.	
Refine swimming skills to improve efficiency and confidence.	Demonstrates swimming skills over greater distances.

INDICATORS AT A GLANCE

Note: *This chart is intended to list the Grade-Span Learning Indicators for grades preK-12. This chart is not intended to show alignment across Grade-Span Learning Indicators. However, some indicators may align across grade spans and some may not due to the content and skills being taught within a specific grade span.*

STANDARD 2	Applies knowledge related to movement and fitness concepts.
RATIONALE	Through learning experiences in physical education, the student uses their knowledge of movement concepts, tactics, and strategies across a variety of environments. This knowledge helps the student become a more versatile and efficient mover. Additionally, the student applies knowledge of health-related and skill-related fitness to enhance their overall well-being. The application of knowledge related to various forms of movement contributes to an individual's physical literacy journey.

Grades preK-2 Learning Indicators	Grades 3-5 Learning Indicators	Grades 6-8 Learning Indicators	Grades 9-12 Learning Indicators
2.2.1 Recognizes personal space and where to move in general space.	2.5.1 Applies movement concepts and strategies for safe movement within dynamic environments.	2.8.1 Identifies the effective use of movement concepts within multiple dynamic environments.	2.12.1 Demonstrates knowledge of tactics and strategies within lifetime sports and activities.
2.2.2 Identifies simple strategies in chasing and fleeing activities.	2.5.2 Demonstrates knowledge of offensive strategies in small-sided invasion practice tasks.	2.8.2 Demonstrates knowledge of offensive tactics to create space with movement in invasion games.	2.12.2 Demonstrates knowledge of tactics and strategies within recreational and backyard games.
2.2.3 Identifies movement concepts related to locomotor, non-locomotor, and manipulative skills.	2.5.3 Demonstrates knowledge of defensive strategies in small-sided invasion practice tasks.	2.8.3 Demonstrates knowledge of reducing open space with movement and denial in invasion games.	2.12.3 Demonstrates knowledge of tactics and strategies within outdoor pursuits.
2.2.4 Demonstrates knowledge of locomotor, non-locomotor, and manipulative skills in movement settings.	2.5.4 Demonstrates knowledge of appropriate movement concepts for efficient performance of manipulative skills.	2.8.4 Selects and applies the appropriate shot and technique in net and wall games.	2.12.4 Applies knowledge of movement sequences to create or participate in one or more forms of dance.
2.2.5 Demonstrates knowledge of locomotor, non-locomotor, and movement concepts used in dance and rhythms.	2.5.5 Demonstrates problem-solving strategies in a variety of games and activities.	2.8.5 Demonstrates knowledge of offensive tactics in striking and fielding games.	2.12.5 Analyzes how health and fitness will impact quality of life after high school.
2.2.6 Identifies physical activities that contribute to fitness.	2.5.6 Applies movement concepts to different types of dances, gymnastics, rhythms, and individual performance activities.	2.8.6 Demonstrates knowledge of defensive positioning tactics in striking and fielding games.	2.12.6 Establishes a goal and creates a practice plan to improve performance for a self-selected skill.
2.2.7 Recognizes the importance of stretching before and after physical activity.	2.5.7 Defines and provides examples of movement activities for developing the health-related fitness components.	2.8.7 Demonstrates problem-solving skills in a variety of games and activities.	2.12.7 Applies the principles of exercise in a variety of self-selected lifetime physical activities.

Grades preK-2 Learning Indicators	Grades 3-5 Learning Indicators	Grades 6-8 Learning Indicators	Grades 9-12 Learning Indicators
2.2.8 Identifies the heart as a muscle that gets stronger with physical activity.	2.5.8 Establishes goals related to enhancing fitness development.	2.8.8 Applies knowledge of movement concepts for the purpose of varying different types of dances and rhythmic activities.	2.12.8 Designs and implements a plan that applies knowledge of aerobic, strength and endurance, and flexibility training exercises.
2.2.9 Recognizes that regular physical activity is good for their health.	2.5.9 Defines and explains how to implement the FITT Principle for fitness development.	2.8.9 Identifies and compares the components of health and skill-related fitness.	2.12.9 Evaluates perceived exertion during physical activity and adjusts effort.
2.2.10 Recognizes physiological changes in their body during physical activities.	2.5.10 Defines and provides examples of movement activities for developing the skill-related fitness components.	2.8.10 Self-selects and monitors physical activity goals based on a self-selected health-related fitness assessment.	2.12.10 Applies heart rate concepts to ensure safety and maximize health-related fitness outcomes.
2.2.11 Recognizes food and hydration choices that provide energy for physical activity.	2.5.11 Identifies the need for warm-up and cool-down relative to various physical activities.	2.8.11 Implements the principles of exercise (progression, overload, and specificity) for different types of physical activity.	2.12.11 Discusses the benefits of a physically active lifestyle as it relates to young adulthood.
2.2.12 Demonstrates knowledge of water safety skills. Demonstrates knowledge of basic swimming skills.	2.5.12 Identifies location of pulse and provides examples of activities that increase heart rate.	2.8.12 Applies knowledge of skill-related fitness to different types of physical activity.	2.12.12 Applies knowledge of rest when planning regular physical activity.
	2.5.13 Explains the benefits of physical activity.	2.8.13 Explains the relationship of aerobic fitness and RPE Scale to physical activity effort.	2.12.13 Applies movement concepts and principles (e.g., force, motion, rotation) to analyze and improve performance of self and/ or others in a selected skill (e.g., overhand throw, back squat, archery).
	2.5.14 Recognizes and explains how physical activity influences physiological changes in their body.	2.8.14 Applies knowledge of dynamic and static stretching to exercise in warm-up, cool-down, flexibility, endurance, etc. physical activities.	2.12.14 Identifies and discusses the historical and cultural roles of games, sports and dance in a society.
	2.5.15 Recognizes the critical elements that contribute to proper execution of a skill.	2.8.15 Demonstrates knowledge of heart rate and describes its relationship to aerobic fitness.	2.12.15 Analyzes and applies technology as tools to support a healthy, active lifestyle.

>continued

STANDARD 2   >continued

Grades preK-2 Learning Indicators	Grades 3-5 Learning Indicators	Grades 6-8 Learning Indicators	Grades 9-12 Learning Indicators
	2.5.16 Identifies technology tools that support physical activity goals.	2.8.16 Identifies ways to be physically active.	2.12.16 Identifies snacks and food choices that help and hinder performance, recovery, and enjoyment during physical activity.
	2.5.17 Describes the impact of food and hydration choices on physical activity.	2.8.17 Examines how rest impacts the body's response to physical activity.	2.12.17 Demonstrates knowledge of water safety skills. Demonstrates knowledge of basic swimming skills.
	2.5.18 Demonstrates knowledge of water safety skills. Demonstrates knowledge of basic swimming skills.	2.8.18 Analyzes skill performance by identifying critical elements.	
		2.8.19 Evaluates usefulness of technology tools to support physical activity and fitness goals.	
		2.8.20 Explains the relationships among nutrition, physical activity, and health factors.	
		2.8.21 Demonstrates knowledge of safety protocols in teacher-selected outdoor activities.	
		2.8.22 Demonstrates knowledge of water safety skills. Demonstrates knowledge of basic swimming skills.	

STANDARD 2	Applies knowledge related to movement and fitness concepts.			
Grades preK-2	**PROGRESSIONS**			

INDICATORS	**TACTICS AND STRATEGIES**			
2.2.1 Recognizes personal space and where to move in general space.	Identifies one's personal space and can maintain their personal space during lesson tasks.	Recognizes how to adhere to boundaries.	Identifies general space and moves through general space while avoiding objects and others.	Recognizes when to change direction and speed when moving through general space.
2.2.2 Identifies simple strategies in chasing and fleeing activities.	Describes how the role of a chaser is different than the role of a fleer.	Identifies specific fleeing strategies (open space, fakes, deception) that prolong fleeing from a chaser.	Identifies specific chasing strategies (limit space, angles, balance) that allow chaser to tag fleer.	
2.2.3 Identifies movement concepts related to locomotor, non-locomotor, and manipulative skills.	Distinguishes among locomotor, non-locomotor, and manipulative skills (i.e., body awareness).	Distinguishes among movement concepts (space, effort, relationships).	Distinguishes among movement concepts as related to various locomotor, non-locomotor, and manipulative skills (i.e., body awareness).	
2.2.4 Demonstrates knowledge of locomotor, non-locomotor, and manipulative skills in movement settings.	Distinguishes among locomotor, non-locomotor, and manipulative skills.	Identifies locomotor, non-locomotor, and manipulative skills as they are utilized across movement settings.	Describes various locomotor, non-locomotor, and manipulative skills across movement.	
	DANCE AND RHYTHMS			
2.2.5 Demonstrates knowledge of locomotor, non-locomotor, and movement concepts used in dance and rhythms.	Identifies different forms of dance (i.e., cultural vs. contemporary).	Identifies how the elements of the movement framework (i.e., body, space, effort and relationship awareness) are used to create dance sequences.		

>continued

STANDARD 2   >continued

STANDARD 2	Applies knowledge related to movement and fitness concepts.			
Grades preK-2	PROGRESSIONS			
	FITNESS CONCEPTS			
2.2.6 Identifies physical activities that contribute to fitness.	Describes the meaning of fitness.	Self-selects physical activities for their fitness journey.	Describes the relationship between physical activity and fitness.	
2.2.7 Recognizes the importance of stretching before and after physical activity.	Describes the difference between stretching and other physical activities.	Describes the importance of warming muscles first before stretching to prevent injuries.	Performs various stretches for different parts of the body.	Describes the benefits of lengthening the muscles before and after a physical activity.
2.2.8 Identifies the heart as a muscle that gets stronger with physical activity.	Locates the heart on both their body and a visual representation of a person.	Identifies the changes in heart rate as a result of physical activity.	Explains the heart as a muscle that grows stronger with physical activity.	
	PHYSICAL ACTIVITY KNOWLEDGE			
2.2.9 Recognizes that regular physical activity is good for their health.	Identifies the components of good health as physical activity (what you do) and nutrition (how you fuel your body).	Describes the importance of physical activity as it relates to good health.		
2.2.10 Recognizes physiological changes in their body during physical activities.	Describes the physiological changes that occur in the body when participating in physical activity.	Selects a physical activity and identifies the physiological changes in their body.		
2.2.11 Recognizes food and hydration choices that provide energy for physical activity.	Describes food and hydration as the basic building blocks for energy.	Identifies nutrient/energy rich foods vs. foods that lack energy-supplying nutrients.		
	AQUATICS			
2.2.12 Demonstrates knowledge of water safety skills. Demonstrates knowledge of basic swimming skills.	Identifies basic water safety skills.	Describes the risk in participating in aquatics without knowledge of water safety skills.	Describes the relationship between floating and sinking.	Describes effective body position when floating.

INDICATORS

STANDARD 2	Applies knowledge related to movement and fitness concepts.				
Grades 3-5	**PROGRESSIONS**				
	TACTICS AND STRATEGIES				
2.5.1 Applies movement concepts and strategies for safe movement within dynamic environments.	Identifies when and how to utilize space, effort, and relationships for safe movement in dynamic environments.	Selects when and how to change direction and speed for safe movement in dynamic environments.			
2.5.2 Demonstrates knowledge of offensive strategies in small-sided invasion practice tasks.	Identifies and selects the specific roles and strategies associated with being on offense.	Identifies and selects specific offensive strategies (e.g., pick and roll) that relate to scoring.			
2.5.3 Demonstrates knowledge of defensive strategies in small-sided invasion practice tasks.	Identifies the specific roles and strategies associated with being on defense.	Identifies specific defensive strategies (zone, press) that prevent the opposition from scoring.			
2.5.4 Demonstrates knowledge of appropriate movement concepts for efficient performance of manipulative skills.	Describes how combining various manipulative, locomotor, and non-locomotor skills can be used to advance toward a target (e.g., executing a gallop prior to a throw-in in soccer to create force on the throw-in; run and dribble a ball; execute a shoulder fake to evade a defender).	Explains where to move in order to execute an appropriate manipulative skill in particular movement settings (e.g., fielding a ball; advancing game object down the field).			
2.5.5 Demonstrates problem-solving strategies in a variety of games and activities.	Identifies the problem within the game or activity.	Identifies potential strategies to the problem within the game or activity.	Creates and executes a plan to solve a problem within the game or activity.	Evaluates and refines a plan to solve the problem within the game or activity.	
	DANCE AND RHYTHMS				
2.5.6 Applies movement concepts to different types of dances, gymnastics, rhythms, and individual performance activities.	Identifies the elements of the movement framework (i.e., body, space, effort, relationship awareness) used to increase the difficulty of different structured dance forms.	Identifies the elements of the movement framework (i.e., body, space, effort, relationship awareness) used to create or modify a dance sequence.			

(Left vertical label: INDICATORS)

>continued

STANDARD 2   >continued

STANDARD 2	Applies knowledge related to movement and fitness concepts.				
Grades 3-5	**PROGRESSIONS**				
	FITNESS CONCEPTS				
2.5.7 Defines and provides examples of movement activities for developing the health-related fitness components.	• Identifies the components of health-related fitness: - Cardiorespiratory endurance, muscular endurance, muscular strength, flexibility, body composition.	• Defines the components of health-related fitness: - Cardiorespiratory endurance, muscular endurance, muscular strength, flexibility, body composition.	Identifies examples of movement activities for each health-related fitness component.	Defines selected skill-related fitness principles including specificity, progression and overload resistance, uniqueness, regularity and reversibility.	Provides an example of selected skill-related fitness principles including specificity, progression and overload resistance, uniqueness, regularity and reversibility.
2.5.8 Establishes goals related to enhancing fitness development.	Describes fitness development as an ongoing cycle that includes self-assessment, goal-setting, practice, and reassessment.	Completes personalized fitness assessments and identifies areas of needed remediation with assistance from the teacher.	Identifies strategies for developing health-related fitness based on individual assessment and individual interests.	Establishes short-term goals for the purpose of developing health-related fitness consistent with personal interests.	
2.5.9 Defines and explains how to implement the FITT Principle for fitness development.	Defines the FITT Principle.	Provides examples of how to use the FITT Principle to enhance fitness development.			
2.5.10 Defines and provides examples of movement activities for developing the skill-related fitness components.	Identifies components of skill-related fitness: agility, balance, coordination, power, reaction time, speed.	Defines the components of skill-related fitness.	Identifies examples of movement activities for each skill-related fitness component.		
2.5.11 Identifies the need for warm-up and cool-down relative to various physical activities.	Defines the concept of warm-up and cool-down.	Identifies effective warm-up and cool-down activities.	Selects warm-up and cool-down activities that maximize participation in selected physical activities.		
2.5.12 Identifies location of pulse and provides examples of activities that increase heart rate.	Defines the concept of pulse and explains its relation to the heart.	Locates the pulse in both wrist and neck.	Identifies types of physical activity that increase heart rate.		

(left vertical label: INDICATORS)

STANDARD 2	Applies knowledge related to movement and fitness concepts.				
Grades 3-5	**PROGRESSIONS**				
	PHYSICAL ACTIVITY KNOWLEDGE				
2.5.13 Explains the benefits of physical activity.	Differentiates between a sedentary lifestyle and physically active lifestyle.	Analyzes participation in various health-related fitness activities and explains benefits of each physical activity.	Analyzes participation in various games and active play situations and examines benefits of each physical activity.		
2.5.14 Recognizes and explains how physical activity influences physiological changes in their body.	Identifies physiological changes that result from participation in physical activity.	Compares and contrasts physiological changes based on the type of physical activities engaged in.			
2.5.15 Recognizes the critical elements that contribute to proper execution of a skill.	Identifies the critical elements of locomotor skills (jumping, galloping, sliding sideways, hopping, skipping, leaping).	Identifies the critical elements of manipulative skills (throwing and catching, striking, kicking, bouncing a ball).			
2.5.16 Identifies technology tools that support physical activity goals.	Distinguishes various technology tools that support physical activity.	Defines own physical activity goals.	Selects technology tool to monitor physical activity goals.		
2.5.17 Describes the impact of food and hydration choices on physical activity.	Identifies food and hydration's connection to participation in physical activity.	Identifies food and hydration choices that enhance participation in physical activity.			
	AQUATICS				
2.5.18 Demonstrates knowledge of water safety skills. Demonstrates knowledge of basic swimming skills.	Identifies water safety skills and the risks associated with aquatics.	Analyzes body positions for floating, glide to kick, and swimming strokes.			

Left vertical label: **INDICATORS**

STANDARD 2	Applies knowledge related to movement and fitness concepts.			
Grades 6-8	PROGRESSIONS			
	TACTICS AND STRATEGIES			
2.8.1 Identifies the effective use of movement concepts within multiple dynamic environments.	Identifies similarities and differences among the application of movement sequences in a number of dynamic environments.			
2.8.2 Demonstrates knowledge of offensive tactics to create space with movement in invasion games.	Exhibits knowledge by describing how or demonstrating how open space can be created by using locomotor movements (e.g., walking, running, jumping and landing) in combination with movement (e.g., varying pathways; change of speed, direction or pace) in a variety of practice tasks.	Exhibits knowledge by describing how or demonstrating how open space can be created by using locomotor movements in combination with movement in small-sided games.	Exhibits knowledge by describing how open space can be created or using offensive tactics (e.g., moves to an open space without the ball; uses a variety of passes, pivots and fakes, give and go) while using locomotor movements in combination with movement in a variety of practice tasks.	Exhibits knowledge of creating open space by describing how to use or using offensive tactics while using locomotor movements in combination with movement in small-sided games.
2.8.3 Demonstrates knowledge of reducing open space with movement and denial in invasion games.	Exhibits knowledge of limiting space by using locomotor movements (e.g., walking, running, jumping and landing, changing size and shape of the body making the body larger, reducing passing angles) staying close to the opponent as they near the goal, and/or prohibits receiving the pass (denial).	Exhibits knowledge of limiting space during small-sided game play by using at least 3 or more defensive tactics like staying on the goal side of the offensive player, reducing the distance to their goal (third-party perspective), prohibiting receiving the pass (denial), and/or anticipating the speed of the object or person for the purpose of interception or deflection (disruption).		
2.8.4 Selects and applies the appropriate shot and technique in net and wall games.	Exhibits knowledge of strategy by returning to midcourt positions in a variety of practice tasks and dynamic environment.	Selects shots based on opponent's location (hit where opponent is not) in a variety of practice tasks and dynamic environment.	Selects shots based on opponent's location (hit where opponent is not) in small games situations.	Exhibits knowledge of varied shot selection based on placement, force, timing, and manipulation to prevent an opponent's anticipation.

INDICATORS

STANDARD 2	Applies knowledge related to movement and fitness concepts.			
Grades 6-8	**PROGRESSIONS**			

TACTICS AND STRATEGIES

INDICATORS				
2.8.5 Demonstrates knowledge of offensive tactics in striking and fielding games.	Identifies open spaces and attempts to strike object into that space in a variety of practice tasks and dynamic environments.	Identifies open spaces and when to strike an object into that space in small-sided games.	Identifies a variety of shots (e.g., slap and run, bunt, line drive, high arc) to hit to open space in a variety of practice tasks and dynamic environments.	Identifies a variety of shots (e.g., slap and run, bunt, line drive, high arc, sacrifice situations) to hit to open space and advance a teammate in small-sided games (e.g., number of outs).
2.8.6 Demonstrates knowledge of defensive positioning tactics in striking and fielding games.	Identifies the correct defensive play based on the situation (e.g., the number of outs) during practice tasks and dynamic environments	Selects the correct defensive play based on the situation (e.g., number of outs) during practice tasks and modified games.	Selects several defensive strategies based on the situation (e.g., number of outs) during modified games.	Identifies how to limit space in the field by working with teammates to maximize coverage during modified games and dynamic environments.
2.8.7 Demonstrates problem-solving skills in a variety of games and activities.	Identifies the problem within the game or activity.	Identifies potential strategies to the problem within the game or activity.	Creates and executes a plan to solve a problem within the game or activity.	Evaluates and refines plan to solve the problem within the game or activity.

DANCE AND RHYTHMS

2.8.8 Applies knowledge of movement concepts for the purpose of varying different types of dances and rhythmic activities.	Replicates varied forms of structured dances (e.g., cultural, contemporary, social).	Utilizes the elements of the movement framework (i.e., body, space, effort and relationship awareness) to modify a structured dance.	Creates a dance sequence based on a theme (e.g., haikus) or with a prop (e.g., a chair).	

FITNESS CONCEPTS

2.8.9 Identifies and compares the components of health and skill-related fitness.	Describes the component of health and skill-related fitness.	Distinguishes between and among the various components of health and skill-related fitness.	Identifies specific physical activities that enhance health and skill-related fitness.	
2.8.10 Self-selects and monitors physical activity goals based on a self-selected health-related fitness assessment.	Assesses current fitness level with a self-selected health-related fitness assessment.	Sets and monitors a self-selected physical activity goal for activity based on current fitness level.	Adjusts physical activity based on quantity of exercise needed for a minimal health standard and/or optimal functioning based on current fitness level.	

>continued

STANDARD 2   >continued

STANDARD 2	Applies knowledge related to movement and fitness concepts.			
Grades 6-8	**PROGRESSIONS**			
FITNESS CONCEPTS				
2.8.11 Implements the principles of exercise (progression, overload, and specificity) for different types of physical activity.	Defines the principles of exercise.	Describes the application of each principle of exercise to different types of physical activity.	Selects a principle of exercise to apply to a self-selected physical activity.	
2.8.12 Applies knowledge of skill-related fitness to different types of physical activity.	Differentiates between the components of skill-related fitness.	Selects a component of skill-related fitness, choosing interested activities associated with selected component.	Creates a plan for participation using selected skill-related fitness component and associated activities.	
2.8.13 Explains the relationship of aerobic fitness and RPE Scale to physical activity effort.	Defines aerobic fitness and describes its relationship to the Borg Rating of Perceived Exertion (RPE) Scale.	Explains how intensity of exercise impact physical activity.	Defines how the RPE Scale can be used to determine the perception of the work effort or intensity of exercise.	Defines how the RPE Scale can be used to adjust workout intensity during physical activity.
2.8.14 Applies knowledge of dynamic and static stretching to exercise in warm-up, cool-down, flexibility, endurance, etc. physical activities	Self-selects a physical activity of interest.	Creates a plan for participation in their physical activity of choice incorporating the concepts of stretching, warm-up, and cool-down.		
2.8.15 Demonstrates knowledge of heart rate and describes its relationship to aerobic fitness.	Defines heart rate principles such as resting heart rate, maximum heart rate, target heart rate, and target heart rate zone.	Explains the relationship among heart rate principles and connection to aerobic fitness.		
PHYSICAL ACTIVITY KNOWLEDGE				
2.8.16 Identifies ways to be physically active.	Analyzes personal environment and lifestyle for physical activity opportunities.			
2.8.17 Examines how rest impacts the body's response to physical activity.	Defines rest in the context of participation in physical activity.	Analyzes the impact of rest versus the lack of rest on the body.	Describes how rest impacts the body in the context of participation in physical activity.	
2.8.18 Analyzes skill performance by identifying critical elements.	Selects a skill of interest and identifies critical elements of skill.	Examines performance based on critical elements of skill.		

(Left margin label: INDICATORS)

STANDARD 2	Applies knowledge related to movement and fitness concepts.			
Grades 6-8	PROGRESSIONS			
PHYSICAL ACTIVITY KNOWLEDGE				
2.8.19 **Evaluates usefulness of technology tools to support physical activity and fitness goals.**	Identifies method for evaluating selected technology tools.	Examines various technology tools based on method for evaluation.		
2.8.20 **Explains the relationships among nutrition, physical activity, and health factors.**	Defines nutrition, physical activity, and health risk factors.	Identifies potential health risk factors both in the present and future.	Describes how nutrition and physical activity can impact various health risk factors.	
OUTDOOR PURSUITS				
2.8.21 **Demonstrates knowledge of safety protocols in teacher-selected outdoor activities.**	Identify safety practices for a specific outdoor activity.	Explain the importance of safety practices for a specific outdoor activity.	Analyzes and makes safe choices to ensure safety of self and others.	
AQUATICS				
2.8.22 **Demonstrates knowledge of water safety skills. Demonstrates knowledge of basic swimming skills.**	Identifies water safety skills.	Identifies life-saving techniques.	Analyzes various swimming skills to improve efficiency, knowledge, and confidence.	

STANDARD 2	Applies knowledge related to movement and fitness concepts.			
Grades 9-12	PROGRESSIONS			
TACTICS AND STRATEGIES				
2.12.1 **Demonstrates knowledge of tactics and strategies within lifetime sports and activities.**	Demonstrates activity-specific tactics and strategies knowledge within a non-dynamic/stationary environment.	Demonstrates activity-specific tactics and strategies knowledge within a structured dynamic environment.	Demonstrates activity-specific tactics and strategies knowledge within a dynamic and game-like environment.	
2.12.2 **Demonstrates knowledge of tactics and strategies within recreational and backyard games.**	Demonstrates activity-specific tactics and strategies knowledge within a non-dynamic/stationary environment.	Demonstrates activity-specific tactics and strategies knowledge within a structured dynamic environment.	Demonstrates activity-specific tactics and strategies knowledge within a dynamic and game-like environment.	
2.12.3 **Demonstrates knowledge of tactics and strategies within outdoor pursuits.**	Demonstrates activity-specific tactics and strategies knowledge within a non-dynamic/stationary environment.	Demonstrates activity-specific tactics and strategies knowledge within a structured dynamic environment.	Demonstrates activity-specific tactics and strategies knowledge within a dynamic and real-world environment.	

>continued

STANDARD 2   >*continued*

STANDARD 2	Applies knowledge related to movement and fitness concepts.			
Grades 9-12	**PROGRESSIONS**			
DANCE AND RHYTHMS				
2.12.4 Applies knowledge of movement sequences to create or participate in one or more forms of dance.	Designs a dance sequence by synthesizing movements from a number of existing dance sequences for self and others.	Designs a dance by generating new movements and applying elements from body, space, effort, and relationship awareness within the dance sequence.		
FITNESS CONCEPTS				
2.12.5 Analyzes how health and fitness will impact quality of life after high school.	Identifies healthy and unhealthy behaviors that should be prioritized to enhance a healthy, active lifestyle transitioning to and through college and career.	Describes the components of skill-related fitness as related to maintaining an active and healthy lifestyle after high school.	Describes the components of health-related fitness as related to maintaining an active and healthy lifestyle after high school.	Develops a personal health and fitness plan for life after high school.
2.12.6 Establishes a goal and creates a practice plan to improve performance for a self-selected skill.	Identifies a goal for improvement in self-selected skill.	Designs a practice plan to improve performance in self-selected skill.		
2.12.7 Applies the principles of exercise in a variety of self-selected lifetime physical activities.	Defines the principles of exercise.	Describes the application of each principle of exercise to various lifetime activities.	Selects a principle of exercise to apply to a self-selected physical activity.	
2.12.8 Designs and implements a plan that applies knowledge of aerobic, strength and endurance, and flexibility training exercises.	Identifies movement activities for aerobic, strength, endurance, and flexibility training exercises.	Create training plan incorporating movement activities for aerobic, strength, endurance, and flexibility.		
2.12.9 Evaluates perceived exertion during physical activity and adjusts effort.	Utilizes the RPE Scale to evaluate exertion during a teacher- and/or self-selected physical activity.	Adjusts effort in subsequent physical activity trials based on evaluation of exertion using RPE Scale.		
2.12.10 Applies heart rate concepts to ensure safety and maximize health-related fitness outcomes.	Identifies multiple health-related fitness activities and examines its effect on the body.	Chooses a health-related fitness activity and analyzes its effect on the body to maximize health-related fitness outcomes.		

INDICATORS

STANDARD 2	Applies knowledge related to movement and fitness concepts.			
Grades 9-12	PROGRESSIONS			

PHYSICAL ACTIVITY KNOWLEDGE

INDICATORS				
2.12.11 Discusses the benefits of a physically active lifestyle as it relates to young adulthood.	Identifies opportunities to participate in physical activities as an adult.	Discusses the benefits (physical, mental, emotional, social) in participating in physical activity into adulthood.		
2.12.12 Applies knowledge of rest when planning regular physical activity.	Defines rest and recovery as it relates to physical activity.	Creates a physical activity plan that incorporates effective rest and recovery.		
2.12.13 Applies movement concepts and principles (e.g., force, motion, rotation) to analyze and improve performance of self and/or others in a selected skill (e.g., overhand throw, back squat, archery).	Defines various movement concepts.	Defines principles of force, motion, and rotation.	Examines performance of self and others, selecting a focus movement concept and/or principle.	
2.12.14 Identifies and discusses the historical and cultural roles of games, sports and dance in a society.	Identifies the various societies present today.	Analyzes society through a historical and cultural lens.	Describes historical and cultural roles of selected games, sports, and dance in society.	
2.12.15 Analyzes and applies technology as tools to support a healthy, active lifestyle.	Chooses a heath and/ or physical activity goal.	Selects a technology tool that supports self-selected health and physical activity goal.		
2.12.16 Identifies snacks and food choices that help and hinder performance, recovery, and enjoyment during physical activity.	Compares and contrasts foods based on nutrients and effect on the body.	Creates a plan that demonstrates knowledge of foods that help performance, recovery, and enjoyment of physical activity.		

AQUATICS

2.12.17 Demonstrates knowledge of water safety skills. Demonstrates knowledge of basic swimming skills.	Identifies water safety skills.	Identifies life-saving techniques.	Examines various swimming skills to improve efficiency, knowledge, and confidence.	Creates and implements a plan to improve efficiency in swimming skills.

INDICATORS AT A GLANCE

Note: *This chart is intended to list the Grade-Span Learning Indicators for grades preK-12. This chart is not intended to show alignment across Grade-Span Learning Indicators. However, some indicators may align across grade spans and some may not due to the content and skills being taught within a specific grade span.*

STANDARD 3	Develops social skills through movement.
RATIONALE	Through learning experiences in physical education, students develop the social skills necessary to exhibit empathy and respect for others and foster and maintain relationships. In addition, students develop skills for communication, leadership, cultural awareness, and conflict resolution in a variety of physical activity settings.

Grades preK-2 Learning Indicators	Grades 3-5 Learning Indicators	Grades 6-8 Learning Indicators	Grades 9-12 Learning Indicators
3.2.1 Recognizes the feelings of others during a variety of physical activities.	3.5.1 Describes the perspective of others during a variety of activities.	3.8.1 Understands and accepts others' differences during a variety of physical activities.	3.12.1 Demonstrates awareness of other people's emotions and perspectives in a physical activity setting.
3.2.2 Demonstrates ability to encourage others.	3.5.2 Uses communication skills to negotiate roles and responsibilities in a physical activity setting.	3.8.2 Demonstrates consideration for others and contributes positively to the group or team.	3.12.2 Exhibits proper etiquette, respect for others, and teamwork while engaging in physical activity.
3.2.3 Uses communication skills to share space and equipment.	3.5.3 Demonstrates respectful behaviors that contribute to positive social interaction in group activities.	3.8.3 Uses communication skills to negotiate strategies and tactics in a physical activity setting.	3.12.3 Encourages and supports others through their interactions in a physical activity setting.
3.2.4 Responds appropriately to directions and feedback from the teacher.	3.5.4 Demonstrates safe behaviors independently with limited reminders.	3.8.4 Implements and provides constructive feedback to and from others when prompted and supported by the teacher.	3.12.4 Implements and provides feedback to improve performance without prompting from the teacher.
3.2.5 Demonstrates respectful behaviors that contribute to positive social interactions in movement.	3.5.5 Solves problems independently, with partners, and in small groups.	3.8.5 Explains the value of a specific physical activity in culture.	3.12.5 Analyzes the value of a specific physical activity in a variety of cultures.

Grades preK-2 Learning Indicators	Grades 3-5 Learning Indicators	Grades 6-8 Learning Indicators	Grades 9-12 Learning Indicators
3.2.6 Describes why following rules is important for safety and fairness.	3.5.6 Makes choices that are fair according to activity etiquette.	3.8.6 Demonstrates the ability to follow game rules in a variety of physical activity situations.	3.12.6 Applies best practices for participating safely in physical activity (e.g., injury prevention, spacing, hydration, use of equipment, implementation of rules, sun protection).
3.2.7 Makes safe choices with physical education equipment.	3.5.7 Describe physical activities that represent a variety of cultures around the world.	3.8.7 Recognizes and implements safe and appropriate behaviors during physical activity and with exercise equipment.	3.12.7 Thinks critically and solves problems in physical activity settings, both as an individual and in groups.
3.2.8 Discusses problems and solutions with teacher support in a physical activity setting.		3.8.8 Solves problems amongst teammates and opponents.	3.12.8 Evaluates the effectiveness of leadership skills when participating in a variety of physical activity settings.
3.2.9 Makes fair choices as directed by the teacher.		3.8.9 Applies and respects the importance of etiquette in a physical activity setting.	
3.2.10 Identifies and participates in physical activities representing different cultures.		3.8.10 Explains how communication, feedback, cooperation, and etiquette relate to leadership roles.	

STANDARD 3	Develops social skills through movement.	
Grades preK-2	**PROGRESSIONS**	
3.2.1 Recognizes the feelings of others during a variety of physical activities.	Recognize that others may have different feelings and abilities.	Uses listening skills to identify what others want or need.
3.2.2 Demonstrates ability to encourage others.	Demonstrates ability to clap, cheer, and congratulate a peer with teacher assistance.	Demonstrates ability to clap, cheer, and congratulate a peer.
3.2.3 Uses communication skills to share space and equipment.	Pays attention to others when they are speaking.	Demonstrates verbal etiquette (e.g., please, excuse me, thank you).
3.2.4 Responds appropriately to directions and feedback from the teacher.	Demonstrates ability to follow directions and incorporate feedback with multiple reminders.	Demonstrates ability to follow directions and incorporate feedback with limited reminders.
3.2.5 Demonstrates respectful behaviors that contribute to positive social interactions in movement.	Praises the movement performance of others both more and less skilled.	Recognizes the role of respectful interactions with others when participating in physical activity.
3.2.6 Describes why following rules is important for safety and fairness.	Recalls safety rules for physical education.	Describes why game rules are important for the safety of others in a physical activity setting.
3.2.7 Makes safe choices with physical education equipment.	Recalls safety rules for use of equipment.	Identifies potential risks using equipment.
3.2.8 Discusses problems and solutions with teacher support in a physical activity setting.	Identifies and describes a problem within a physical activity setting.	Selects and justifies use of an appropriate solution when options are provided by the teacher.
3.2.9 Makes fair choices as directed by the teacher.	Identifies fair choices for a selected activity.	Demonstrates fair behavior (e.g., being honest, taking turns, letting others go first, trading equipment, respecting personal space) directed by the teacher.
3.2.10 Identifies and participates in physical activities representing different cultures.	Participates in a physical activity from another culture.	Provides examples of activities that are different from our own culture.

INDICATORS

Recognizes when a classmate needs help and takes action.	Can describe how their words and actions can affect others.	
Appropriately communicates praise for effort or completion of a skill.	Appropriately communicates encouragement during fatigue or after unsuccessful attempts.	
Demonstrates the ability to cooperate with one or two classmates.	Demonstrates the ability to cooperate with multiple classmates.	Appropriately communicates needs, wants and ideas in a respectful manner.
Recognizes and demonstrates elements of cooperation and teamwork with partner(s), small group, and whole group.	Describes why following game rules is important in a physical activity setting.	
Justifies why it is important for students to follow the rules in relation to fairness and cooperation during participation in a physical activity.		
Demonstrates the ability to make safe choices with equipment for self.	Demonstrates the ability to make safe choices with equipment for self and others.	
Develops and justifies possible solutions to a problem, within a physical activity, with limited teacher support.		
Independently demonstrates fair behavior (e.g., being honest, taking turns, letting others go first, trading equipment, respecting personal space).		
Identifies an activity from another culture and provides additional details about that culture.		

STANDARD 3	Develops social skills through movement.			
Grades 3-5	**PROGRESSIONS**			
3.5.1 Describes the perspective of others during a variety of activities.	Recognize that others may have a different perspective.	Uses listening skills to identify the perspectives of others.	Describe how their words and actions can impact the perspective of others.	
3.5.2 Uses communication skills to negotiate roles and responsibilities in a physical activity setting.	Identifies needed roles and responsibilities in a physical activity setting.	Describes desired behaviors that promote teamwork and cooperation.	Appropriately communicates needs, wants and ideas in a respectful manner.	Demonstrates cooperative communication in a group (e.g., listen, encourage, problem solve, compromise and reach consensus).
3.5.3 Demonstrates respectful behaviors that contribute to positive social interaction in group activities.	Praises the movement performance of others both more and less-skilled.	Recognizes the role of respectful interactions with others when participating in physical activity.	Demonstrates teamwork with partner(s), small group, and whole group.	Describes why following game rules is important in a physical activity setting.
3.5.4 Demonstrates safe behaviors independently with limited reminders.	Works safely with equipment in physical activity settings with teacher guidance.	Works independently and safely in physical activity settings.	Works safely with peers and equipment in physical activity settings.	
3.5.5 Solves problems independently, with partners, and in small groups.	Identifies a problem in a physical activity setting.	Identifies a problem in a relationship and seeks appropriate assistance.	Demonstrates the steps of the conflict resolution process (i.e., listen, express feelings, discuss solutions, make amends, etc.).	
3.5.6 Makes choices that are fair according to activity etiquette.	Identifies characteristics of fair choices within an activity.	Demonstrates fair behavior (e.g., being honest, taking turns, following rules, sharing roles, respecting personal space) directed by the teacher.	Independently demonstrates fair behavior (e.g., being honest, taking turns, following rules, sharing roles, respecting personal space).	
3.5.7 Describes physical activities that represent a variety of cultures around the world.	Identifies and describes characteristics of a self-selected activity from another culture.	Selects an activity that is unique to a culture; provides details of the relevance to that culture.	Selects an activity that is played across multiple cultures from around the world; cites the similarities or differences of how it is played.	

INDICATORS

STANDARD 3	Develops social skills through movement.			
Grades 6-8	**PROGRESSIONS**			
3.8.1 **Understands and accepts others' differences during a variety of physical activities.**	Accepts differences amongst peers (i.e., physical development, maturation, and varying skill levels) in a physical education setting.	Establishes supportive relationships by encouraging and providing positive feedback to peers (i.e., physical development, maturation, and varying skill levels) in a physical education setting.		
3.8.2 **Demonstrates consideration for others and contributes positively to the group or team.**	Describes how respectful behaviors contribute to positive social interaction in movement.	Evaluates the role of respectful interactions with others when participating in physical activity.	Articulates how respectful behaviors may vary among populations.	
3.8.3 **Uses communication skills to negotiate strategies and tactics in a physical activity setting.**	Describes possible strategies and tactics in a physical activity setting.	Appropriately communicates needs, wants, and ideas in a respectful manner.	Demonstrates cooperative communication in a group (e.g., listen, encourage, problem solve, compromise and reach consensus).	
3.8.4 **Implements and provides constructive feedback to and from others when prompted and supported by the teacher.**	**Receiving feedback**	Listens respectfully to corrective feedback from others (e.g., peers, adults).	Accepts and implements specific corrective teacher feedback.	
	Provides feedback	Provides corrective feedback to peers using prompting from the teacher (i.e., teacher-generated guidelines, incorporating appropriate tone and other communication skills).	Demonstrates encouragement and corrective feedback to peers without prompting from the teacher.	
3.8.5 **Explains the value of a specific physical activity in culture.**	Identifies the rules, history, customs and/or significance of engaging in physical activities from various cultures (e.g., dance, music, games).	Compares physical activities in various cultures with those practiced in their own culture.	Describes the significance of cultural and historical context associated with participation in a specific physical activity (e.g., attire, rituals, tradition, etiquette).	
3.8.6 **Demonstrates the ability to follow game rules in a variety of physical activity situations.**	Identifies rules for a selected activity.	Demonstrates ability to follow activity or game rules directed by the teacher.	Independently demonstrates ability to follow activity or game rules.	

INDICATORS

>continued

STANDARD 3 >*continued*

STANDARD 3	Develops social skills through movement.			
Grades 6-8	**PROGRESSIONS**			
INDICATORS				
3.8.7 Recognizes and implements safe and appropriate behaviors during physical activity and with exercise equipment.	Recognizes the importance of using physical activity and exercise equipment appropriately and safely, with the teacher's guidance.	Demonstrates the use of physical activity and exercise equipment appropriately and safely, with the teacher's guidance.	Implements use of physical activity and exercise equipment appropriately and safely while identifying safety concerns associated with the activity, without the teacher's guidance.	Identifies potential safety concerns associated with the activity and/or equipment.
3.8.8 Solves problems amongst teammates and opponents.	Lists potential conflicts and resolutions that could arise during physical activity.	Works with peers to establish rules and guidelines for resolving conflicts.	Responds appropriately to conflict with peers by using rules and guidelines for resolving conflicts.	
3.8.9 Applies and respects the importance of etiquette in a physical activity setting.	Recognizes etiquette in physical education.	Describes the importance of etiquette for physical activities, games, and dance activities.	Demonstrates knowledge of etiquette by self-officiating modified physical activities and games or following parameters to create or modify a dance.	Applies etiquette by acting as an official for modified physical activities and games and creating dance routines within a given set of parameters.
3.8.10 Explains how communication, feedback, cooperation, and etiquette relate to leadership roles.	Identifies characteristics of an effective leader.	Describes how the actions of an effective leader might impact a group in a physical activity setting.	Assesses personal leadership skills based on the characteristics of an effective leader within a physical activity.	

STANDARD 3	Develops social skills through movement.			
Grades 9-12	**PROGRESSIONS**			
INDICATORS				
3.12.1 Demonstrates awareness of other people's emotions and perspectives in a physical activity setting.	Acknowledges others' feelings or emotions.	Listens to other perspectives and seeks to understand.	Demonstrates positive tone and body language consistent with cultural norms during disagreements.	Demonstrates strategies for collaborating with teammates and opponents to move group efforts forward.
3.12.2 Exhibits proper etiquette, respect for others, and teamwork while engaging in physical activity.	Describes the importance of etiquette, respect for others, and teamwork during physical activities, games, and dance activities.	Evaluates and demonstrates appropriate respectful behaviors that contribute to positive social interaction in movement.	Acknowledges the difference between foul play and fair play in a competition setting (e.g., intentional fouls, performance-enhancing substances, gambling, current events in sport). This includes understanding of intentional fouls that are strategic, accidental, or malicious.	

STANDARD 3	Develops social skills through movement.			
Grades 9-12	**PROGRESSIONS**			
3.12.3 Encourages and supports others through their interactions in a physical activity setting.	Uses communication skills that promote team and group cooperation.	Demonstrates positive body language while engaging in physical activity that promote team and group cooperation.	Analyzes personal behaviors to improve support for others.	
3.12.4 Implements and provides feedback to improve performance without prompting from the teacher.	**Receiving feedback**	Listens respectfully to corrective feedback from others (e.g., peers, adults).	Accepts and implements specific corrective feedback to improve performance.	
	Provides feedback	Provides corrective feedback to peers (incorporating appropriate tone and other communication skills).	Provides encouragement and corrective feedback to peers.	
3.12.5 Analyzes the value of a specific physical activity in a variety of cultures.	Explains the rules, history, customs and/or significance of engaging in physical activities from various cultures (e.g., dance, music, games).	Compares and contrasts elements of various cultures with those practiced in their own personal culture in physical activity.	Researches and cites the significance of cultural and historical context associated with participation in various physical activities (e.g., attire, rituals, tradition, etiquette).	
3.12.6 Applies best practices for participating safely in physical activity (e.g., injury prevention, spacing, hydration, use of equipment, implementation of rules, sun protection).	Recognizes best practices of using physical activity and exercise equipment appropriately and safely.	Demonstrates best practices of physical activity and exercise equipment appropriately and safely.	Identifies potential safety concerns associated with the activity and/or equipment.	
3.12.7 Thinks critically and solves problems in physical activity settings, both as an individual and in groups.	Works with peers to establish rules and guidelines for resolving conflicts.	Collaborates with peers to solve a problem or task designed by the teacher to promote critical thinking and cooperation.	Responds appropriately with peers by independently resolving conflicts.	
3.12.8 Evaluates the effectiveness of leadership skills when participating in a variety of physical activity settings.	Compares and contrasts different leadership styles within a physical activity setting.	Evaluates the role of leadership characteristics to explain various outcomes within a physical activity.	Analyzes the role of leadership characteristics after high school and its application to multiple settings.	

INDICATORS

INDICATORS AT A GLANCE

Note: *This chart is intended to list the Grade-Span Learning Indicators for grades preK-12. This chart is not intended to show alignment across Grade-Span Learning Indicators. However, some indicators may align across grade spans and some may not due to the content and skills being taught within a specific grade span.*

STANDARD 4	Develops personal skills, identifies personal benefits of movement, and chooses to engage in physical activity.		
RATIONALE	Through learning experiences in physical education, the student develops an understanding of how movement is personally beneficial and subsequently chooses to participate in physical activities that are personally meaningful (e.g., activities that offer social interaction, cultural connection, exploration, choice, self-expression, appropriate levels of challenge, and added health benefits). The student develops personal skills including goal setting, identifying strengths, and reflection to enhance their physical literacy journey.		
Grades preK-2 Learning Indicators	**Grades 3-5 Learning Indicators**	**Grades 6-8 Learning Indicators**	**Grades 9-12 Learning Indicators**
4.2.1 Identifies physical activities that can meet the need for self-expression.	4.5.1 Explains how preferred physical activities meet the need for personal self-expression.	4.8.1 Describes how self-expression impacts individual engagement in physical activity.	4.12.1 Selects and participates in physical activities (e.g., dance, yoga, aerobics) that meet the need for self-expression.
4.2.2 Identifies physical activities that can meet the need for social interaction.	4.5.2 Explains how preferred physical activities meet the need for social interaction.	4.8.2 Describes how social interaction impacts individual engagement in physical activity.	4.12.2 Selects and participates in physical activities that meet the need for social interaction.
4.2.3 Lists ways that movement positively affects personal health.	4.5.3 Describes how movement positively affects personal health.	4.8.3 Participates in a variety of physical activities that can positively affect personal health.	4.12.3 Identifies and participates in physical activity that positively affects health.
4.2.4 Identifies preferred physical activities based on personal interests.	4.5.4 Explains the rationale for one's choices related to physical activity based on personal interests.	4.8.4 Connects how choice and personal interests impact individual engagement in physical activity.	4.12.4 Chooses and participates in physical activity based on personal interests.
4.2.5 Recognizes individual challenges through movement.	4.5.5 Recognizes group challenges through movement.	4.8.5 Examines individual and group challenges through movement.	4.12.5 Chooses and successfully participates in self-selected physical activity at a level that is appropriately challenging.

Grades preK-2 Learning Indicators	Grades 3-5 Learning Indicators	Grades 6-8 Learning Indicators	Grades 9-12 Learning Indicators
4.2.6 Sets observable short-term goals.	4.5.6 Sets observable long-term goals.	4.8.6 Sets goals to participate in physical activities based on examining individual ability.	4.12.6 Sets and develops movement goals related to personal interests.
4.2.7 Recognizes movement strengths and the need for practice for individual improvement.	4.5.7 Identifies movement strengths and opportunities for practice for individual improvement.	4.8.7 Examines opportunities and barriers to participating in physical activity outside of physical education class.	4.12.7 Analyzes factors on regular participation in physical activity after high school (e.g., life choices, economics, motivation, accessibility).
4.2.8 Recognizes the opportunity for physical activity within physical education class.	4.5.8 Identifies physical activity opportunities outside of physical education class.	4.8.8 Utilizes a variety of techniques to manage one's emotions and behaviors in a physical activity setting.	4.12.8 Analyzes and applies self-selected techniques to manage one's emotions in a physical activity setting.
4.2.9 Demonstrates techniques (e.g., breathing, counting) to assist with managing emotions and behaviors in a physical activity.	4.5.9 Recognizes personally effective techniques that assist with managing one's emotions and behaviors in a physical activity setting.	4.8.9 Reflects on movement experiences during physical education to develop understanding of how movement is personally meaningful.	4.12.9 Reflects on movement experiences during physical education to develop understanding of how movement is personally meaningful.
4.2.10 Reflects on movement experiences during physical education to develop understanding of how movement is personally meaningful.	4.5.10 Reflects on movement experiences during physical education to develop understanding of how movement is personally meaningful.		

STANDARD 4	Develops personal skills, identifies personal benefits of movement, and chooses to engage in physical activity.			
Grades preK-2	**PROGRESSIONS**			
4.2.1 Identifies physical activities that can meet the need for self-expression.	Describes ways to express oneself through physical activity.	Identifies one activity that meets the need for self-expression.	Explains that sometimes people engage in physical activities to express themselves.	
4.2.2 Identifies physical activities that can meet the need for social interaction.	Describes ways one might socially interact in physical activity.	Identifies one activity that meets the need for social interaction.	Explains that sometimes people engage in physical activities as a way to socially interact with others.	
4.2.3 Lists ways that movement positively affects personal health.	Describes one way that movement positively affects personal health.	Describes ways movement positively affects personal health.	Describes ways movement positively affects personal health.	
4.2.4 Identifies preferred physical activities based on personal interests.	Identifies one activity that is of personal interest within physical education.	Identifies three activities that are of personal interest within physical education.		
4.2.5 Recognizes individual challenges through movement.	Explains that some physical activities can be hard or challenging in physical education.	Identifies one physical activity that is challenging for them to perform.		
4.2.6 Sets observable short-term goals.	Defines what a goal is in their own words.	Defines what a short-term goal is in their own words.	Articulates a short-term goal that is realistic to achieve during a class period.	Sets and accomplishes a short-term goal during the physical education class period.
4.2.7 Recognizes movement strengths and the need for practice for individual improvement.	Explains that everyone has skills they are good at and skills they need work on in physical education.	Explains, in their own words, things/skills that they are good at in physical education.		
4.2.8 Recognizes the opportunity for physical activity within physical education class.	Identifies various ways to be physically active.	Explains that physical education is one opportunity to be physically active throughout the day.		
4.2.9 Demonstrates techniques (e.g., breathing, counting) to assist with managing emotions and behaviors in a physical activity.	Identifies emotions related to engagement in physical activity.	Explains the importance of managing emotions and behaviors in physical activity.	Recognizes there are several techniques they can use to manage emotions and behaviors during physical activity.	Demonstrates one technique they can use to manage emotions and behaviors during physical activity.
4.2.10 Reflects on movement experiences during physical education to develop understanding of how movement is personally meaningful.	Identifies what was enjoyable or not enjoyable during physical education class.	Articulates one reason why an activity was enjoyable or not enjoyable.		

INDICATORS

STANDARD 4	Develops personal skills, identifies personal benefits of movement, and chooses to engage in physical activity.			
Grades 3-5	PROGRESSIONS			
4.5.1 Explains how preferred physical activities meet the need for personal self-expression.	Defines self-expression as a way to express one's creativity, identity, or culture.	Identifies one activity they prefer that meets the need to express their creativity, identity, or culture.	Describes how their preferred physical activity meets the need to express their creativity, identity, or culture.	
4.5.2 Explains how preferred physical activities meet the need for social interaction.	Identifies one activity they prefer that meets the need for social interaction.	Describes how their preferred physical activity meets the need for social interaction.	Explains a benefit of interacting with others during physical activity.	
4.5.3 Describes how movement positively affects personal health.	Explains the differences between physical health and mental health.	Describes how movement can positively affect physical health.	Describes how movement can positively affect mental health.	
4.5.4 Explains the rationale for one's choices related to physical activity based on personal interests.	Identifies one reason they chose to participate in a specific physical activity in physical education.	Identifies two or more reasons they chose to participate in a specific physical activity in physical education.	Compares and contrasts why they chose or didn't choose one activity over another.	
4.5.5 Recognizes group challenges through movement.	Discusses advantages and disadvantages of working in groups.	Identifies physical activities that require working with others that are personally challenging.	Reflects on what went well and challenges that were faced during a group activity.	
4.5.6 Sets observable long-term goals.	Identifies what a long-term goal is.	Explains the difference between a short-term and long-term goal.	Articulates something realistic they want to achieve over several class periods or unit.	Sets and accomplishes a long-term goal over several physical education class periods or a unit.
4.5.7 Identifies movement strengths and opportunities for practice for individual improvement.	Lists skills or activities they feel they are good at.	Explains in their own words how practice can help them improve their skills.	Lists opportunities for practice in order to improve on a skill or activity.	
4.5.8 Identifies physical activity opportunities outside of physical education class.	Identifies ways to be physically active within school, but not in physical education.	Identifies ways to be physically active before or after school.	Identifies ways to be physically active at home.	Identifies opportunities for physical activity they can do on their own and opportunities that require an adult.
4.5.9 Recognizes personally effective techniques that assist with managing one's emotions and behaviors in a physical activity setting.	Identifies technique that is personally effective to manage emotions and behaviors during physical activity.	Demonstrates 1-3 techniques that are personally effective they can use to manage emotions and behaviors.	Recognizes the relationship between one's emotions and physical activity.	
4.5.10 Reflects on movement experiences during physical education to develop understanding of how movement is personally meaningful.	Identifies basic emotions before and after participating in activities during physical education class.	Identifies activities that affect emotions positively.	Recognizes how feelings/emotions change after engagement in physical activity/physical education.	Ranks activities/skills within physical education based on how they meet the need for self-expression, challenge, health, joy, and social interaction.

INDICATORS

STANDARD 4	Develops personal skills, identifies personal benefits of movement, and chooses to engage in physical activity.				
Grades 6-8	**PROGRESSIONS**				
4.8.1 **Describes how self-expression impacts individual engagement in physical activity.**	Identifies examples of movement opportunities that support creativity, identity, and cultural expression.	Participates in various movement opportunities that support creativity, identity, and cultural expression.	Reflects on movement opportunities that support creativity, identity, and cultural expression.	Explains the importance of movement related to creativity, identity, and cultural expression.	
4.8.2 **Describes how social interaction impacts individual engagement in physical activity.**	Identifies examples of movement opportunities that support social interaction preferences (e.g., large group, small group, paired, or alone).	Participates in various movement opportunities that support social interaction preferences (e.g., large group, small group, paired, or alone).	Reflects on movement opportunities that support social interaction preferences (e.g., large group, small group, paired, or alone).	Explains the importance of movement opportunities that support the need for social interaction (e.g., large group, small group, paired, or alone).	
4.8.3 **Participates in a variety of physical activities that can positively affect personal health.**	Identifies examples of movement opportunities that enhance well-being.	Participates in movement opportunities that enhance well-being.	Reflects on movement opportunities that enhance well-being.	Explains the importance of movement opportunities that enhance well-being.	
4.8.4 **Connects how choice and personal interests impact individual engagement in physical activity.**	Identifies examples of movement opportunities that are personally relevant.	Participates in movement opportunities that are personally relevant.	Reflects on movement opportunities that are personally relevant.	Explains the importance of movement opportunities that are personally relevant.	
4.8.5 **Examines individual and group challenges through movement.**	**Group challenge**	Identifies challenges when working with others in a group.	Reflects on group challenges and identifies what can be done to avoid those challenges in the future.		
	Individual challenge	Rates physical activities on how challenging they are and explains why the physical activity is challenging.	Analyzes how challenges related to physical activity or movement can affect participation in physical activity.		

INDICATORS (vertical label)

STANDARD 4	Develops personal skills, identifies personal benefits of movement, and chooses to engage in physical activity.				
Grades 6-8	PROGRESSIONS				
4.8.6 Sets goals to participate in physical activities based on examining individual ability.	Identifies what a SMART goal is.	Identify strengths and areas of improvement, with teacher guidance, in a teacher-selected activity/skill/unit.	Create a SMART goal related to the teacher-selected activity/unit/skill.	Engages in activities that target their SMART goal related to the teacher-selected activity/unit/skill.	Assesses progress toward their personal SMART goal and adjusts as necessary.
4.8.7 Examines opportunities and barriers to participating in physical activity outside of physical education class.	Lists opportunities to participate in physical activity outside of physical education class.	Lists barriers to participating in physical activity outside of physical education class.	Identifies a time and place where they could be active outside of physical education class.	Compares and contrasts opportunities and barriers to participating in physical activity outside of physical education class.	Correlates how access to opportunities and barriers affect participation in physical activity outside of physical education class.
4.8.8 Utilizes a variety of techniques to manage one's emotions and behaviors in a physical activity setting.	Connects how emotions can impact one's physical activity experiences.	Applies techniques that are personally effective to manage emotions and behaviors as needed.			
4.8.9 Reflects on movement experiences during physical education to develop understanding of how movement is personally meaningful.	Connects movement experiences within physical education class with thoughts and feelings after participation.	Reflects on movement experiences after a unit of instruction in physical education class by answering provided questions.	Determines how/if movement experiences in physical education class can be applied outside of physical education class.		

STANDARD 4	Develops personal skills, identifies personal benefits of movement, and chooses to engage in physical activity.			
Grades 9-12	**PROGRESSIONS**			
4.12.1 Selects and participates in physical activities (e.g., dance, yoga, aerobics) that meet the need for self-expression.	Identifies movement opportunities that support the student's creativity, identity, and cultural expression.	Participates in movement opportunities that support the student's creativity, identity, and cultural expression.	Reflects on movement opportunities that support the student's creativity, identity, and cultural expression.	Evaluates the need for self-expression for relevance and significance in relation to future activity choices.
4.12.2 Selects and participates in physical activities that meet the need for social interaction.	Identifies movement opportunities that support the student's social interaction preferences (e.g., large group, small group, paired, or alone).	Participates in movement opportunities that support the student's social interaction preferences (e.g., large group, small group, paired, or alone).	Reflects on movement opportunities that support the student's social interaction preferences (e.g., large group, small group, paired, or alone).	Evaluates different levels of social interaction for relevance and significance in relation to future activity choices.
4.12.3 Identifies and participates in physical activity that positively affects health.	Identifies movement opportunities that enhance well-being.	Participates in movement opportunities that enhance well-being.	Reflects on movement opportunities that enhance well-being.	Evaluates movement opportunities that enhance well-being for relevance and significance in relation to future activity choices.
4.12.4 Chooses and participates in physical activity based on personal interests.	Identifies movement opportunities that are personally relevant.	Participates in movement opportunities that are personally relevant.	Reflects on movement opportunities that are personally relevant.	Evaluates movement opportunities that are personally meaningful for relevance and significance in relation to future activity choices.
4.12.5 Chooses and successfully participates in self-selected physical activity at a level that is appropriately challenging.	Identifies movement opportunities that are appropriately challenging (not too easy, not too hard, just right).	Participates in movement opportunities that are appropriately challenging.	Reflects on movement opportunities that are appropriately challenging (not too easy, not too hard, just right).	Evaluates movement opportunities that are appropriately challenging (not too easy, not too hard, just right) for relevance and significance in relation to future activity choices.
4.12.6 Sets and develops movement goals related to personal interests.	Identifies strengths and areas of improvement in an activity of their choice.	Creates a SMART goal related to their activity of their choice.	Plans and engages in activities that target their personal SMART goal.	Monitors progress toward their personal SMART goal and adjusts as necessary.

INDICATORS

STANDARD 4	Develops personal skills, identifies personal benefits of movement, and chooses to engage in physical activity.			
Grades 9-12	**PROGRESSIONS**			
4.12.7 Analyzes factors on regular participation in physical activity after high school (e.g., life choices, economics, motivation, accessibility).	Identifies potential barriers, factors, and opportunities to participation in physical activity after high school.	Compares and contrasts opportunities and barriers to participating in physical activity after high school.	Correlates how access to opportunities and barriers affect participation in physical activity after high school.	Examines how one's access to participation in physical activity can potentially affect health after high school.
4.12.8 Analyzes and applies self-selected techniques to manage one's emotions in a physical activity setting.	Identifies techniques that are effective in managing one's emotions.	Identifies feelings and situations when managing one's emotions is necessary.	Applies a technique for managing one's emotion as needed.	Reflects on effectiveness of the self-selected technique in managing one's emotions.
4.12.9 Reflects on movement experiences during physical education to develop understanding of how movement is personally meaningful.	Reflects regularly on movement experiences in physical education class through a medium of their choice (e.g., journal, blog, provided questions, etc.).	Connects movement experiences in physical education class with what is relevant or to what they consider important.	Supports a positive relationship with physical activity citing evidence from participation in a broad range of physical activities using reflections, photos, videos, or other supporting documents.	

(INDICATORS label shown vertically at left of table rows)

Conclusion

The Learning Progressions are a useful tool in guiding teachers in developing physical education learning experiences that support differentiated levels of learning. Teachers are empowered and encouraged to make adjustments to the Learning Progressions to meet the individual needs of their students, with respect to access to resources, and that take into account their unique settings.

FUNDAMENTAL MOVEMENT SKILLS

CRITICAL ELEMENTS

MANIPULATIVE

Catching
- Move to get behind oncoming ball or anticipate ball position
- Keep eyes on ball
- Reach out for ball with hands
- Thumbs together above head
- Pinkies together below waist
- Catch with hands only
- Give with body
- Pull the ball into the body

Underhand Throw

Preparation
- Chest faces target
- Hold ball in both hands at waist level and off center toward throwing side

Execution
- Swing throwing arm back behind bottom
- Non-throwing arm reaches for target
- As throwing arms swings forward, step toward target with opposite foot
- Release ball at the level of the target

Follow-Through
- Throwing arm extends toward target

Overhand Throw

Preparation
- Side to target
- Hold ball in both hands at waist level and off center toward throwing side

Execution
- Across the body
- Wind up, bringing throwing arm back behind head with elbow bent at a 90-degree angle (i.e., "L" shape)
- Step toward target on opposite foot
- Rotate chest and hips toward target as throwing arm is extended toward target

Follow-Through
- Across the body
- Toward target

Striking With a Short-Handled Implement

Preparation
- Turn the side body to the target
- Start with bringing the paddle or racket back behind bottom
- Firm wrist and elbow

Execution
- Extend the racket arm and swing slightly from low to high
- Step with opposite foot during swing

Follow-Through
- Extend racket arm toward target

Striking With a Long-Handled Implement

Preparation
- Side to target (side stance)
- Bat prepared behind shoulder

Execution
- Level swing
- Some weight shifts toward forward foot

Follow-Through
- Across the body

Dribbling With Hands
- Use finger pads to push ball down
- Keep ball in front and slightly to side of body (to right if bouncing with right hand; to left if bouncing with left hand)
- Keep elbow of bouncing arm flexed
- Keep wrist firm
- Bounce ball waist high
- Keep chest and head up

>continued

FUNDAMENTAL MOVEMENT SKILLS   >continued

CRITICAL ELEMENTS

MANIPULATIVE

Instep Kick

Preparation
- Eyes focus on ball
- Two- to three-step approach with last step being non-kicking foot
- Non-kicking foot is placed beside and slightly behind the ball

Execution
- Leg action is from knee on down
- Contact ball with shoelaces
- Contact ball in middle of ball for low kick (trunk leans forward)
- Contact bottom of ball for lofted kick (trunk leans backward)
- Body weight forward over ball

Follow-Through
- Leg extends toward target at a low level

Rolling a Ball

Preparation
- Non-dominant hand placed in middle and front of playground ball
- Dominant (rolling hand) placed in middle and back of ball
- Swing arms back along dominant side of body to behind bottom

Execution
- Swing arms forward while stepping and shifting weight forward on opposite foot
- Bend knee of opposite leg to lower body toward floor level
- Release ball at a low level while taking non-dominant hand off of the ball

Follow-Through
- Reach with dominant or rolling hand and arm toward target
- Weight stays forward on opposite foot

Volleying: Striking Underhand

Preparation
- Pinkies are close together
- Fingers of hands are spread out
- Hands are positioned below waist with arms extended in front of body

Execution
- Contact ball with finger pads of all five fingers
- Lift arms from low to high (chest or face level)

Follow-Through
- Extend hands and arms toward target

Volleying: Striking Overhead

Preparation
- Thumbs are close together
- Fingers of hands are spread out
- Hands are positioned above head
- Elbows are bent

Execution
- Contact ball with finger pads of all five fingers
- Extend arms upward, straightening elbows

Follow-Through
- Extend hands and arms toward target

LOCOMOTOR

Run
- Preparation
- Push off of one foot; arm swing in opposition

Main action
- Definite flight phase; stride length at a maximum; complete extension of support leg; arms bent at right angle; heels kick buttocks
- Recourse with feet; arms swing forward in a coordinated fashion with legs to achieve distance and height

Recovery
- Lands on ball of lead foot with trail foot behind lead foot
- Entire action is step-together-step with a flight phase during "together"

Slide
- Preparation
- Turn body so side is leading action; arms extended at shoulder level

Main action
- Step with lead foot to side; step together with opposite/trail foot pushing off ground with lead foot and trail foot to attain a flight phase; step on lead foot; arms stay extended out to sides

Recovery
- Thigh parallel to ground; land on ball of foot; arms bent at right angle at sides; body is balanced

CRITICAL ELEMENTS

LOCOMOTOR

Gallop

Preparation
- Step forward on lead foot; arms begin back and bent at elbows

Main action
- Step together with trail leg touching the heel of lead foot; push-off of trail foot is forceful enough to achieve a flight phase

Recovery
- Land on lead foot with knee slightly bent; body stays upright

Hop

Preparation
- Non-hopping leg bent at 90 degrees

Main action
- Non-hopping leg swings in a pendular fashion to produce upward and forward force and distance; arms bent at elbows swing from back to front in coordination with the hopping action; well timed

Recovery
- Lands on hopping leg with bent knee and overall body control

Skip

Preparation
- Step on one foot; raise opposite knee

Main action
- Alternate stepping and hopping and right and left feet; lift knees to waist height; arms alternate and swing up and forward; left arm forward when right knee is up

Recovery
- Bend knee slightly on landing leg

Leap

Preparation
- Run with forceful push-off from one foot and forward extension of the opposite leg

Main action
- Legs are fully extended, arms are stretched out for balance; full extension of legs during flight; forward trunk lean

Recovery
- Land on ball of lead foot; bend knee slightly to absorb force; can recover and step out of leap into a standing position

Jumping and Landing
Two- to Two-Foot Jump

Preparation
- Take-off crouch and arm position appropriate for height and distance of jump; swings arms back

Main action
- Quick extension of legs and arms

Recovery
- Land on balls of feet with crouch appropriate to absorb height and distance of jump; arms reach out in front for balance

Jumping and Landing
One- to Two-Foot Jump

Preparation
- Step and push off of one foot with slight knee bend

Main action
- Push off by extending knee and swinging foot forward; bring push-off foot to meet and land on both feet simultaneously

Recovery
- Land on balls of feet with crouch appropriate to absorb height and distance of jump; arms reach out in front for balance

SPECIALIZED MOVEMENT SKILLS

CRITICAL ELEMENTS

GYMNASTICS

Inverted Balances

Tripod
- Triangle with head and hands
- Walk hips over triangle
- Knees on back of upper arms

Headstand
- Triangle with head and hands

Tripod
- Straighten legs toward ceiling

Scissor Kick Handstand
- Stand with arms raised
- Step forward; place hands on mat
- Scissor kick extended legs up and down
- Attempt to get body beyond 45-degree angle (close to 90 degrees with shoulders over hands)

Pencil Roll
- Start on back; legs are extended straight
- Arms are extended straight overhead and touching the mat
- Roll on to the stomach and continue in the same direction to roll on to the back

Rocker
- Sit on mat in tucked sitting position with chin tucked to chest and palms on the mat
- Back should be rounded, knees should be bent, and toes touch the floor
- Holding this shape, lean backward and rock backward and forward on their back

Side-to-Side Roll in a Tuck Position
- Start on all fours with hands and knees on the mat
- Bend the arm on one side and keep forearms bent and palms of hands flat
- Lean into the direction of the bent arm and roll onto back with knees tucked tight into chest
- Return to all fours position

Safety Roll
- One foot in front of other
- Bend knees to lower body toward one side
- Roll on the lower part of the arm on the same side
- Tuck chin to side into chest
- Legs stay bent but not tucked
- Roll on a diagonal

Forward Roll
- Start in a squat and push hard against the mat (with feet) to generate force for the roll
- Straighten the legs into a pike position, which will lift the bottom over the head
- Place the hands in front of the body and tuck the head
- Keep knees tucked into chest

Backward Roll
- Crouch, chin tucked, overbalance, and roll back on rounded back; thumbs placed by ear
- Keep knees tucked to chest and chin to chest
- As hands contact mat push up forcefully, extend hips, and land on feet

CRITICAL ELEMENTS

INVASION GAMES

Maintain Possession
Offense

Faking
- Move head, shoulders; jab step in one direction and move in opposite direction

Jab Step
- Step to right or left of defender and pivot or turn away from defender

Block or Pick
- One offensive player uses body by standing close to an offensive teammate, thus creating a block or pick; this protects the blocked offensive player and prevents defense from taking their flag

Faking With Dribbling—Feet or Hands
- Push ball slightly to one direction using the outside of the foot and then quickly use the inside of the foot to dribble ball in the opposite direction
- When dribbling with hands step in one direction with same foot as dribbling hand and then quickly step on diagonal with opposite foot to avoid obstacle

Avoiding Obstacles
- Make quick directional changes (use zig-zag pathways) when approaching a stationary obstacle
- Use different parts of foot to manipulate ball with feet to change directions quickly (soccer)
- Use different parts of the face of the hockey stick to push puck in direction away from obstacle (hockey)
- When dribbling with hands use outside hand to dribble to keep ball away from stationary obstacle; protect ball with non-dribbling hand by extending it toward the obstacle (basketball); keep body between the obstacle and the ball
- When dribbling with hands use a crossover dribble (left to right hand or right to left hand) to avoid obstacles (basketball)

Maintain Possession
Defense

Defense Body Position
- Vary body position (moving high, low, right, left) so that actions are unpredictable
- Fake by moving head or shoulders, or use a jab step pretending to move toward one offensive player but instead moving toward a different offensive player
- Try to deny space and prevent offense from moving forward toward endline

Chest Pass

Preparation
- Hold basketball on sides
- Ball is chest level
- Elbows flexed

Execution
- Step toward target
- Extend arms
- Release at chest level of target

Follow-Through
- Pronate hands upon release

Bounce Pass

Preparation
- Hold basketball on sides
- Ball is chest level
- Elbows flexed

Execution
- Step into pass
- Push ball down toward the floor on an angle
- Extend arms
- Position pass to land halfway between self and receiver

Follow-Through
- Pronate hands upon release

>continued

SPECIALIZED MOVEMENT SKILLS   >continued

CRITICAL ELEMENTS

INVASION GAMES

Inside-of-Foot Soccer Pass

Preparation
- Push ball slightly ahead of body
- Draw leg back by bending at knee
- Arms out for balance

Execution
- Swing toward middle of ball from knee on down
- Use big toe area of inside of foot to contact ball
- Head down

Follow-Through
- Low follow-through (below waist) toward target

Receiving in soccer
- Present trapping surface to the ball
- Cushion the ball (drawing body part back as ball is received)

Hockey Push-Pass

Hockey stance
- Form a triangle with feet and stick, knees slightly bent, stick flat on floor
- Non-dominant hand on top of stick
- Dominant hand halfway down stick
- Puck starts at heel of blade
- Blade sweeps puck forward with a cupping motion
- See target, then puck, then pass
- Roll wrists toward target (Fronske & Wilson, 2002, p.120)

Receiving in hockey
- Hockey stance
- Reach toward oncoming puck
- Watch puck into blade
- Absorb puck by pulling blade back to back foot

TARGET GAMES

Short Swing Iron Shot

Preparation
- Baseball grip: Dominant hand on bottom
- Square stance with ball positioned about 10-12 inches (25-30 cm) in front of and in middle of stance ("Make a Y" with arms and club; Fronske & Wilson, 2002)
- Line up ball and club head with target

Execution
- Backswing initiated with shoulders keeping club low to ground
- Slow backswing, taking weight on back leg
- Limit backswing, swinging club so hands are chest high
- Non-dominant arm stays straight during backswing
- Head down, eyes on ball
- Contact the ball below its center to make it travel upward
- Swing arms forward to hit through the ball

Follow-Through
- Low toward target

Bowling
- Step: Step forward with the foot that is on the same side as the hand holding the bowling ball; say "Step"
- Step: Continue holding the ball in front of the body when taking second step; use a normal stride; say "Step"
- Swing: On the third step, the rolling arm comes straight down at the side and back; say "Swing"
- Roll: On the fourth step, squat when bringing the rolling arm forward to release the ball on the ground; say "Roll"
- Follow-Through: After releasing the ball the palm should be up as the arm continues in an arc and in line with pins; say "Follow through"

CRITICAL ELEMENTS

NET AND WALL GAMES

Tennis

Forehand Strike

Grip
- Non-racket hand on throat of racket
- "Shake hands" Eastern grip; make a "V"

Preparation
- Turn shoulder and pivot feet
- Bring racket back and down

Execution
- Step with opposite foot
- Swing racket from low to high
- Contact ball in front of opposite foot

Follow-Through
- Beginning at 12 o'clock

Backhand Strike
- Two-handed grip

Preparation
- Turn shoulders and pivot feet
- Bring racket back to "thumb on thigh"

Execution
- Swing from low to high
- Contact ball in front of opposite foot

Follow-Through
- Follow-through for beginner is 12 o'clock

Serve
- Feet shoulder-width apart (right-handed player)
- Toes point at the right net post (45-degree angle)
- Elbow up and racket touching the back (imagine scratching the back)
- Tossing arm straight and in front of the body
- Toss ball up and slightly in front (younger kids can toss it on top of their head)
- Reach up high with racket and high five the ball; strings look at the target when making contact with the ball

Forehand Volley (Right-Handed)
- "Face the net": Body faces the net
- "Racket in front": Both hands hold racket in front of body; racket head should be at height of the player's head
- "Move racket to the right of body": Quickly move racket to the right of body by pivoting feet and turning shoulders; racket head should be at 45-degree angle
- "Step with left foot": Left foot steps forward and slightly to the right
- "High five the ball": Contact is slightly in front of body; hold racket and allow ball to bounce off strings; may allow a slight push
- "No follow-through": Valleys should not contain a follow-through
- Punch or tap the ball

Volleyball

Forearm Pass
- Make a flat surface with arms by placing back of one hand in palm of the other
- Move feet to get under the ball
- One foot in front of the other with knees bent
- Extend arms, body, and knees to the ball
- Do not swing arms; meet the ball with arms
- Aim arms toward the top of the net, not to the ceiling

Overhead Set
- Elbows high
- Make a diamond shape with hands using thumb and index fingers
- Bend knees
- Quick "catch" and push with fingers
- Extend arms and wrist
- Imagine catching a water balloon to learn the feeling of not stabbing at the ball

>continued

SPECIALIZED MOVEMENT SKILLS   *>continued*

CRITICAL ELEMENTS

NET AND WALL GAMES

Volleyball

Underhand Serve

- Side to target
- Forward and backward strike with non-hitting shoulder facing the net
- Hold the ball in medium space with non-striking hand (imagine the ball sitting on a batting tee)
- Use a bowling motion (step with the opposite foot and bring striking hand back)
- As the open hand comes forward, strike the ball with the heel of the hand
- Do not toss the ball in the air during the striking motion
- Follow through toward the target

Overhead Serve

- Align shoulders square to the net facing the target area. Step forward with the foot opposite the striking or serving hand
- Toss the ball 3-4 feet (90-120 cm) above the head and in front of the serving shoulder
- Strike the ball with an open hand in one continuous motion ("Swing through the ball")
- Keep eyes on the ball ("See actual contact take place")
- Follow through with the striking hand in the direction of the ball
- Transfer weight from the back foot to the front foot

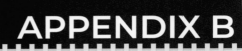

Movement Framework

Body		
the what		
Shapes	**Non-locomotor**	**Locomotor**
Straight	Stretch	Walk
Curved	Bend	Run
Angular	Twist	Skip
Twisted	Spin	Leap
Tilted		Gallop
Wide		Slide
Narrow		Jump
		Hop
Manipulative		
Throwing		
Catching		
Kicking		
Dribbling		
Striking		

Effort	
the how	
Energy qualities	**Effort actions**
Sustained	Float
Percussive	Punch
Vibratory	Glide
Suspended	Slash
Collapsed	Dab
Swinging	Wring
Explosive	Flick
	Press

Space				
the where				
Directions	**Levels**	**Pathways**	**Personal space**	**General space**
Forward	Low	Straight		
Backward	Middle	Curved		
Diagonal	High	Zigzag		
Sideways		Spiral		
Up				
Down				

Time		
the when		
Measured time	**Free rhythm**	**Freezing**
Rhythm	No	"Preserving"
Accent	discernable	a moment
Tempo	beat or	in time
Fast	rhythmic	
Slow	pattern	
Moderate		
Accelerate		
Decelerate		

Relationships	
the interaction	
Unison	Act and react
Shadow	Weave
Ripple	Cannon
Contrast	Mirror
Link	Lift
Support	Meet and part
Sculpt	Over and under
Magnetic sculpting	Around

Based on Laban's Movement Principles.

Reprinted by permission from F.E. Cleland Donnelly and V.F. Millar, "Moving Green, Going Green: An Interdisciplinary Creative Dance Experience," *Journal of Physical Education, Recreation & Dance* 90, no. 8 (2019), reprinted by permission of Taylor & Francis Ltd, https://www.tandfonline.com/ on behalf of https://www.shapeamerica.org/.

APPENDIX C

Scope and Sequence

STANDARD 1: DEVELOPS A VARIETY OF MOTOR SKILLS.				
	Grades preK-2 Learning Indicators	**Grades 3-5 Learning Indicators**	**Grades 6-8 Learning Indicators**	**Grades 9-12 Learning Indicators**
Locomotor	1.2.1 Demonstrates a variety of locomotor skills with the concepts of space, effort, and relationship awareness.	1.5.1 Combines varied locomotor skills in a variety of practice tasks.	*Applies prior skills and concepts to other contexts, within this grade span.*	*Applies prior skills and concepts to other contexts, within this grade span.*
	1.2.2 Demonstrates jumping and landing in a non-dynamic environment.	1.5.2 Demonstrates transferring weight from feet to hands and hands to feet in a non-dynamic environment.		
	1.2.3 Demonstrates transferring weight on multiple body parts.	1.5.3 Demonstrates rolling with the body in a non-dynamic environment.		
		1.5.4 Combines jumping and landing, rolling, balancing and transfer of weight from feet to hands in a non-dynamic environment.		
Non-locomotor	1.2.4 Demonstrates non-locomotor skills with the concepts of space, effort, and relationship awareness.	1.5.7 Demonstrates jumping and landing in a non-dynamic environment.	*Applies prior skills and concepts to other contexts, within this grade span.*	*Applies prior skills and concepts to other contexts, within this grade span.*
	1.2.5 Demonstrates balancing on different body parts in a non-dynamic environment.	1.5.8 Demonstrates balancing on different body parts in a non-dynamic environment.		

>continued

STANDARD 1   >continued

STANDARD 1: DEVELOPS A VARIETY OF MOTOR SKILLS.

	Grades preK-2 Learning Indicators	Grades 3-5 Learning Indicators	Grades 6-8 Learning Indicators	Grades 9-12 Learning Indicators
Manipulative	1.2.6 Demonstrates bouncing a ball in a variety of non-dynamic practice tasks.	1.5.9 Demonstrates rolling a ball in a non-dynamic environment.		
	1.2.7 Demonstrates rolling a ball in a variety of non-dynamic practice tasks.	1.5.10 Demonstrates throwing in a variety of practice tasks.		
	1.2.8 Demonstrates catching in a variety of non-dynamic practice tasks.	1.5.11 Demonstrates striking with a long-handled implement in a variety of practice tasks.		
	1.2.9 Demonstrates throwing in a variety of non-dynamic practice tasks.	1.5.12 Demonstrates catching in a variety of practice tasks.		
	1.2.10 Demonstrates kicking a ball in a variety of non-dynamic practice tasks.	1.5.13 Demonstrates striking with hands above waist in a variety of practice tasks.		
	1.2.11 Demonstrates dribbling with feet in a variety of non-dynamic practice tasks.	1.5.14 Demonstrates striking with hands below waist in a variety of practice tasks.		
	1.2.12 Demonstrates striking with hands in a variety of non-dynamic practice tasks.	1.5.15 Demonstrates serving an object in a non-dynamic environment.	*Applies prior skills and concepts to other contexts, within this grade span.	*Applies prior skills and concepts to other contexts, within this grade span.
	1.2.13 Demonstrates striking with a short-handled implement in a variety of non-dynamic practice tasks.	1.5.16 Demonstrates striking a ball with a short-handled implement in a variety of practice tasks.		
	1.2.14 Demonstrates striking with a long-handled implement in a variety of non-dynamic practice tasks.	1.5.17 Demonstrates sending and receiving an object in a variety of practice tasks.		
		1.5.18 Demonstrates kicking a ball using the instep in a variety of practice tasks.		
		1.5.19 Demonstrates dribbling with hands in a variety of practice tasks.		
		1.5.20 Demonstrates dribbling with feet in a variety of practice tasks.		
		1.5.21 Combines manipulative skills and traveling for execution to a target in a variety of practice tasks.		

STANDARD 1: DEVELOPS A VARIETY OF MOTOR SKILLS.

	Grades preK-2 Learning Indicators	Grades 3-5 Learning Indicators	Grades 6-8 Learning Indicators	Grades 9-12 Learning Indicators
Dance and rhythms	1.2.15 Demonstrates locomotor, non-locomotor, and manipulative movements based on a variety of dance forms.	1.5.5 Combines locomotor, non-locomotor, and manipulative movements based on a variety of dance forms.	1.8.2 Demonstrates movement sequences within varied dance forms.	1.12.4 Demonstrates and creates movement sequences based on one or more forms of dance.
	1.2.16 Demonstrates jumping rope in a non-dynamic environment.	1.5.6 Demonstrates jumping rope in a variety of practice tasks.		
Outdoor pursuits	*Developmentally appropriate outcomes first appear in grades 6-8.	*Developmentally appropriate outcomes first appear in grades 6-8.	1.8.1 Demonstrates correct technique in a variety of outdoor activities.	1.12.3 Demonstrates activity-specific movement skills in a variety of outdoor pursuits.
Fitness activities	*Developmentally appropriate outcomes first appear in grades 6-8.	*Developmentally appropriate outcomes first appear in grades 6-8.	1.8.3 Demonstrates appropriate form in a variety of health-related fitness activities.	1.12.5 Demonstrates appropriate technique in cardiovascular training.
			1.8.4. Demonstrates appropriate form in a variety of skill-related fitness activities.	1.12.6 Demonstrates appropriate technique in muscular strength and endurance training.
				1.12.7 Demonstrates appropriate technique in flexibility training.
				1.12.8 Demonstrates appropriate technique in skill-related fitness training.
Target	*Developmentally appropriate outcomes first appear in grades 3-5.	1.5.9 Demonstrates rolling a ball in a non-dynamic environment.	1.8.5 Demonstrates a striking motion with a long-handled implement.	1.12.2 Demonstrates activity-specific movement skills in a variety of recreational and backyard games.
			1.8.6 Demonstrates a correct rolling and throwing (underhand, sidearm, overhand) technique in a variety of practice tasks and modified target games.	

>continued

STANDARD 1   >continued

STANDARD 1: DEVELOPS A VARIETY OF MOTOR SKILLS.				
	Grades preK-2 Learning Indicators	**Grades 3-5 Learning Indicators**	**Grades 6-8 Learning Indicators**	**Grades 9-12 Learning Indicators**
Striking and fielding	*Developmentally appropriate outcomes first appear in grades 3-5.*	1.5.10 Demonstrates throwing in a variety of practice tasks.	1.8.7 Demonstrates striking a self-tossed/pitched ball with an implement to open space in a variety of practice tasks and small-sided games.	1.12.1 Demonstrates activity-specific movement skills in a variety of lifetime sports and activities.
		1.5.11 Demonstrates striking with a long-handled implement in a variety of practice tasks.	1.8.8 Demonstrates a proper catch with or without an implement in a variety of practice tasks and small-sided games.	
		1.5.12 Demonstrates catching in a variety of practice tasks.	1.8.9 Demonstrates throwing for accuracy, distance, and power in a variety of practice tasks and small-sided games.	
Net and wall	*Developmentally appropriate outcomes first appear in grades 3-5.*	1.5.13 Demonstrates striking with hands above waist in a variety of practice tasks.	1.8.10 Demonstrates a proper underhand and overhand serve using the hand in a variety of practice tasks and modified small-sided games.	1.12.1 Demonstrates activity-specific movement skills in a variety of lifetime sports and activities.
		1.5.14 Demonstrates striking with hands below waist in a variety of practice tasks.	1.8.11 Demonstrates a proper underhand and overhand serve using a short- or long-handled implement in a variety of practice tasks and modified small-sided games.	
		1.5.15 Demonstrates serving an object in a non-dynamic environment.	1.8.12 Demonstrates the correct form of a forehand and backhand stroke with a short-handled and long-handled implement in a variety of practice tasks and modified small-sided games.	
		1.5.16 Demonstrates striking an object with a short-handled implement in a variety of practice tasks.	1.8.13 Demonstrates a volley using a short-handled and long-handled implement in a variety of practice tasks and modified net and wall games.	

STANDARD 1: DEVELOPS A VARIETY OF MOTOR SKILLS.

	Grades preK-2 Learning Indicators	Grades 3-5 Learning Indicators	Grades 6-8 Learning Indicators	Grades 9-12 Learning Indicators
Invasion	*Developmentally appropriate outcomes first appear in grades 3-5.*	**1.5.17** Demonstrates sending and receiving an object in a variety of practice tasks.	**1.8.14** Demonstrates sending and receiving in combination with locomotor skills in a variety of small-sided games.	**1.12.1** Demonstrates activity-specific movement skills in a variety of lifetime sports and activities.
		1.5.18 Demonstrates kicking a ball using the instep in a variety of practice tasks.	**1.8.15** Demonstrates a dribbling skill in a variety of practice tasks and small-sided games.	
		1.5.19 Demonstrates dribbling with hands in a variety of practice tasks.	**1.8.16** Demonstrates dribbling an object with an implement in a variety of practice tasks and small-sided games.	
		1.5.20 Demonstrates dribbling with feet in a variety of practice tasks.	**1.8.17** Demonstrates a shot on goal with and without an implement in a variety of practice tasks and small-sided games.	
			1.8.18 Demonstrates multiple techniques to create open space during a variety of practice tasks and small-sided games (offense).	
			1.8.19 Demonstrates a defensive ready position in a variety of practice tasks and small-sided games.	
Aquatics	**1.2.17** Demonstrates water safety skills. If a pool facility is available, demonstrates water safety and basic swimming skills.	**1.5.22** Demonstrates water safety skills. If a pool facility is available, demonstrates water safety and basic swimming skills.	**1.8.20** Demonstrates water safety skills. If a pool facility is available, demonstrates water safety and basic swimming skills.	**1.12.9** Demonstrates water safety skills. If a pool facility is available, demonstrates water safety and basic swimming skills.

STANDARD 2: APPLIES KNOWLEDGE RELATED TO MOVEMENT AND FITNESS CONCEPTS.

	Grades preK-2 Learning Indicators	Grades 3-5 Learning Indicators	Grades 6-8 Learning Indicators	Grades 9-12 Learning Indicators
Tactics and strategies	2.2.1 Recognizes personal space and where to move in general space.	2.5.1 Applies movement concepts and strategies for safe movement within dynamic environments.	2.8.1 Identifies the effective use of movement concepts within multiple dynamic environments.	2.12.1 Demonstrates knowledge of tactics and strategies within lifetime sports and activities.
	2.2.2 Identifies simple strategies in chasing and fleeing activities.	2.5.2 Demonstrates knowledge of offensive strategies in small-sided invasion practice tasks.	2.8.2 Demonstrates knowledge of offensive tactics to create space with movement in invasion games.	2.12.2 Demonstrates knowledge of tactics and strategies within recreational and backyard games.
	2.2.3 Identifies movement concepts related to locomotor, non-locomotor, and manipulative skills.	2.5.3 Demonstrates knowledge of defensive strategies in small-sided invasion practice tasks.	2.8.3 Demonstrates knowledge of reducing open space with movement and denial in invasion games.	2.12.3 Demonstrates knowledge of tactics and strategies within outdoor pursuits.
	2.2.4 Demonstrates knowledge of locomotor, non-locomotor, and manipulative skills in movement settings.	2.5.4 Demonstrates knowledge of appropriate movement concepts for efficient performance of manipulative skills.	2.8.4 Selects and applies the appropriate shot and technique in net and wall games.	
		2.5.5 Demonstrates problem-solving strategies in a variety of games and activities.	2.8.5 Demonstrates knowledge of offensive tactics in striking and fielding games.	
			2.8.6 Demonstrates knowledge of defensive positioning tactics in striking and fielding games.	
			2.8.7 Demonstrates problem-solving skills in a variety of games and activities.	
Dance and rhythms	2.2.5 Demonstrates knowledge of locomotor, non-locomotor, and movement concepts used in dance and rhythms.	2.5.6 Applies movement concepts to different types of dances, gymnastics, rhythms, and individual performance activities.	2.8.8 Applies knowledge of movement concepts for the purpose of varying different types of dances and rhythmic activities.	2.12.4 Applies knowledge of movement sequences to create or participate in one or more forms of dance.

STANDARD 2: APPLIES KNOWLEDGE RELATED TO MOVEMENT AND FITNESS CONCEPTS.

	Grades preK-2 Learning Indicators	Grades 3-5 Learning Indicators	Grades 6-8 Learning Indicators	Grades 9-12 Learning Indicators
Fitness concepts	2.2.6 Identifies physical activities that contribute to fitness.	2.5.7 Defines and provides examples of movement activities for developing the health-related fitness components.	2.8.9 Identifies and compares the components of health and skill-related fitness.	2.12.5 Analyzes how health and fitness will impact quality of life after high school.
	2.2.7 Recognizes the importance of stretching before and after physical activity.	2.5.8 Establishes goals related to enhancing fitness development.	2.8.10 Self-selects and monitors physical activity goals based on a self-selected health-related fitness assessment.	2.12.6 Establishes a goal and creates a practice plan to improve performance for a self-selected skill.
	2.2.8 Identifies the heart as a muscle that gets stronger with physical activity.	2.5.9 Defines and explains how to implement the FITT Principle for fitness development.	2.8.11 Implements the principles of exercise (progression, overload, and specificity) for different types of physical activity.	2.12.7 Applies the principles of exercise in a variety of self-selected lifetime physical activities.
		2.5.10 Defines and provides examples of movement activities for developing the skill-related fitness components.	2.8.12 Applies knowledge of skill-related fitness to different types of physical activity.	2.12.8 Designs and implements a plan that applies knowledge of aerobic, strength and endurance, and flexibility training exercises.
		2.5.11 Identifies the need for warm-up and cool-down relative to various physical activities.	2.8.13 Explains the relationship of aerobic fitness and RPE Scale to physical activity effort.	2.12.9 Evaluates perceived exertion during physical activity and adjusts effort.
		2.5.12 Identifies location of pulse and provides examples of activities that increase heart rate.	2.8.14 Applies knowledge of dynamic and static stretching to exercise in warm-up, cool-down, flexibility, endurance, etc. physical activities.	2.12.10 Applies heart rate concepts to ensure safety and maximize health-related fitness outcomes.
			2.8.15 Demonstrates knowledge of heart rate and describes its relationship to aerobic fitness.	

>continued

STANDARD 2   >continued

STANDARD 2: APPLIES KNOWLEDGE RELATED TO MOVEMENT AND FITNESS CONCEPTS.				
	Grades preK-2 Learning Indicators	**Grades 3-5 Learning Indicators**	**Grades 6-8 Learning Indicators**	**Grades 9-12 Learning Indicators**
Physical activity knowledge	2.2.9 Recognizes that regular physical activity is good for their health.	2.5.13 Explains the benefits of physical activity.	2.8.16 Identifies ways to be physically active.	2.12.11 Discusses the benefits of a physically active lifestyle as it relates to young adulthood.
	2.2.10 Recognizes physiological changes in their body during physical activities.	2.5.14 Recognizes and explains how physical activity influences physiological changes in their body.	2.8.17 Examines how rest impacts the body's response to physical activity.	2.12.12 Applies knowledge of rest when planning regular physical activity.
	2.2.11 Recognizes food and hydration choices that provide energy for physical activity.	2.5.15 Recognizes the critical elements that contribute to proper execution of a skill.	2.8.18 Analyzes skill performance by identifying critical elements.	2.12.13 Applies movement concepts and principles (e.g., force, motion, rotation) to analyze and improve performance of self and/or others in a selected skill (e.g., overhand throw, back squat, archery).
		2.5.16 Identifies technology tools that support physical activity goals.	2.8.19 Evaluates usefulness of technology tools to support physical activity and fitness goals.	2.12.14 Identifies and discusses the historical and cultural roles of games, sports and dance in a society.
		2.5.17 Describes the impact of food and hydration choices on physical activity.	2.8.20 Explains the relationships among nutrition, physical activity, and health factors.	2.12.15 Analyzes and applies technology as tools to support a healthy, active lifestyle.
				2.12.16 Identifies snacks and food choices that help and hinder performance, recovery, and enjoyment during physical activity.
Outdoor pursuits	*Developmentally appropriate outcomes first appear in grades 6-8.*	*Developmentally appropriate outcomes first appear in grades 6-8.*	2.8.21 Demonstrates knowledge of safety protocols in teacher-selected outdoor activities.	2.12.13 Applies movement concepts and principles (e.g., force, motion, rotation) to analyze and improve performance of self and/or others in a selected skill (e.g., overhand throw, back squat, archery).
Aquatics	2.2.12 Demonstrates knowledge of water safety skills. Demonstrates knowledge of basic swimming skills.	2.5.18 Demonstrates knowledge of water safety skills. Demonstrates knowledge of basic swimming skills.	2.8.22 Demonstrates knowledge of water safety skills. Demonstrates knowledge of basic swimming skills.	2.12.17 Demonstrates knowledge of water safety skills. Demonstrates knowledge of basic swimming skills.

STANDARD 3: DEVELOPS SOCIAL SKILLS THROUGH MOVEMENT.

	Grades preK-2 Learning Indicators	Grades 3-5 Learning Indicators	Grades 6-8 Learning Indicators	Grades 9-12 Learning Indicators
Social awareness	3.2.1 Recognizes the feelings of others during a variety of physical activities.	3.5.1 Describes the perspective of others during a variety of activities.	3.8.1 Understands and accepts others' differences during a variety of physical activities.	3.12.1 Demonstrates awareness of other people's emotions and perspectives in a physical activity setting.
	3.2.5 Demonstrates respectful behaviors that contribute to positive social interactions in movement.	3.5.7 Describes physical activities that represent a variety of cultures around the world.	3.8.2 Demonstrates consideration for others and contributes positively to the group or team.	3.12.5 Analyzes the value of a specific physical activity in a variety of cultures.
	3.2.10 Identifies and participates in physical activities representing different cultures.		3.8.5 Explains the value of a specific physical activity in culture.	
Communication	3.2.3 Uses communication skills to share space and equipment.	3.5.2 Uses communication skills to negotiate roles and responsibilities in a physical activity setting.	3.8.3 Uses communication skills to negotiate strategies and tactics in a physical activity setting.	3.12.3 Encourages and supports others through their interactions in a physical activity setting.
	3.2.4 Responds appropriately to directions and feedback from the teacher.		3.8.4 Implements and provides constructive feedback to and from others when prompted and supported by the teacher.	3.12.4 Implements and provides feedback to improve performance without prompting from the teacher.
Working with others	3.2.2 Demonstrates ability to encourage others.	3.5.4 Demonstrates respectful behaviors that contribute to positive social interaction in group activities.	3.8.8 Solves problems amongst teammates and opponents.	3.12.2 Exhibits proper etiquette, respect for others, and teamwork while engaging in physical activity.
	3.2.8 Discusses problems and solutions with teacher support in a physical activity setting.	3.5.5 Solves problems independently, with partners, and in small groups.	3.8.9 Applies and respects the importance of etiquette in a physical activity setting.	3.12.7 Thinks critically and solves problems in physical activity settings, both as an individual and in groups.
	3.2.9 Makes fair choices as directed by the teacher.	3.5.6 Makes choices that are fair according to activity etiquette.	3.8.10 Explains how communication, feedback, cooperation, and etiquette relate to leadership roles.	3.12.8 Evaluates the effectiveness of leadership skills when participating in a variety of physical activity settings.
Safety	3.2.6 Describes why following rules is important for safety and fairness.	3.5.4 Demonstrates safe behaviors independently with limited reminders.	3.8.6 Demonstrates the ability to follow game rules in a variety of physical activity situations.	3.12.6 Applies best practices for participating safely in physical activity (e.g., injury prevention, spacing, hydration, use of equipment, implementation of rules, sun protection).
	3.2.7 Makes safe choices with physical education equipment.		3.8.7 Recognizes and implements safe and appropriate behaviors during physical activity and with exercise equipment.	

STANDARD 4: DEVELOPS PERSONAL SKILLS, IDENTIFIES PERSONAL BENEFITS OF MOVEMENT, AND CHOOSES TO ENGAGE IN PHYSICAL ACTIVITY.

	Grades preK-2 Learning Indicators	Grades 3-5 Learning Indicators	Grades 6-8 Learning Indicators	Grades 9-12 Learning Indicators
Self-expression and social interaction	4.2.1 Identifies physical activities that can meet the need for self-expression.	4.5.1 Explains how preferred physical activities meet the need for personal self-expression.	4.8.1 Describes how self-expression impacts individual engagement in physical activity.	4.12.1 Selects and participates in physical activities (e.g., dance, yoga, aerobics) that meet the need for self-expression.
	4.2.2 Identifies physical activities that can meet the need for social interaction.	4.5.2 Explains how preferred physical activities meet the need for social interaction.	4.8.2 Describes how social interaction impacts individual engagement in physical activity.	4.12.2 Selects and participates in physical activities that meet the need for social interaction.
Self-management and personal health	4.2.3 Lists ways that movement positively affects personal health.	4.5.3 Describes how movement positively affects personal health.	4.8.3 Participates in a variety of physical activities that can positively affect personal health.	4.12.3 Identifies and participates in physical activity that positively affects health.
	4.2.9 Demonstrates techniques (e.g., breathing, counting) to assist with managing emotions and behaviors in a physical activity.	4.5.9 Recognizes personally effective techniques that assist with managing one's emotions and behaviors in a physical activity setting.	4.8.8 Utilizes a variety of techniques to manage one's emotions and behaviors in a physical activity setting.	4.12.8 Analyzes and applies self-selected techniques to manage one's emotions in a physical activity setting.
Choice	4.2.4 Identifies preferred physical activities based on personal interests.	4.5.4 Explains the rationale for one's choices related to physical activity based on personal interests.	4.8.4 Connects how choice and personal interests impact individual engagement in physical activity.	4.12.4 Chooses and participates in physical activity based on personal interests.
				4.12.5 Chooses and successfully participates in self-selected physical activity at a level that is appropriately challenging.
Goal setting	4.2.5 Recognizes individual challenges through movement.	4.5.5 Recognizes group challenges through movement.	4.8.5 Examines individual and group challenges through movement.	4.12.6 Sets and develops movement goals related to personal interests.
	4.2.6 Sets observable short-term goals.	4.5.6 Sets observable long-term goals.	4.8.6 Sets goals to participate in physical activities based on examining individual ability.	
	4.2.7 Recognizes movement strengths and the need for practice for individual improvement.	4.5.7 Identifies movement strengths and opportunities for practice for individual improvement.		

STANDARD 4: DEVELOPS PERSONAL SKILLS, IDENTIFIES PERSONAL BENEFITS OF MOVEMENT, AND CHOOSES TO ENGAGE IN PHYSICAL ACTIVITY.				
	Grades preK-2 Learning Indicators	Grades 3-5 Learning Indicators	Grades 6-8 Learning Indicators	Grades 9-12 Learning Indicators
Reflection	4.2.8 Recognizes the opportunity for physical activity within physical education class.	4.5.8 Identifies physical activity opportunities outside of physical education class.	4.8.7 Examines opportunities and barriers to participating in physical activity outside of physical education class.	4.12.7 Analyzes factors on regular participation in physical activity after high school (e.g., life choices, economics, motivation, accessibility).
	4.2.10 Reflects on movement experiences during physical education to develop understanding of how movement is personally meaningful.	4.5.10 Reflects on movement experiences during physical education to develop understanding of how movement is personally meaningful.	4.8.9 Reflects on movement experiences during physical education to develop understanding of how movement is personally meaningful.	4.12.9 Reflects on movement experiences during physical education to develop understanding of how movement is personally meaningful.

Curriculum Map and Planning Guide

DOCUMENT GUIDANCE

This document provides a source of reference for teachers to consider the use of the 2024 SHAPE America National Physical Education Standards when planning and preparing for instruction. The information provided does not encompass all instructional opportunities but can be used as a guide of consideration.

All schools have differences in scheduling, grade-based groupings, equipment, student demographics, and facility space. This guide is not prescriptive but was written as a support for teachers to consider how they may create their own instructional plan to meet the unique needs of their students at each school site. Educators can use these instructional focus, unit or activities, skills, and guiding questions as they see fit to meet those needs.

Time frame: The preK-5 time frame is categorized monthly because many elementary schools have students for the whole year within a course. The grades 6-12 time frame reflects most semester-based schedules. We encourage educators to make time frame changes to meet their own school site needs.

Instructional focus: This document uses concepts to assist in planning from the lens of the big idea and using the academic standards to assist in breaking down that big idea.

Unit or activities: The unit ideas are foundational considerations of what a unit focus could be based on the academic standards and the skills or outcomes of what students can do. Educators can use their own creativity in adding unique unit ideas to their own instructional plan.

Skills: The skills listed are not comprehensive but suggestions on what the physical, cognitive, or affective skills could be when creating lessons for each concept.

Guiding questions: The essential questions in this guide are written to reflect student-facing language and can be used to prime the curiosity of students to lead them to discovering connections to the big ideas within each unit or concept.

NATIONAL PHYSICAL EDUCATION STANDARDS	
STANDARD 1: DEVELOPS A VARIETY OF MOTOR SKILLS.	**STANDARD 2: APPLIES KNOWLEDGE RELATED TO MOVEMENT AND FITNESS CONCEPTS.**
Through learning experiences in physical education, the student develops motor skills across a variety of environments. Motor skills are a foundational part of child development and support the movements of everyday life. The development of motor skills contributes to an individual's physical literacy journey.	Through learning experiences in physical education, the student uses their knowledge of movement concepts, tactics, and strategies across a variety of environments. This knowledge helps the student become a more versatile and efficient mover. Additionally, the student applies knowledge of health-related and skill-related fitness to enhance their overall well-being. The application of knowledge related to various forms of movement contributes to an individual's physical literacy journey.
STANDARD 3: DEVELOPS SOCIAL SKILLS THROUGH MOVEMENT.	**STANDARD 4: DEVELOPS PERSONAL SKILLS, IDENTIFIES PERSONAL BENEFITS OF MOVEMENT, AND CHOOSES TO ENGAGE IN PHYSICAL ACTIVITY.**
Through learning experiences in physical education, students develop the social skills necessary to exhibit empathy and respect for others, and foster and maintain relationships. In addition, students develop skills for communication, leadership, cultural awareness, and conflict resolution in a variety of physical activity settings.	Through learning experiences in physical education, the student develops an understanding of how movement is personally beneficial and subsequently chooses to participate in physical activities that are personally meaningful (e.g., activities that offer social interaction, cultural connection, exploration, choice, self-expression, appropriate levels of challenge, and added health benefits). The student develops personal skills including goal setting, identifying strengths, and reflection to enhance their physical literacy journey.

GRADES PREK-2					
Time frame	National Physical Education Standards	Instructional focus	Unit or activities	Skills	Guiding questions
August *This instructional focus will be revisited throughout the course.*	Standard 3 3.2.1-3.2.10 Standard 4 4.2.1-4.2.7	Personal and social responsibility	• Routines and rituals • Relationship building • Cooperative activities • Parachute unit • Obstacle course unit	• Understands rules and etiquette • Communicates effectively • Makes safe choices • Respects self, others, and equipment • Receives feedback from teacher • Engages in self-expression and social interaction • Reflects on movement experiences • Uses collaboration and problem-solving skills	1. Why is it important to use rules and safety in the classroom? 2. How can you become a good teammate to others? 3. What does it look or sound like to show respect to others and follow directions?
September	Standard 1 1.2.1, 1.2.4 Standard 2 2.2.1-2.2.3 Standard 4 4.2.4, 4.2.10	Spatial relationships	• Body shapes unit • Obstacle course unit • Animal movements unit • Mirror or Simon says unit • Directional activities • Cross-lateral activities • Tag activities	• Travels with knowledge of personal and general space • Engages in speeds, levels, pathways • Demonstrates beginner locomotor and non-locomotor skills • Engages in chasing and fleeing • Travels under, through, over, next to, or behind objects • Transitions between movements • Identifies preferred activities based on personal interest	1. What is the difference between personal and general space? 2. What does it look like to demonstrate good spacing? 3. How does your body change from when you walk or run?

GRADES PREK-2					
Time frame	National Physical Education Standards	Instructional focus	Unit or activities	Skills	Guiding questions
October	Standard 1 1.2.1-1.2.5 Standard 2 2.2.3 Standard 3 3.2.4 Standard 4 4.2.10	Locomotor and non-locomotor	• Locomotor activities • Non-locomotor activities • Balancing activities • Yoga • Obstacle course unit • Transfer of weight from feet to hands, rolling, jumping, and landing • Twisting and turning activities • Bending and stretching activities	• Balances with body parts and levels • Combines locomotor skills with levels, speeds, and pathways • Identifies movement concepts • Engages in non-locomotor skills: bending, twisting, stretching, swaying, turning • Responds to teacher feedback and direction • Reflects on movement experiences • Focuses on weight transfer skills • Responds to feedback and direction from teacher	1. How are jumping, hopping, and leaping similar or different? 2. What activities require you to quickly change a skill or direction? 3. What activities can you do to bend, twist, stretch, or turn?
October	Standard 1 1.2.1-1.25 Standard 2 2.2.3 Standard 3 3.2.4 Standard 4 4.2.10	Movement competence	• Locomotor activities • Non-locomotor activities • Balancing activities • Yoga • Directional activities • Cross-lateral activities	• Travels forward, backward, and sideways • Changes directions quickly • Balances with body parts and levels • Travels under, through, over, next to, or behind objects • Combines locomotor skills with levels, speeds, and pathways • Demonstrates non-locomotor skills (e.g., bending, twisting, stretching, swaying, turning)	1. How are jumping, hopping, and leaping similar or different? 2. What activities require you to change a skill or direction quickly? 3. What activities can you do to bend, twist, stretch, or turn?

>continued

	National Physical Education Standards	Instructional focus	Unit or activities	Skills	Guiding questions
Time frame					
November and December	Standard 1 *1.2.15, 1.2.16* Standard 2 *2.2.5* Standard 3 *3.2.3* Standard 4 *4.2.1*	Dance and rhythms	• Dance activities • Jumping and landing activities • Jump rope activities • Mirroring activities • Create a small dance sequence • Yoga • Fitness drumming	• Jumps with timing and patterns • Moves the body to music using locomotor skills • Moves in sequence to dance steps • Moves in a variety of rhythms • Demonstrates and identifies locomotor, non-locomotor, and manipulative movement within dance • Uses communication with peers effectively to share space • Identifies activities that support self-expression	1. What movements do you use to jump rope? Please describe. 2. What does it mean to have rhythm? 3. What are some activities outside of school that you can use to work on rhythm?
January	Standard 1 *1.2.6-1.2.9* Standard 2 *2.2.3, 2.2.4* Standard 3 *3.2.2* Standard 4 *4.2.9*	Manipulative Throwing and catching	• Throwing and catching stations • Bouncing and hand dribbling activities • Skill stations • Variable manipulatives (bean bag toss, balloon toss) • Juggling unit • Circus unit • Modified bowling unit	• Bounces and rolls an implement • Demonstrates underhand and overhand throw • Catches an object either self-tossed or from a partner • Dribbles with hands while moving • Demonstrates ability to encourage and work with others • Demonstrates and identifies movement concepts related to locomotor, non-locomotor, and manipulative skills • Demonstrates managing emotion and behavior	1. What are similarities and differences between an overhand and underhand throw? 2. What are some ways that you can dribble a ball with a hand? Please describe to a partner.

GRADES PREK-2					
Time frame	National Physical Education Standards	Instructional focus	Unit or activities	Skills	Guiding questions
February	Standard 1 1.2.12-1.2.14 Standard 2 2.2.3, 2.2.4 Standard 3 3.2.6 Standard 4 4.2.8	Manipulative Striking and volleying	• Striking activities • Volleying activities • Skill combination stations • Modified paddle activities • Hula hoop target unit • Variable manipulatives (balloon volleying, beach ball striking)	• Strikes with hand and short-handled implement • Strikes a ball off of a tee or stand • Demonstrates underhand volley with light object • Demonstrates and identifies movement concepts related to locomotor, non-locomotor, and manipulative skills • Discusses the importance of why following rules can affect safety and fairness	1. What is a good strategy you can use to keep a ball in the air (volley)? 2. What activities use striking? Please describe.
March	Standard 1 1.2.10, 1.2.11 Standard 2 2.2.3, 2.2.4 Standard 3 3.2.8 Standard 4 4.2.7	Manipulative Kicking and dribbling	• Kicking unit • Skill stations • Movement combination unit • Skill refinement activities • Modified target activities • Foot skills unit	• Dribbles with feet while moving • Kicks both a stationary and moving ball toward a target • Demonstrates basic combinations of locomotor, non-locomotor, and manipulative skills • Demonstrates basic understanding of strategy • Recognizes improvement opportunities and strengths in skill • Demonstrates and identifies movement concepts related to locomotor, non-locomotor, and manipulative skills	1. What are some ways that you can dribble a ball with a hand? Please describe to a partner with cues. 2. What movement or activity do you find to be the most difficult? Why? How can you improve? 3. What would be a good strategy for improving your kicking ability?

>continued

GRADES PREK-2   >continued

GRADES PREK-2					
Time frame	National Physical Education Standards	Instructional focus	Unit or activities	Skills	Guiding questions
April and May	Standard 2 2.2.6-2.2.10 Standard 4 4.2.3, 4.2.8	Fitness concepts	• Body awareness and identification • Yoga • Perceived exertion identification • Heart rate identification	• Recognizes personal health and safety practices • Participates in activities that increase heart rate • Identifies heart rate through rest and physical activity • Identifies the body's reaction to moderate to vigorous physical activity • Identifies healthy habits for personal wellness (i.e., movement, stretching, warm-up and cool-down, hydration) • Recognizes that food provides energy • Recognizes activities that enhance fitness levels	1. Why is it important to know about your body? 2. How does your body react to various activities? Why? 3. What are some healthy habits that you can use to feel good about yourself? 4. What are some ways you can continue to move outside of school? What activities would you choose? Why?

	National Physical Education Standards	Instructional focus	Unit or activities	Skills	Guiding questions
Time frame					

GRADES 3-5

Time frame	National Physical Education Standards	Instructional focus	Unit or activities	Skills	Guiding questions
August *This instructional focus will be revisited throughout the course.*	Standard 2 2.5.1, 2.5.5 Standard 3 3.5.2, 3.5.5 Standard 4 4.5.9	Personal and social responsibility	• Routines and rituals • Team building • Cooperative games • Relationship building • Character traits activities • Social and self-awareness activities	• Understands and describes rules and etiquette • Communicates effectively with others • Demonstrates personal responsibility • Receives feedback from teacher and independently uses it to modify behavior or movement concepts • Engages in self-reflection • Identifies problem-solving strategies within an activity • Uses effective communication skills to determine roles and responsibility of self or others • Identifies techniques that assist in managing emotions and behaviors • Engages in self-reflection	1. What does it look or sound like to encourage others in an activity? 2. What impact did showing cooperative traits have on the activity and your group? 3. What are some ways one can resolve a conflict in an activity?
September	Standard 1 1.2.1, 1.2.4 Standard 3 3.5.6 Standard 4 4.5.4, 4.5.10	Locomotor and non-locomotor	• Locomotor activities • Non-locomotor activities • Obstacle course creation unit • Yoga • Cross-lateral activities • Obstacle course unit • Tag activities • Basic dance introduction activities • Circus unit	• Demonstrates locomotor and non-locomotor skills and describes their physical cues to others • Combines movement concepts with connection to speed, direction, and force • Combines and applies movement and space concepts with various motor skills • Gives feedback to peers using basic motor skill cues • Changes directions quickly and with fluidity • Makes fair choices that are related to the etiquette within an activity • Provides rationale for personal choices and interest in physical activity	1. What does it mean to give good feedback to others? Why is it important? 2. What activities include balance, speed, and agility? How are they used in the activity? 3. What would it look like to create an activity with your favorite movements? Describe in detail using locomotor and non-locomotor vocabulary.

>continued

GRADES 3-5   >continued

	National Physical Education Standards	Instructional focus	Unit or activities	Skills	Guiding questions
Time frame					
October and November	Standard 1 1.5.5, 1.5.6 Standard 2 2.5.6 Standard 3 3.5.5, 3.5.7 Standard 4 4.5.1	Dance and rhythms	• Dance activities • Jump rope activities • Group small dance creation task • Yoga vinyasa sequence • Create a gymnastic sequence to music • Fitness drumming • Tinikling	• Performs a jump rope routine with small group or partner • Combines skills to engage in fluid movement to music with rhythmic beat or tempo • Combines locomotor and non-locomotor movement to create short sequential dance steps • Engages in cultural and creative dance sequences with appropriate beat or tempo • Identifies and uses dance-related vocabulary when engaging in dance and rhythm activities • Solves problems independently and with others in a group setting • Explains how or why an activity meets the need for personal self-expression	1. What is the difference between beat and tempo? Please compare and contrast. 2. Why is it important to learn about the cultures of others in dance? 3. How would you create a small dance or gymnastic sequence? Justify the use of a step or move.

December and January	Standard 1
	1.5.9-1.5.16, 1.5.18-1.5.20
	
	Standard 2
	2.5.15, 2.5.16
	
	Standard 3
	3.5.7
	
	Standard 4
	4.5.7
		Manipulative	• Net and wall activities (small sided)
			• Baseball and softball activities (small sided)
			• Spikeball unit
			• Combined skill stations
			  - Throwing
			  - Catching
			  - Striking
			  - Passing
			• Target activities
			  - Bowling
			  - Can/jam
			  - Frisbee golf
			• Foot-based small-sided activities
			  - Soccer
			  - Sepak takraw
			  - Foot tennis
			• Combined skill stations
			  - Dribbling
			  - Kicking
			  - Volleying
			  - Passing
			• Volleying activities (small sided)
				• Throws underhand and overhand for accuracy
				• Catches a thrown object from a partner
				• Strikes with short- and long-handled implements
				• Combines use of skills in various activities and small-sided tasks
				• Dribbles with hands and feet in personal and general space with control and speed changes
				• Passes and receives an object with feet
				• Demonstrates kicking a ball using the instep toward a stationary and moving target
				• Volleys an object both underhand and overhead
				• Serves an object in a non-dynamic setting
				• Combines manipulative skills to execute shots on a target
				• Recognizes skill cues that contribute to proper execution of the skill and opportunity for improvement
				• Identifies physical activity that represents other cultures
					1. Think about your favorite activity in this unit. Can you identify the skill-related components of fitness connected to it?
					2. Define and describe the use of a basic strategy or tactic in an activity. Why did you choose this strategy or tactic?
					3. What does the word accuracy mean? How can we improve accuracy in a task?

	GRADES 3-5				
Time frame	National Physical Education Standards	Instructional focus	Unit or activities	Skills	Guiding questions
February and March	Standard 1 1.5.17-1.5.20 Standard 2 2.5.1-2.5.5, 2.5.15 Standard 3 3.5.5, 3.5.7 Standard 4 4.5.7	Invasion	• Basketball activities (small sided) • Hockey and lacrosse activities (small sided) • Net and wall activities (small sided) • Components of a game • Introductory offensive activities • Introductory defensive activities • Sport-specific skill stations	• Demonstrates basic offensive and defensive strategy within invasion activity • Combines use of manipulative skills in invasion-based small-sided tasks • Uses change of speed, direction, and force to control offensive possession • Displays spatial awareness when defending in small-sided task • Recognizes type of skill or action needed to achieve a task in small-sided activity • Combines skills with passing and receiving while traveling in a small-sided task • Demonstrates and justifies basic use of strategy and tactics in small-sided tasks • Shows respectful behavior to others in a social or group activity • Identifies cues of a skill and how to improve upon that skill	1. Think about your favorite activity in this unit. Can you identify the health-related components of fitness connected to it? How do you know? 2. Describe the use of a strategy or tactic on offense or defense. Why did you choose this strategy or tactic? 3. How does one use the elements of speed, direction, force, and accuracy in invasion activities? How could you modify their use to improve your impact in the activity?
April and May	Standard 2 2.5.7-2.2.14, 2.5.16, 2.5.17 Standard 3 3.5.6 Standard 4 4.5.3, 4.5.6	Fitness concepts	• Body awareness and identification • Yoga • Perceived exertion identification • Heart rate identification • Nutrition concepts	• Identifies, demonstrates, and provides examples of health and skill-related components of fitness • Identifies the FITT principle and how it relates to personal improvement • Locates pulse and measures and records heart rate before, during, and after moderate to vigorous activity • Develops short-term and long-term goals • Identifies and describes the need for warm-up and cool-down movements • Describes importance of hydration and food choice in relation to physical activity and health • Identifies technology tools that enhance personal goal setting • Recognizes the benefit of physical activity and how it influences healthy changes in the body	1. Why is collecting your heart rate important? Compare your heart rate in different activities. 2. What happens to your heart and body when you engage in vigorous activity? 3. Can you identify the health-related component of fitness to the exercise in which you just engaged? What evidence do you have? 4. What impact will making progress toward a goal have on you and others?

GRADES 6-8					
Time frame	National Physical Education Standards	Instructional focus	Unit or activities	Skills	Guiding questions
Weeks 1 and 2 *This instructional focus will be revisited throughout the course.*	Standard 2 2.5.1, 2.5.5 Standard 3 3.5.2, 3.5.5 Standard 4 4.5.9	Personal and social responsibility	• Routines and rituals • Team building • Cooperative games • Relationship building • Reflective journals • Effective feedback activities • Conflict resolution activities • Sportsmanship activities • Goal-setting activities	• Demonstrates encouragement and inclusivity toward others in class setting • Applies rules, etiquette, and safety to physical activity • Explains the value of understanding culture in physical activities • Demonstrates respect for safety, teamwork, and sportsmanship • Provides constructive feedback to peers in cooperative environments • Examines how self-expression affects the desire to engage in physical activity • Uses problem-solving skills independently and with others • Explains how specific skills relate to leadership roles	1. How can one show respect for peers with various abilities? 2. What changes could you make to the activity today to enhance teamwork? 3. How might participating in an activity today affect how you feel emotionally, mentally, and physically? Please describe your reasoning.

Weeks 3 and 4	Standard 1
	1.8.1
	
	Standard 2
	2.8.7, 2.8.21
	
	Standard 3
	3.8.1-3.8.4, 3.8.7-3.8.9
	
	Standard 4
	4.8.2, 4.8.3, 4.8.5
		Outdoor pursuits	• Nature scavenger hunt unit
			• Orienteering
			• Geocaching
			• Outdoor survival skills
			• Outdoor activities
			  - Hiking
			  - Biking
			  - Climbing
				• Applies effective strategy, tactics, and safety practices
				• Identifies personal preference of outdoor activity to engage for a lifetime
				• Uses cooperation and problem solving in personal and group efforts within outdoor pursuits
				• Researches and selects community resources in outdoor pursuits for effective use
				• Demonstrates effective technique in skill while participating in a variety of outdoor activities
				• Demonstrates consideration for others and contributes to group effort
				• Uses effective communication to discuss challenges and problem-solving strategies with others
					1. Reflect on the problem-solving strategies you used today. What worked well, and what could be improved?
					2. How does one balance taking risks and ensuring safety for self or others? Please explain.
					3. What are some ways you can engage in outdoor pursuits after school? Research and provide sources for your response.

	National Physical Education Standards	Instructional focus	Unit or activities	Skills	Guiding questions

Time frame	National Physical Education Standards	Instructional focus	Unit or activities	Skills	Guiding questions
Weeks 5 and 6	Standard 1 1.8.5, 1.8.6 Standard 2 2.8.1, 2.8.18 Standard 3 3.8.3, 3.8.8, 3.8.9 Standard 4 4.8.6, 4.8.7, 4.8.9	Target	• Golf activities • Archery activities • Bowling, bocce, croquet • Frisbee golf • Create a target game • Sport science unit (speed, force, accuracy, trajectory) • Video skill analysis unit • Lawn games unit	• Identifies and analyzes components of a game • Selects variation in speed, force, and trajectory of an object to affect accuracy • Identifies connections of skill-related components of fitness to use in target activities • Demonstrates offensive and defensive skills in target activities • Consistently demonstrates a mature underhand throw and striking pattern in target activities • Analyzes skill performance of self or others and provides useful feedback for improvement • Uses effective communication to discuss tactics, strategies, problem-solving, and etiquette with others	1. What are the components of a game? How can you justify use of such components when creating your own game? 2. What are some modifications you could make to a game or activity to enhance various components of fitness? Justify your prediction. 3. How can one improve their accuracy by using variations in speed, force, or trajectory? Please explain your reasoning.

Weeks 7-9	Standard 1 1.8.14-1.8.19
	
	Standard 2 2.8.2, 2.8.3, 2.8.9, 2.8.18
	
	Standard 3 3.8.2, 3.8.3, 3.8.8
	
	Standard 4 4.8.5
		Invasion	• Ultimate Frisbee
			• Team sports
			  - Basketball
			  - Hockey
			  - Lacrosse
			  - Soccer
			• Skill video analysis unit
			• Sport science unit (speed, force, accuracy, trajectory)
				• Demonstrates and describes how to create open space on offense
				• Reduces open space on defense
				• Dribbles with control using change of speed and direction in small-sided tasks
				• Identifies health and skill-related components of fitness to use in invasion activities
				• Describes cues and demonstrates how to throw a pass to a receiver
				• Describes cues and demonstrates how to shoot with power or accuracy on goal
				• Explains basis for use of various strategies and tactics within small-sided games
				• Uses effective problem-solving and communication skills in group efforts
					1. Evaluate the use of strategies and tactics in invasion activities. What do you notice about their use? Justify your answer.
					2. What skill cues are being used in this activity and in what order? What is the most effective use for improvement? How do you know?
					3. How does one effectively create and reduce space in invasion offensive and defensive scenarios? How do you know?

>continued

GRADES 6-8   >continued

GRADES 6-8					
Time frame	**National Physical Education Standards**	**Instructional focus**	**Unit or activities**	**Skills**	**Guiding questions**

Weeks 10-12	Standard 1 *1.8.6-1.8.9*
	
	Standard 2 *2.8.5, 2.8.6, 2.8.12, 2.8.18*
	
	Standard 3 *3.8.2-3.8.4, 3.8.9*
	
	Standard 4 *4.8.9*
		Striking and fielding	• Sport science unit (speed, force, accuracy, trajectory)
			• Video skill analysis unit
			• Peer teaching unit
			• Fielding activities
			• Baseball and softball activities (small-sided)
			• World/cultural games unit
			  - Cricket
			  - Kilikiti
				• Demonstrates and describes proper cues of throwing and catching
				• Demonstrates striking a ball with an implement to open space
				• Selects variation in speed, force, and trajectory of an object to affect accuracy, distance, and power
				• Demonstrates offensive and defensive skills in striking and fielding activities
				• Identifies connections of skill-related components of fitness to use in striking and fielding activities
				• Implements and provides constructive feedback to and from peers
				• Reflects on movement experiences in physical education
					1. How can one improve their accuracy by using variations in speed, force, or trajectory? Please explain your reasoning.
					2. What skill cues are being used in this activity and in what order? What is the most effective use for improvement? How do you know?
					3. What positive movement experiences have you had during this unit? What aspects of the experience were positive? Why?

Weeks 13 and 14	Standard 1 *1.8.10-1.8.13*
	
	Standard 2 *2.8.4*
	
	Standard 3 *3.8.1-3.8.3*
	
	Standard 4 *4.8.7*
		Net and wall	• Net games
			  - Tennis
			  - Volleyball
			  - Table tennis
			  - Badminton
			• World/cultural games unit
			  - Sepak takraw
			  - Squash
			  - Team handball
			• Skill video analysis unit
			• Sport science unit (speed, force, accuracy, trajectory)
				• Demonstrates and provides rationale for offensive and defensive scheme
				• Chooses various shot selections based on strategy within net and wall activities
				• Demonstrates and describes cues of volleying with effective form and control, overhand striking pattern, forehand and backhand strokes
				• Accepts the differences of others in physical activity
				• Examines barriers to participating in activity outside of school
				• Uses effective communication to discuss tactics and strategies and to contribute positively to the group
					1. How does one effectively defend in net and wall scenarios? How do you know?
					2. What is the importance of various shot selections in offense within net and wall activities? Justify your answer.
					3. Evaluate the use of strategies and tactics in net and wall activities. What do you notice about their use? Justify your answer.
					4. What skill cues are being used in this activity and in what order? What is the most effective use for improvement? How do you know?

				GRADES 6-8		
Time frame	**National Physical Education Standards**	**Instructional focus**	**Unit or activities**	**Skills**	**Guiding questions**	
Weeks 15 and 16	Standard 1 *1.8.2* Standard 2 *2.8.8* Standard 3 *3.8.4, 3.8.5* Standard 4 *4.8.1, 4.8.9*	Dance and rhythms	• Group and individual dance creation task • Yoga • Fitness drumming • Folk, social, creative, world dance activities • Video skill analysis unit	• Demonstrates rhythm and movement patterns in various forms of dance • Creates a dance sequence individually and with a group • Identifies and describes how self-expression affects desire to engage in physical activity • Engages in cultural and creative dance sequences with appropriate beat or tempo • Describes the value of physical activity and culture • Learns and demonstrates a basic 16-count dance sequence • Provides effective feedback to and from others	1. Why is it important to learn various forms of dance? What about dances from other cultures? 2. How does your opportunity to express yourself through movement affect your desire to continue to engage in dance? 3. What dance steps or cues were included in the activity today? Describe and demonstrate with a peer.	
Weeks 17 and 18	Standard 1 *1.8.3, 1.8.4* Standard 2 *2.8.9-2.8.15, 2.8.19, 2.8.20* Standard 3 *3.8.7* Standard 4 *4.8.3, 4.8.6*	Fitness concepts	• Identification • Yoga • Perceived exertion identification • Heart rate identification • Nutrition concepts • Activities with nutrition elements	• Identifies, defines, and describes how to use the principles of exercise (FITT, progression overload, and specificity) for various physical activities • Demonstrates appropriate form in health-related and skill-related fitness activities • Identifies resting, active, and target heart rate • Identifies and applies knowledge of dynamic and static stretching in various activities • Sets and monitors physical activity goals based on personal results • Describes the connections between nutrition, physical activity, and health factors • Compares and contrasts health and skill-related components of fitness within various physical activities • Implements safe behaviors for use of exercise equipment	1. Based on the analysis of fitness data, what types of exercises do you think you should improve upon? Please justify your answer using the FITT principle and health-related components of fitness. 2. What do you notice about your heart rate when participating in cardiovascular endurance and muscular strength activities? Why are they different or similar? 3. What is the relationship between nutrition, physical activity, and the risks associated with one's health? How could this affect you, your family, and your community?	

GRADES 9-12					
Time frame	National Physical Education Standards	Instructional focus	Unit or activities	Skills	Guiding questions
Week 1 *This instructional focus will be revisited throughout the course.	Standard 3 3.12.1-3.12.5, 3.12.7, 3.12.8 Standard 4 4.12.2, 4.12.4, 4.12.6, 4.12.8	Personal and social responsibility	• Routines and rituals • Team building • Cooperative games • Relationship building • Leadership skill-building activities • Peer feedback unit • Conflict resolution activities • Sportsmanship activities • Goal-setting activities • Self-awareness • Social awareness activities • Self-management activities	• Demonstrates awareness, encouragement, and inclusivity toward others in class setting • Demonstrates and evaluates respectful behaviors and communicates effectively with peers • Uses critical thinking skills within individual and group tasks • Applies rules, etiquette, safety, and teamwork to physical activity • Analyzes culture and describes value in relation to various physical activities • Provides constructive feedback to peers in cooperative environments • Examines how self-expression and personal interest affect the desire to engage in physical activity • Applies learned techniques in managing emotions within a physical activity setting	1. How does one display empathy to others? What is an example of using empathy, and how did it affect the scenario? 2. What impact can positive social interactions have on an activity or game? How can one avoid negative interactions? 3. What are some positive aspects of learning about cultures of others and within various physical activities?

Weeks 2 and 3	Standard 1
	1.12.3
	
	Standard 2
	2.12.3,
	2.12.11
	
	Standard 3
	3.12.1-3.12.4,
	3.12.6,
	3.12.7
	
	Standard 4
	4.12.2,
	4.12.3,
	4.12.5,
	4.12.9
		Outdoor pursuits	• Nature scavenger hunt
			• Navigation
			  - Orienteering
			  - Geocaching
			• Canoeing and kayaking
			• Conservation and environmental education
			• Skating and balance
			  - Ice-skating
			  - Snowboarding
			  - Skateboarding
			  - Surfing
			• Outdoor survival skills and first aid
			• Outdoor activities
			  - Hiking
			  - Backpacking
			  - Biking
			  - Climbing
			• Self-reflection portfolio
			• Create outdoor safety public service announcement
				• Demonstrates movement skills in various sports and activities
				• Adapts and applies effective strategy, tactics, and safety practices to real-world scenarios in outdoor pursuits
				• Uses critical thinking skills within individual and group tasks
				• Defends the benefits of a physically active lifestyle relating to outdoor pursuits
				• Analyzes leadership skills and how they apply to participating in a variety of physical activity settings
				• Self-selects physical activity opportunities that are appropriately challenging
				• Plans, executes, and evaluates effective skill technique while participating in a variety of outdoor activities
				• Uses peer and self-evaluation, critique, and analysis of outdoor skills
				• Uses evidence to justify selection of specified equipment, strategies, and tactics in various outdoor scenarios
				• Reflects on experiences in outdoor pursuits
					1. In what ways can our outdoor experiences influence our commitment to environmental conservation? Please justify your answer.
					2. Reflect on the importance of building an inclusive team environment. What elements are included to create this outcome?
					3. How can the mindset of persevering through challenges in outdoor pursuits contribute to your personal success outside of school?
					4. What attributes must one have to be an effective leader? Reflect on a time when you have taken a leadership role. How did you deal with the responsibility?

			GRADES 9-12		
Time frame	**National Physical Education Standards**	**Instructional focus**	**Unit or activities**	**Skills**	**Guiding questions**

Weeks 4 and 5	Standard 1 *1.12.1, 1.12.2*
	
	Standard 2 *2.12.1, 2.12.2, 2.12.12*
	
	Standard 3 *3.12.1-3.12.4*
	
	Standard 4 *4.12.2, 4.12.9*
		Target	• Creates a skill-enhancement plan
			• Target activities
			  - Bowling
			  - Can/jam
			  - Frisbee golf
			• World/cultural games unit
			  - Sepak takraw
			  - Squash
			  - Team handball
			• Strategies and tactics portfolio
			• Create a game
			• Career exploration
			• Sport science unit (speed, force, accuracy, trajectory)
			• Video skill analysis unit
				• Self-selects engagement in activity for enjoyment and lifelong connection
				• Encourages and supports others during engagement in activity
				• Demonstrates movement skills in various sports and activities
				• Analyzes, tests, and hypothesizes the use of strategies and tactics in various physical activities
				• Demonstrates and describes the progressive use of specific cues and technique in manipulative skills
				• Decides when rest is appropriate when planning regular physical activity
				• Reflects on personal experiences in physical education to make connections to how movement is meaningful
					1. Evaluate the technique and skill cues of a peer. What are the steps to understanding and demonstrating a motor skill? What recommendations would you have for improvement?
					2. How do speed, force, trajectory, and accuracy affect specific skills and outcomes in a game or activity? Research and create an improvement plan based on modifications of these elements.

Weeks 6 and 7	Standard 1 *1.12.1*
	
	Standard 2 *2.12.11*
	
	Standard 3 *3.12.2, 3.12.7*
	
	Standard 4 *4.12.2, 4.12.6*
		Invasion	• Sport science unit (speed, force, accuracy, trajectory)
			• Video skill analysis unit
			• Create a skill-enhancement plan
			• Invasion activities
			• World/cultural games unit
			  - Sepak takraw
			  - Squash
			  - Team handball
			• Strategies and tactics portfolio
			• Create a game
			• Career exploration
				• Analyzes, tests, and hypothesizes the use of strategies and tactics in various physical activities
				• Critiques and demonstrates various uses of offensive and defensive strategy and how to create and reduce open space in various activities
				• Analyzes heart rate and fitness data while participating in invasion activities
				• Demonstrates movement skills in various sports and activities
				• Describes the benefits of a physically active lifestyle
				• Uses critical thinking skills within individual and group tasks
				• Develops a movement- or skill-focused goal related to an activity that is personally interesting
				• Displays proper etiquette and respect for others while engaging in physical activity
					1. Analyze the use of specific strategies or tactics in an activity. What are effective and ineffective ways they can be used? Create a playbook.
					2. How do speed, force, trajectory, and accuracy affect specific skills and outcomes in a game or activity? Research and create an improvement plan based on modifications of these elements.
					3. Critique the use of offensive and defensive spacing in an activity. What elements and moves are effective in the use of spacing? How do you know?

>continued

GRADES 9-12   >continued

	GRADES 9-12				
Time frame	National Physical Education Standards	Instructional focus	Unit or activities	Skills	Guiding questions

Weeks 7 and 8	Standard 1 *1.12.1*
	
	Standard 2 *2.12.6, 2.12.13*
	
	Standard 3 *3.12.1, 3.12.6, 3.12.7*
	
	Standard 4 *4.12.5*
		Striking and fielding	• Sport science unit (speed, force, accuracy, trajectory)
			• Video skill analysis unit
			• Create a skill-enhancement plan
			• World/cultural games unit
			  - Sepak takraw
			  - Squash
			  - Team handball
			• Strategies and tactics portfolio
			• Create a game
			• Career exploration
				• Demonstrates and describes the progressive use of specific cues and technique in manipulative skills
				• Evaluates technique and skill cues of a specific skill and provides feedback to a peer for improvement
				• Demonstrates movement skills in various sports and activities
				• Creates a practice plan with a focus on improvement of a self-selected skill
				• Uses critical thinking skills within individual and group tasks
				• Self-selects physical activity opportunities that are appropriately challenging
					1. Evaluate the technique and skill cues of a peer. What are the steps to understanding and demonstrating a motor skill? What recommendations would you have for improvement?
					2. How do speed, force, trajectory, and accuracy affect specific skills and outcomes in a game or activity? Research and create an improvement plan based on modifications of these elements.
					3. Why is it important to challenge yourself when engaging in physical activity? Please explain your answer.

Weeks 9 and 10	Standard 1 *1.12.1*
	
	Standard 2 *2.12.6, 2.12.13*
	
	Standard 3 *3.12.1, 3.12.3, 3.12.6, 3.12.7*
	
	Standard 4 *4.12.2, 4.12.6*
		Net and wall	• Net games
			  - Tennis
			  - Volleyball
			  - Table tennis
			  - Badminton
			• World/cultural games unit
			  - Sepak takraw
			  - Squash
			  - Team handball
			• Create a skill-enhancement plan
			• Strategies and tactics portfolio
			• Video skill analysis unit
			• Sport science unit (speed, force, accuracy, trajectory)
				• Analyzes components of a game and creates a game that can be played a real-life scenario
				• Explains and demonstrates how to use and enhance various physical skills and how they transfer from one activity to another
				• Uses critical thinking skills within individual and group tasks
				• Demonstrates movement skills in various sports and activities
				• Demonstrates awareness, encouragement, and inclusivity toward others in class setting
				• Sets and develops goals related to personal development and interest
					1. What are the essential skills of a specific net or wall activity? How can those skills transfer to another activity? To what activities do they transfer?
					2. What are the components of one game? How can you justify use of such components when creating your own net and wall game?
					3. Why are strategies relating to shot selection so important in net and wall activities? Analyze net and wall game videos and explain the use of specific strategies.

GRADES 9-12

Time frame	National Physical Education Standards	Instructional focus	Unit or activities	Skills	Guiding questions
Weeks 11 and 12	Standard 1 *1.12.4* Standard 2 *2.12.4* Standard 3 *3.12.3-3.12.5* Standard 4 *4.12.1, 4.12.3, 4.12.4*	Dance and rhythms	• Group and individual dance creation task • Yoga • Fitness drumming • Social, cultural, and relevant dance activities • Skill video analysis unit • Elements of dance unit	• Creates a dance sequence and justifies use of various elements of dance and self-expression within the routine • Demonstrates, describes, and justifies the progressive use of specific cues and technique in various forms of dance • Researches and recommends community resources that focus on dance and rhythm activities for future use in the real world • Investigates and describes the historical and cultural roles of various dance forms in society • Demonstrates fluid skills and appropriate cues in various social and cultural dance forms • Selects specific activities that meet the need for self-expression	1. What do you notice about the similarities and differences in various dance types? What are the historical and cultural implications of these dances in society? 2. Why is creative expression important? What feelings, physical responses, and emotions do you experience after expressing yourself through dance? 3. What would you consider to be an effective practice in improving your own skill set in dance? How does feedback from others affect that process?

Weeks 13 and 14	Standard 1 *1.12.9*
	
	Standard 2 *2.12.5, 2.12.6, 2.12.11, 2.12.17*
	
	Standard 3 *3.12.4, 3.12.6, 3.12.7*
	
	Standard 4 *4.12.3, 4.12.5, 4.12.9*
		Aquatics	• Basic and intermediate swim skills unit
			• Lifeguard training unit
			• CPR training unit
			• Aquatic activity unit
			  - Water polo
			  - Swimming
			  - Diving
			• Create aquatic aerobics routine
			• Career exploration
			• Create water safety PSA
			• Skill video analysis unit
				• Identifies and analyzes the components and use of aerobic and anaerobic activities and their health benefit
				• Demonstrates and describes the progressive use of specific cues and technique in various aquatic skills
				• Critiques, demonstrates, and recommends aquatic activities that enhance physical health and wellness and the reaction of the body to those activities
				• Researches various life-saving skills and recommends actionable tactics based on data from multiple cited sources
				• Demonstrates and justifies the use of specific life-saving skills based on real-life scenarios
					1. What are the fundamental cues associated with various basic swimming strokes? How are they similar or different?
					2. What are the ways that aquatic exercise can contribute to overall fitness and wellness? What types of health-related fitness components can be targeted during swimming? Justify your answer.
					3. What are the essential elements of water rescue and CPR techniques? How will you know when to use life-saving procedures? Research and cite your answer.

>continued

GRADES 9-12   *>continued*

			GRADES 9-12		
Time frame	National Physical Education Standards	Instructional focus	Unit or activities	Skills	Guiding questions
Weeks 15 and 16	Standard 1 *1.12.5-1.12.8* Standard 2 *2.12.5-2.12.10, 2.12.16* Standard 3 *3.12.6* Standard 4 *4.12.3, 4.12.6, 4.12.7*	Fitness concepts	• Anatomy unit • Heart rate identification • Nutrition concepts • Heart rate monitoring unit • Fitness for enjoyment unit • Fitness science lab unit • Personal fitness plan • Career exploration • Yoga and Pilates unit • Strength and body resistance training unit • Mindfulness and stress reduction • Dimensions of wellness • Personal training scenario unit • Skill video analysis unit	• Demonstrates appropriate technique in cardiovascular, muscular strength, endurance, and flexibility training • Identifies healthy food choices and their relationship to performance and recovery • Applies best practice in injury prevention and safety • Sets and develops goals related to personal development and interest • Identifies, researches, and creates a plan for healthy habits and lifetime activity in community and at home • Records resting, active, and target heart rate within activity and interprets how to use it to enhance health-related fitness outcomes • Participates in health-enhancing physical activity • Identifies the components of principles of exercise and applies to a fitness plan • Creates, analyzes, and monitors a personal fitness plan that applies knowledge of aerobic, strength and endurance, and flexibility exercises	1. Document and determine the use of specific exercises to develop specific muscle groups. What type of strength exercises would you use to enhance fitness development? 2. When one experiences a plateau in their fitness plan's results, what changes could be made to continue improvement? How could you use the principles of exercise to determine the answer? 3. Create a personalized fitness plan for self or a peer using all learned aspects of fitness and wellness. What would you include? How can you determine it will be effective?

GRADES 9-12					
Time frame	National Physical Education Standards	Instructional focus	Unit or activities	Skills	Guiding questions
Weeks 17 and 18	Standard 1 *1.12.1, 1.12.2* Standard 2 *2.12.11-2.12.14* Standard 3 *3.12.5* Standard 4 *4.12.1, 4.12.2, 4.12.9*	Lifetime activities	• Martial arts • Cycling • Basic swimming skills unit • Yoga and Pilates unit • Tai chi • Social dancing • Golf • Walking or jogging • Career exploration • Holistic wellness practices	• Applies movement principles to improve performance of self or others • Discusses the historical and cultural contexts in games, sport, and society • Reflects on movement experiences that can be personally meaningful and also meet the need for self-expression • Researches and plans use of resources for choice of lifetime activities outside of school • Researches and explains the health implications of participating in lifetime activities throughout adulthood • Analyzes heart rate and fitness data while participating in lifetime activity	1. What are the health benefits of engaging in a lifetime activity as an adult? What are ways you can overcome barriers to participation? Research and cite your answer. 2. Trace the historical and societal evolution of martial arts. What did you learn about the journey of this activity? Research and cite your evidence. 3. What are some lifetime activities and holistic wellness practices that you can engage in outside of school? Create a plan for the future.

accommodation—Adapting responses to new information.

adaptation—Includes both accommodation (adapting responses to new information) and assimilation (interpreting new information within present cognitive structures).

adapted physical education—Specially designed instruction in physical education that has been adapted or modified so that it is as appropriate for the person with a disability as it is for a person without a disability (NCPEID, 2022).

affective domain—The affective domain is one of the three domains in Bloom's Taxonomy. It involves feelings, attitudes, and emotions. It includes the ways in which people deal with external and internal phenomena emotionally, such as values, enthusiasms, and motivations.

age-related, not age-dependent—Motor skill development is related to a child's age but is not dependent on their age. For example, seven-year-olds are not all at the same stage of motor development.

application stage—Form, precision, accuracy, and standards of good performance are especially important to the learner at the application stage. Therefore, the child practices more complex skills, and strategies and rules take on greater importance. Children at the application stage have begun to select types of sports that they prefer. This stage spans approximately from ages 11 to 13.

assimilation—Interpreting new information within present cognitive structures.

augmented feedback—Information that comes from a source other than the performer (e.g., teacher, heart rate monitor, time-delayed video feedback).

body-scaled—Equipment that has been modified (e.g., size, weight, length, texture) and task requirements whose conditions within the environment have been varied (i.e., spatial, temporal, relationships).

closed skills—Skills that take place in a stable, predictable environment in which objects or events are stationary.

cognitive domain—How students acquire, process, and use knowledge.

competence motivation— Represents the fundamental desire of humans to be competent (i.e., successful and skillful).

concrete operations stage—A stage of cognitive development in which thinking is logical; however, it is still dependent on events that are personally experienced, seen, or heard. Children are also less egocentric and realize that they must learn to consider the perspective of others if they want to be understood.

conserve—The awareness that physical quantities do not change in amount when they are altered in appearance.

constant practice—Repeating a skill using the same movement characteristics (i.e., spatial, temporal, and relationship variables).

critical elements—The biomechanical features of motor skills that lead to efficient performance. Typically organized by preparation, execution or force phase, and follow-through or recovery.

dance and rhythmic activities—Activities that focus on dance or rhythms. Dance and rhythmic activities might include but are not limited to dance forms such as creative movement or dance, ballet, modern, ethnic or folk, hip-hop, Latin, line, ballroom, social and square, and jumping rope.

demonstrate—An act of showing someone how to use or perform something.

descriptive feedback—Information provided by physical educators that verbally describes what students did correctly (e.g., "Great job; you stepped with your opposite foot during your throw").

developmental milestone theory—A conceptual framework describing the characteristics of learners over time.

differentiated instruction—Tailoring instruction to meet the needs of the student. Teachers can modify the content (i.e., what the student needs to learn), the process (i.e., activities in which the student engages to learn the content), and the learning environment.

dynamic environment—An environment with unanticipated variables; an environment in which objects, people, and events are changing and unpredictable.

egocentric—Children are unable to view the world from a perspective other than their own.

emerging elementary stage—Performers in this stage gain greater control of their movements but still appear somewhat awkward and lacking in fluidity. During this period the increases in strength with growth and gradual lengthening of the trunk and limbs allow moderate ranges of flexion, extension, and rotation, although short, stubby fingers still hamper object handling.

feedback—Information performers receive about their movement responses.

fitness activities—Activities with a focus on improving or maintaining fitness. Fitness activities might include but are not limited to yoga, Pilates, resistance training, spinning, running, fitness walking, fitness swimming, kickboxing, cardio-kick, Zumba, and exergaming.

formal operations stage—A stage of cognitive development in which children are able to systematically look at possible solutions to a problem and, through rational and abstract reasoning, choose the best solutions for the problem. Prediction and planning are also characteristic of the formal operational thinker.

fundamental movement phase—A period of time characterized by a remarkable change in children's abilities to perform the fundamental stability (non-locomotor), locomotor, and manipulative motor skills. Children begin unable to produce the ranges of motion, balance, and speed to perform the fundamental movement skills and end with the potential for producing biomechanically efficient movement patterns for running, skipping, rolling, kicking, catching, and so on. This metamorphosis between the ages of two and seven is based in part on maturation of the neuromuscular system and changes in body proportion brought about through growth.

generalized motor program—A representation of a pattern of movements that is modifiable to produce a movement outcome. A generalized motor program can be thought of as a set of instructions stored in the brain. When we perform a particular skill, we retrieve this set of instructions, sending the message to the appropriate muscles. The time needed to organize a motor program depends on the complexity of the task; more complex tasks require more time to organize than less complex tasks do.

Grade-Span Learning Indicators—The indicators unpack the standard statement and articulate the specific content areas within that standard.

growth-oriented feedback—Feedback focused on the process of developing skills that emphasizes effort and motivates individuals to persist when learning.

Hourglass Model—A heuristic for conceptualizing, describing, and explaining the process of motor development.

identity versus role confusion stage—Younger adolescents begin to develop more masculine or feminine identity as they experience rapid changes in physical and sexual maturation. Additionally, perceived peer acceptance and rejection starts to take a significant precedence.

individualized education program (IEP)—A written statement of the educational program designed to meet a child's individual needs (CPIR, 2022).

industry versus inferiority stage—The stage of psychosocial development attributed to children ages 6 to 12 years. During this stage of development, children are learning to relate to others. Through social interactions, children begin to develop a sense of pride in their accomplishments and abilities.

intimacy versus isolation stage—Healthy and intimate relationships begin to outweigh or supersede other social factors. This stage is marked by one's ability to accept the identity established in the previous stages of development and begin to accept and synthesize the identities formed by others with their own.

intrinsic feedback—Information that comes from the performer's senses (i.e., proprioceptors).

knowledge of performance (KP)—Augmented feedback about the process or movement characteristics of the performance, including information about the location, speed, direction, or coordination of body actions.

knowledge of results (KR)—Either intrinsic or augmented feedback about the outcome or end results of the movement performance.

Learning Progressions—Sequential learning tasks that address a range of skill abilities within each grade span.

lifelong utilization stage—The final stage within the specialized movement phase begins at age 14 and continues throughout adolescence and into adulthood. At this stage, individuals are encouraged to select activities they particularly enjoy and can pursue throughout their lifetime for fun, fitness, and fulfillment. High interest in specific activities is evidenced through active participation on a regular basis, whether on a performance, competitive, or recreational level.

mature stage—The mature stage is characterized by progress in gaining a well-coordinated and biomechanically efficient movement performance. By six years of age, children can move through full ranges of flexion, extension, and rotation because their body proportions are more similar to adults.

meaningful physical education—Meaningful physical education (MPE) includes an emphasis on democratic (e.g., providing autonomy support; involving students in decision making) and reflective pedagogies (e.g., goal-setting and verbal and written reflection) and highlights the value of six provisional features of meaningfulness (social interaction, fun, challenge, motor competence, personally relevant learning, and delight) (Beni, Fletcher, & Chróinín, 2022, p. 570).

non-dynamic environment—A stable, predictable environment in which objects or events are stationary.

open skills—An environment in which there are unanticipated variables; an environment in which objects, people, and events are changing and unpredictable.

outcome goals—Address the product of the movement and focus on end results such as how high, how far, how accurate, or how fast.

outdoor pursuit activities—The outdoor environment is an important factor in student engagement in activity. Outdoor pursuits might include but are not limited to recreational boating (e.g., kayaking, canoeing, sailing, rowing), hiking, backpacking, fishing, orienteering or geocaching, ice skating, skateboarding, snow or water skiing, snowboarding, snowshoeing, surfing, bouldering, traversing or climbing, mountain biking, adventure activities, and ropes courses. The selection of activities depends on the environmental opportunities within the geographical region.

physical literacy journey—The physical literacy journey involves the ongoing acquisition and application of knowledge, skills, and dispositions necessary for engagement in a lifetime of healthful and meaningful physical activity.

present level of academic achievement and functional performance (PLAAFP)—A part of an IEP that summarizes "how the child's disability affects the child's involvement and progress in the general education curriculum (i.e., the same curriculum as for nondisabled children)" (IDEA, 2017). It is "objective data that describe what [a] child knows and is able to do. They describe [a] child's strengths, challenges, and needs. The present levels include baseline data" (Wrightslaw, 2024).

practice—To perform a skill regularly or repeatedly in order to become better at it.

prescriptive feedback—Information provided to the performer that focuses on what performers specifically need to do to correct their movements.

pre-operational stage—"The child uses elementary logic and reasoning as they learn to use past experiences and the beginning use of symbols to represent objects in their environment. This process leads to oral communication" (Nichols, 1994, p. 23).

process goals—Address the pattern of the movement and focus on biomechanical efficiency of the critical elements of the skill.

psychomotor domain—Physical movement and use of motor skills.

relationship awareness—Involves the ability to establish and maintain healthy and supportive relationships and to effectively navigate settings with diverse individuals and groups (CASEL, 2023).

responsible decision-making—The ability to make caring and constructive choices about one's personal behavior and social interactions across diverse situations.

self-awareness—Defined as the ability to understand one's own emotions, thoughts, and values and how they influence behavior across contexts.

self-determination—A theory postulating that humans have basic needs to feel competent, autonomous, and connected with other people (i.e., relatedness).

self-efficacy—An individual's confidence in their ability to be physically active in a given physical activity situation.

self-expression—Expressing one's thoughts and feelings through words, choices, or actions; self-expression can be related to one's creativity, identity, and culture.

self-management—Defined as the ability to manage one's emotions, thoughts, and behaviors effectively in different situations and to achieve goals and aspirations (CASEL, 2023).

short-term goals—Observable goals that can be achieved over a brief period of time (e.g., during a physical education class or within a few days).

social awareness—Involves the ability to understand the perspectives of and empathize with others, including those from diverse backgrounds, cultures, and contexts (CASEL, 2023).

social competence—Involves both social awareness and relationship awareness.

social domain—The domain of learning that involves the ability to interact with others.

specialized movement phase—The period of motor development beginning around age seven and lasting through adolescence and beyond. During this time children progress from performing stability, locomotor, and manipulative skills in the fundamental phase to performing corresponding combinations of motor skills within culturally appropriate movement activities in the specialized phase.

specialized movement skills—Combination motor skills used in specific movement forms (e.g., basketball or tennis).

transition stage—The transition stage of specialized movement skill development occurs from about age 7 to about age 10. During this period of prepubescence, children's slow and steady growth gives them a chance to get used to their more adult-like body proportions, and the completion of myelination affords increased complexity in movement skills. These changes pave the way for children to transition from biomechanically efficient performance of the fundamental motor skills to the corresponding specialized skills in cultural games, sports, and dances.

variable practice—Practice that includes variations of the skill itself or the context of the skill in variable order such as varying an underhand toss to targets at different levels, distances, or directions. The parameters (i.e., space, temporal, relationship parameters) of skill practice are changed.

REFERENCES

Azzarito, L., & Ennis, C.D. (2003). A sense of connection: Toward social constructivist physical education. *Sport, Education and Society, 8*(2), 179-197.

Bailey, R., Armour, K., Kirk, D., Jess, M., Pickup, I., Sandford, R., & Education, B.P. (2009). The educational benefits claimed for physical education and school sport: An academic review. *Research Papers in Education, 24*(1), 1-27.

Bandura, A. (1997). *Self-efficacy: The exercise of control.* W H Freeman/Times Books/Henry Holt.

Beach, P., Perreault, M., Brian, A., & Collier, D. (2024). *Motor development and learning* (3rd ed.). Human Kinetics.

Beni, S., Fletcher, T., & Chróinín, D.N. (2019). Using features of meaningful experiences to guide primary physical education practice. *European Physical Education Review, 25*(3), 599-615.

Beni, S., Fletcher, T., & Chróinín, D. (2022). Teachers' engagement with professional development to support implementation of meaningful physical education. *Journal of Teaching in Physical Education, 2022*(41), 570-579.

Bishop, P.A., Downes, J.M., & Farber, K. (2019). *Personalized learning in the middle grades: A guide for classroom teachers and school leaders.* Harvard Education Press.

Braga, L., Elliott, E., Jones, E., & Bulger, S. (2015). Middle school students' perceptions of culturally and geographically relevant content in physical education. *International Journal of Kinesiology and Sports Science, 3*(4), 62-73.

Brinegar, K., & Caskey, M. (2022). *Developmental characteristics of young adolescents: Research summary.* Association for Middle Level Education. www.amle.org/developmental-characteristics-of-young-adolescents

CASEL. (2023, August 10). *Advancing social and emotional learning.* CASEL. https://casel.org/

CAST. (2018). *Universal Design for Learning Guidelines version 2.2.* http://udlguidelines.cast.org

Castelli, D.M., Barcelona, J.M., & Bryant, L. (2015). Contextualizing physical literacy in the school environment: The challenges. *Journal of Sport and Health Science, 4*(2), 156-163.

Chen, W., Zhu, W., Mason, S., Hammond-Bennett, A., & Colombo-Dougovito, A. (2016). Effectiveness of quality physical education in improving students' manipulative skill competency. *Journal of Sport and Health Science, 5*(2), 231-238.

Cleland Donnelly, F. (2021). Meaningful physical education. *SHAPE PA Journal,* Spring Issue 2.

Cleland Donnelly, F., Mueller, S., & Gallahue, D. (2017). *Developmental physical education for all children—Theory into practice* (5th ed.). Human Kinetics.

Coker, C. (2004). *Motor learning and control for practitioners.* McGraw-Hill.

CPIR. (2022, April). *The short-and-sweet IEP overview.* CPIR. https://parentcenterhub.org/iep-overview/

Dettmer, P. (2005). New blooms in established fields: Four domains of learning and doing. *Roeper Review, 28*(2), 70-78.

Dismore, H., & Bailey, R. (2011). Fun and enjoyment in physical education: Young people's attitudes. *Research papers in education*, *26*(4), 499-516.

Dyson, B.P. (1995). Students' voices in two alternative elementary physical education programs. *Journal of teaching in physical education*, *14*(4), 394-407.

Ennis, C.D. (2017). Educating students for a lifetime of physical activity: Enhancing mindfulness, motivation, and meaning. *Research Quarterly for Exercise and Sport, 88*(3), 241-250.

Enright, E., & O'Sullivan, M. (2010). Carving a new order of experience with young people in physical education. In M. O'Sullivan & A. MacPhail (Eds.), *Young people's voices in physical education and youth sport* (pp. 163-180). Routledge.

Erikson, E.H. (1963). *Youth: Change and challenge*. Basic Books.

Erikson, E.H. (1968). *Identity: youth and crisis*. W. W. Norton & Company, Inc.

Erikson, E.H. (1980). *Identity and the life cycle*. W. W. Norton & Company, Inc.

Estevan, I., Bardid, F., Utesch, T., Menescardi, C., Barnett, L.M., & Castillo, I. (2021). Examining early adolescents' motivation for physical education: Associations with actual and perceived motor competence. *Physical Education and Sport Pedagogy, 26*(4), 359-374.

Farrey, T., & Isard, R. (2015). *Physical literacy in the United States: A model, strategic plan, and call to action*. The Aspen Institute.

Fletcher, T., Chróinín, D.N., Gleddie, D., & Beni, S. (2021). The why, what, and how of Meaningful Physical Education. In S. Beni, D. N. Chróinín, D. Gleddie, and T. Fletcher (Eds.), *Meaningful physical education: An approach for teaching and learning* (pp. 3-19). Routledge.

Fronske, H., & Wilson, R., (2002). *Teaching cues for fundamental sport skills and activities for elementary and middle school*. Benjamin Cummings.

Gleddie, D., & Harding-Kuriger, J. (2021 July 3). Meaningful development of professionals. Lampe. https://meaningfulpe.wordpress.com/2021/07/21/meaningful-development-of-professionals-doug-gleddie-jodi-harding-kuriger

Goodway, J.D., Crowe, H., & Ward, P. (2003). Effects of motor skill instruction on fundamental motor skill development. *Adapted physical activity quarterly, 20*(3), 298-314.

Goodway. J., Ozmun, J., & Gallahue, D. (2021). *Understanding motor development: Infants, children, adolescents, adults*. Jones & Bartlett Learning.

Harrison, L.M., Brinegar, K.M., & Hurd, E. (2019). Exploring the convergence of developmentalism and cultural responsiveness. In K.M. Brinegar, L.M. Harrison, & E. Hurd (Eds.), *Equity and cultural responsiveness in the middle grades* (pp. 3-21). Information Age.

Harter, S. (1999). *The construction of self: A developmental perspective*. Guilford.

Hopple, C.J. (2018). Top 10 reasons why children find physical activity to be "unfun." *Strategies, 31*(3), 32-39.

Houser, N., & Kriellaars, D. (2023). "Where was this when I was in physical education?" Physical literacy enriched pedagogy in a quality physical education context. *Frontiers in Sports and Active Living, 5*, 1185680.

IDEA. (2017, July 12). Sec. 300.320 (a) (1). IDEA. https://sites.ed.gov/idea/regs/b/d/300.320/a/1

Kober, N., & Rentner, D.S. (2020). History and evolution of public education in the US. *Center on Education Policy*.

Kretchmar, R.S. (2006). Ten more reasons for quality physical education. *Journal of Physical Education, Recreation and Dance, 77*(9), 6-8.

Ladwig, M.A., Vazou, S., & Ekkekakis, P. (2018). "My best memory is when I was done with it": PE memories are associated with adult sedentary behavior. *Translational Journal of the American College of Sports Medicine, 3*(16), 119-129.

Logan, S., Webster, E.K., Getchell, N., Pfeiffer, K., & Robinson, L. (2015). Relationship between fundamental motor skill competence and physical activity during childhood & adolescence: A systematic review. *Kinesiology Review, 4*(4), 418-426.

Lubans, D.R., Morgan, P.J., Cliff, D.P., Barnett, L.M., & Okely, A.D. (2010). Fundamental movement skills in children and adolescents. *Sports Med, 40*, 1019–1035. https://doi.org/10.2165/11536850-000000000-00000

Lynch, S., & Sargent, J. (2020) Using the meaningful physical education features as a lens to view student experiences of democratic pedagogy in higher education. *Physical Education and Sport Pedagogy, 25*(6), 629-642. https://doi.org/10.1080/17408989.2020.1779684

Lyngstad, I., Bjerke, Ø., & Lagestad, P. (2020). Students' views on the purpose of physical education in upper secondary school. Physical education as a break in everyday school life—Learning or just fun? *Sport, Education and Society, 25*(2), 230-241.

McCarthy, K., Brady, M., & Hallman, K. (2016). *Investing when it counts: Reviewing the evidence and charting a course of research and action for very young adolescents.* Population Council. www.popcouncil.org/uploads/pdfs/2016PGY_InvestingWhenItCounts.pdf

Mercier, R., & Hutchinson, G. (2003). Social psychology. In B. Mohnsen (Ed.), *Concepts and principles of physical education: What every student should know* (2nd ed., pp. 245-307). National Association for Sport and Physical Education.

Mosston, M., & Ashworth, S. (2008). *Teaching physical education.* Spectrum Institute for Teaching and Learning. https://spectrumofteachingstyles.org/index.php?id=16

NCPEID. (2022). *The national consortium for physical education for individuals with disabilities.* NCPEID. https://ncpeid.org/

Nichols, B. (1994). *Moving and learning: The elementary school physical education experience* (3rd ed.). Mosby.

Chróinín, D.N., Fletcher, T., Beni, S., Griffin, C., & Coulter, M. (2023). Children's experiences of pedagogies that prioritise meaningfulness in primary physical education in Ireland. *Education 3-13, 51*(1), 41-54.

Patton, G.C., Sawyer, S.M., Santelli, J.S., Ross, D.A., Afifi, R., Allen, N.B., Arora, M., Azzopardi, P., Baldwin, W., Bonell, C., Kakuma, R., Kennedy, E., Mahon, J., McGovern, T., Mokdad, A.H., Patel, V., Petroni, S., Reavley, N., Taiwo, K., . . . Viner, R.M. (2016). Our future: A Lancet commission on adolescent health and wellbeing. *The Lancet, 387*(10036), 2423-2478. https://doi.org/10.1016/S0140-6736(16)00579-1

Piaget, J. (1952). *The origins of intelligence in children.* (M. Cook, Trans.). W. W. Norton & Company, Inc. https://doi.org/10.1037/11494-000

Piaget, J. (1954). *The construction of reality in the child.* (M. Cook, Trans.). Basic Books. https://doi.org/10.1037/11168-000

Piaget, J. (1974). *The origins of intelligence in children.* International Universities Press.

Piaget, J., Inhelder, B., & Weaver, H. (1969). *The psychology of the child.* Basic Books.

Rink, J.E. (2004). It's okay to be a beginner. *Journal of Physical Education, Recreation & Dance, 75*, 31-34.

Ryan, R.M., & Deci, E.L. (2000). Intrinsic and extrinsic motivations: Classic definitions and new directions. *Contemporary Educational Psychology, 25*(1), 54-67.

Scales, P.C. (2010). Characteristics of young adolescents. In *This we believe: Keys to educating young adolescents* (pp. 63-62). National Middle School Association.

SHAPE America. (2014). *National standards & grade-level outcomes for K-12 physical education.* Human Kinetics.

Smart, J. (2019). *Disability across the developmental lifespan: An introduction for the helping professions.* Springer.

Snowman, J., & McCown, R. (2014). *Psychology applied to teaching*. Cengage Learning.

Stodden, D., Langendorfer, S., & Roberton, M.A. (2009). The association between motor skill competence and physical fitness in young adults. *Research Quarterly for Exercise and Sport, 80*(2), 223-229. https://doi.org/10.1080/02701367.2009.10599556

Teixeira, P.J., Carraça, E.V., Markland, D., Silva, M.N., & Ryan, R.M. (2012). Exercise, physical activity, and self-determination theory: A systematic review. *International Journal of Behavioral Nutrition and Physical Activity, 9*, 78-107. https://doi.org/10.1186/1479-5868-9-78

Walseth, K., Engebretsen, B., & Elvebakk, L. (2018). Meaningful experiences in PE for all students: An activist research approach. *Physical Education and Sport Pedagogy, 23*(3), 235-249.

Wood, C.L., Lane, L.C., & Cheetham, T. (2019). Puberty: Normal physiology (brief overview). *Best Practice & Research Clinical Endocrinology & Metabolism, 33*(3), 101265.

Wrightslaw. (2024). *Developing your child's IEP present levels, goals & services, accommodations*. Wrightslaw. https://wrightslaw.com/info/iep.develop.popup.resp1.htm

Young, D., LaCourse, M. & Husak, W. (2000). *A practical guide to motor learning* (2nd ed.). Eddie Bowers Publishing.

Zittel, L.L., & Houston-Wilson, C. (2000). Early childhood adapted physical education. In J.P. Winnick (Ed.), *Adapted physical activity and sport* (3rd ed., pp. 303-314). Human Kinetics.

PHOTO CREDITS

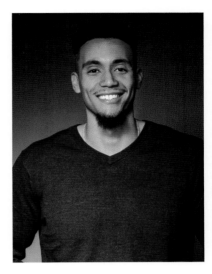

Cory Dixon, PhD, is an assistant professor in the department of content area teacher education. His current research foci are centered on the educator preparation of physical education students at predominantly white institutions (PWIs) and the racialized experiences of students and faculty of color in higher education. He seeks to advocate for equitable educational opportunities for all by critically examining higher education, physical education pedagogy, and teacher preparation, in addition to better understanding the recruitment, retention, and experiences of faculty and students of color in higher education. Dixon's research has been presented and published at various national and international conferences and in leading academic journals.

Dixon earned his PhD and MEd in kinesiology and physical education teacher education from Auburn University. He holds a bachelor's degree in kinesiology, sports studies, and physical education from Morehouse College, a historically Black college in Atlanta, Georgia.

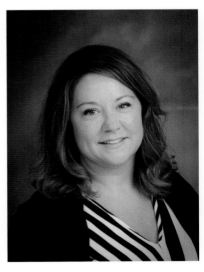

Suzanna Dillon, PhD, CAPE, is a professor of kinesiology at Texas Woman's University (TWU). Dillon has over 20 years of experience in teaching, researching, and mentoring in the fields of physical education, adapted physical education, adapted physical activity, and special education. At both TWU and Wayne State University, she has been awarded U.S. Department of Education grants, through which she conducts interdisciplinary personnel preparation and collaborative physical activity interventions for children and young adults with disabilities. Dillon is passionate about preparing future educators and physical activity professionals so that they are prepared to deliver interdisciplinary services to people with disabilities and are skilled in advocating for equitable physical activity opportunities within their communities. Through her grants and service on various boards, committees, and professional associations, particularly the National Consortium for Physical Education for Individuals With Disabilities, she aims to leverage her years of experience and content expertise to advance the field of adapted physical activity and make an impact within her local community and beyond.

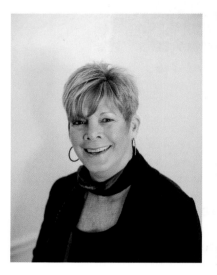

Fran Cleland, PED, is a professor emeritus of health and physical education within the College of Health Sciences at West Chester University (WCU) in West Chester, Pennsylvania. Cleland taught for 28 years at WCU, where she also served as assistant chair of the Health and Physical Education Teacher Certification Program. She earned her bachelor of science degree in health and physical education at Purdue University and her doctoral degree in motor development, child development, and adapted physical education at Indiana University in Bloomington, Indiana.

Prior to her years at WCU, Cleland taught at the University of New Hampshire and East Stroudsburg University in Pennsylvania, after beginning her career as a K-12 health and physical education teacher. She has served at the state, district, and national levels, including as SHAPE PA president (2009) and SHAPE America president (2017-2018). She is the lead author of *Developmental Physical Education for All Children: Theory Into Practice*. She has received numerous state, district, and national awards in recognition of her outstanding contributions to the profession, including the Elmer B. Cottrell Award from SHAPE PA, the Honor Award from SHAPE America, and the Tilia J. Fantasia Service Award from SHAPE America Eastern District. She was inducted into the North American Society of Health, Physical Education, Recreation, Sport and Dance Professionals by SHAPE America. In 2023, she was honored with the SHAPE America Hall of Fame Award.

SHAPE America – Society of Health and Physical Educators serves as the voice for more than 200,000 health and physical education professionals across the United States. The organization's extensive community includes

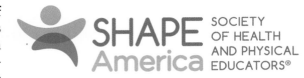

a diverse membership of health and physical educators, as well as advocates, supporters, and over 50 state affiliate organizations.

Since its founding in 1885, the organization has defined excellence in physical education. For decades, SHAPE America's National Standards for K-12 Physical Education have served as the foundation for well-designed physical education programs across the country, just as SHAPE America's National Health Education Standards serve as the foundation for effective skills-based health education. Together, these national standards provide a comprehensive framework for educators to deliver high-quality instruction and make a positive difference in the health and well-being of every preK-12 student.

SHAPE America provides programs, resources, and advocacy that support an inclusive, active, and healthier school culture, and the organization's newest program—health. moves. minds.©—helps teachers and schools incorporate social and emotional learning so students can thrive physically and emotionally.

Our Vision

A nation where all children are prepared to lead healthy, physically active lives.

Our Mission

To advance professional practice and promote research related to health and physical education, physical activity, dance, and sport.

To learn more, visit **www.shapeamerica.org**.

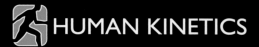
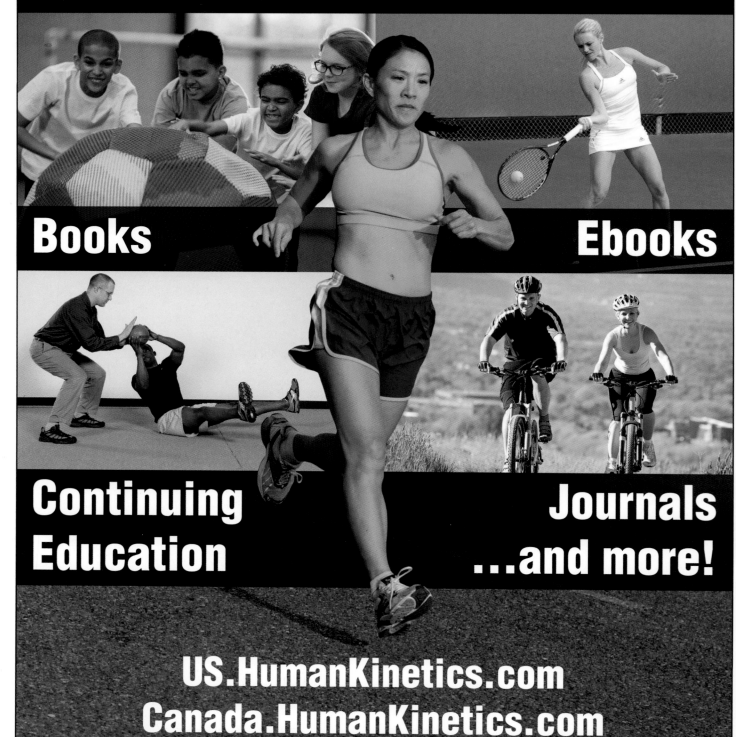

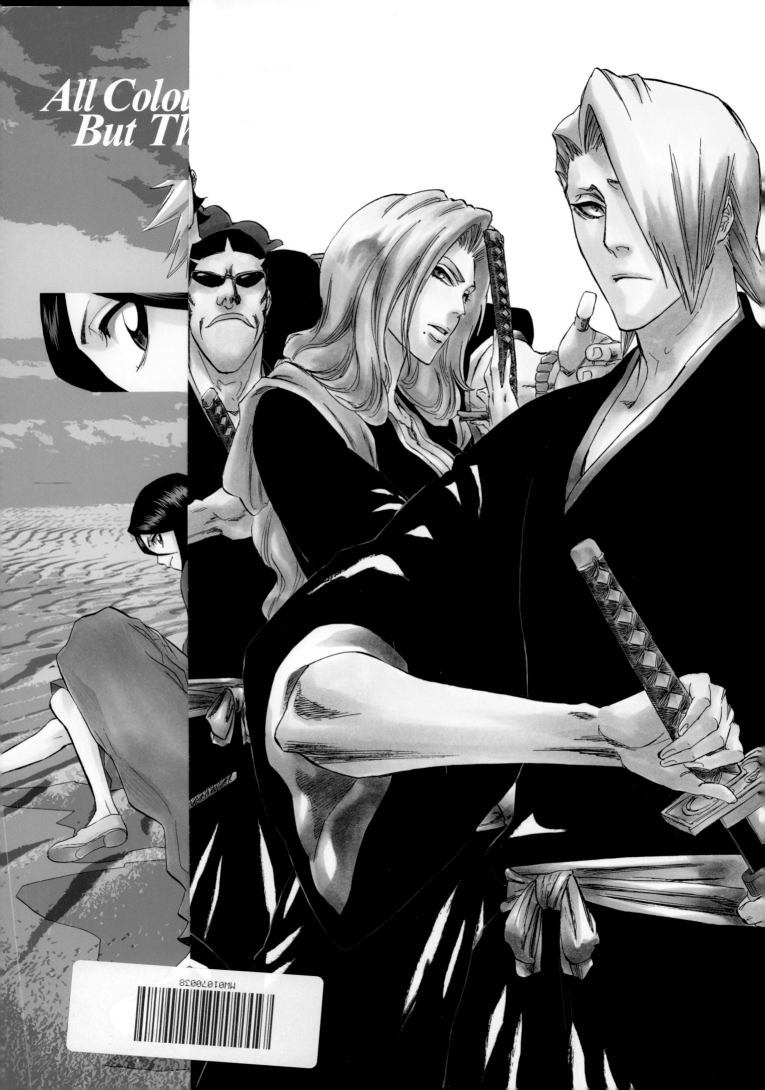

All Colou
But Th

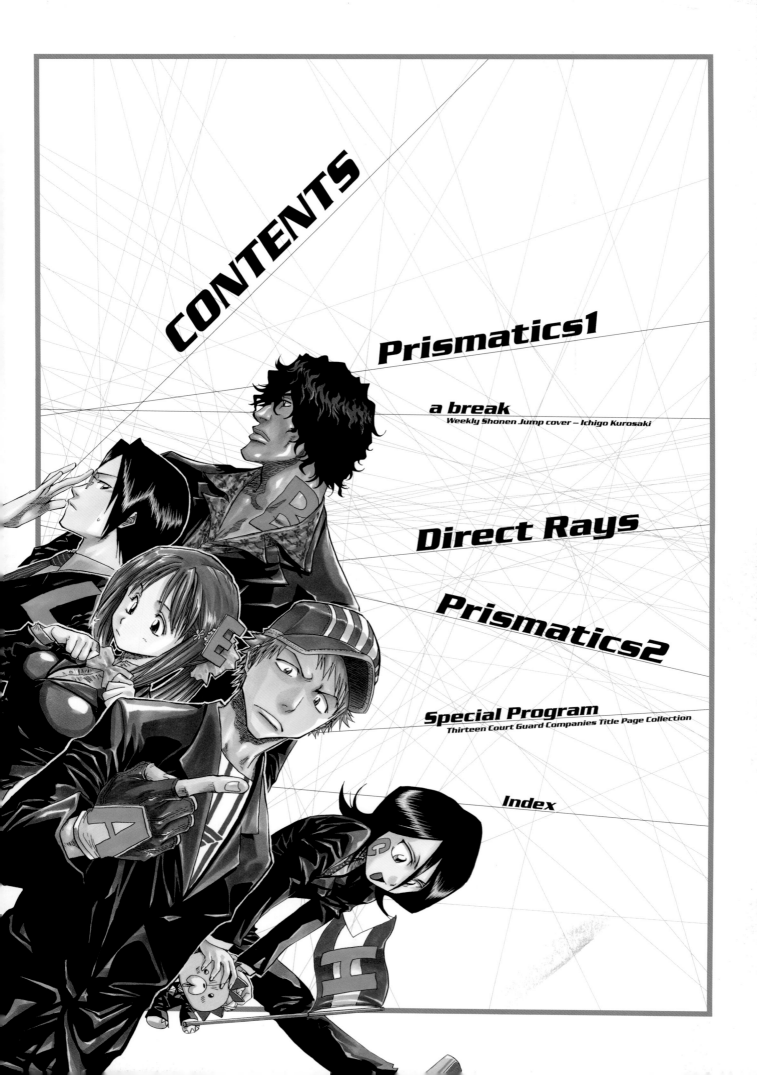

CONTENTS

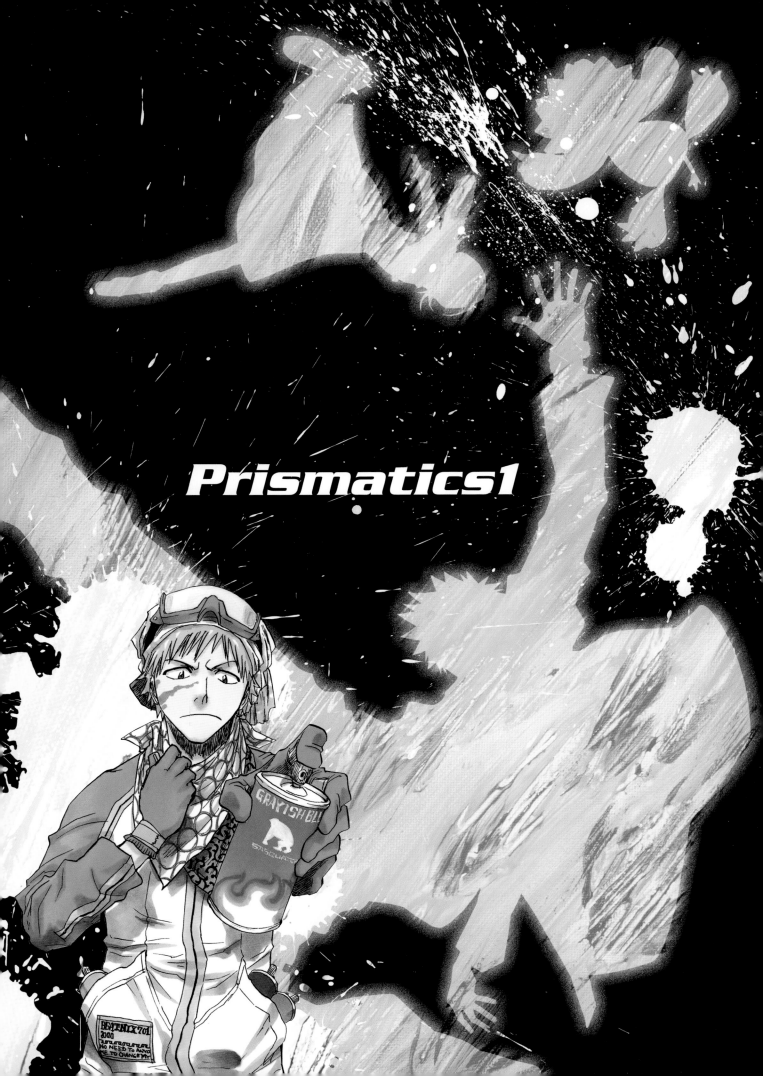

Prismatics1

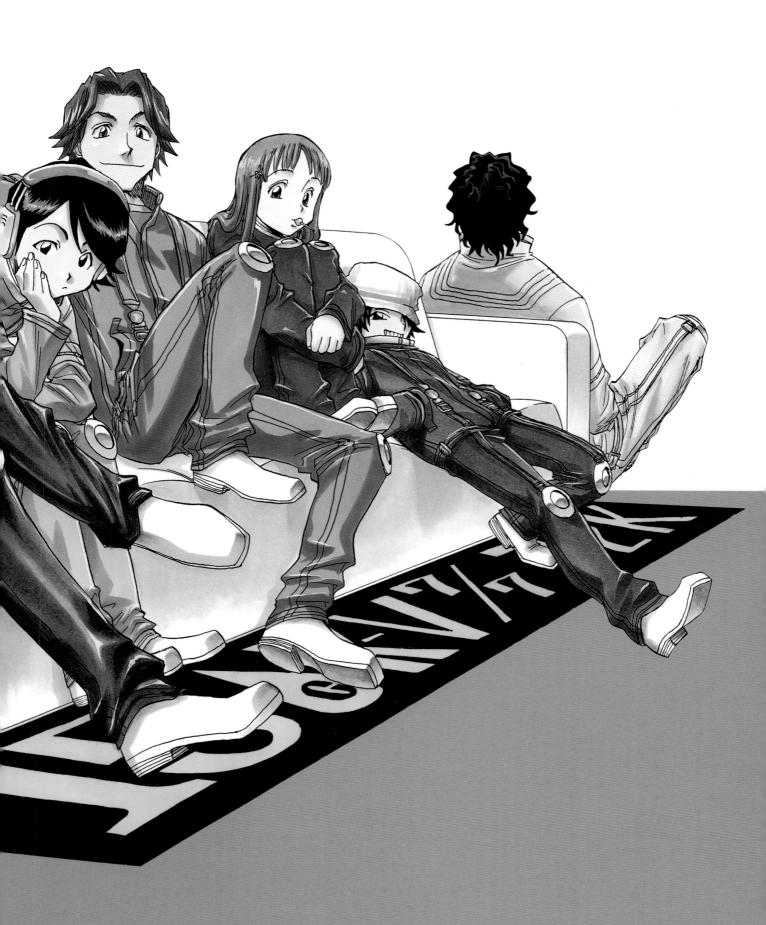

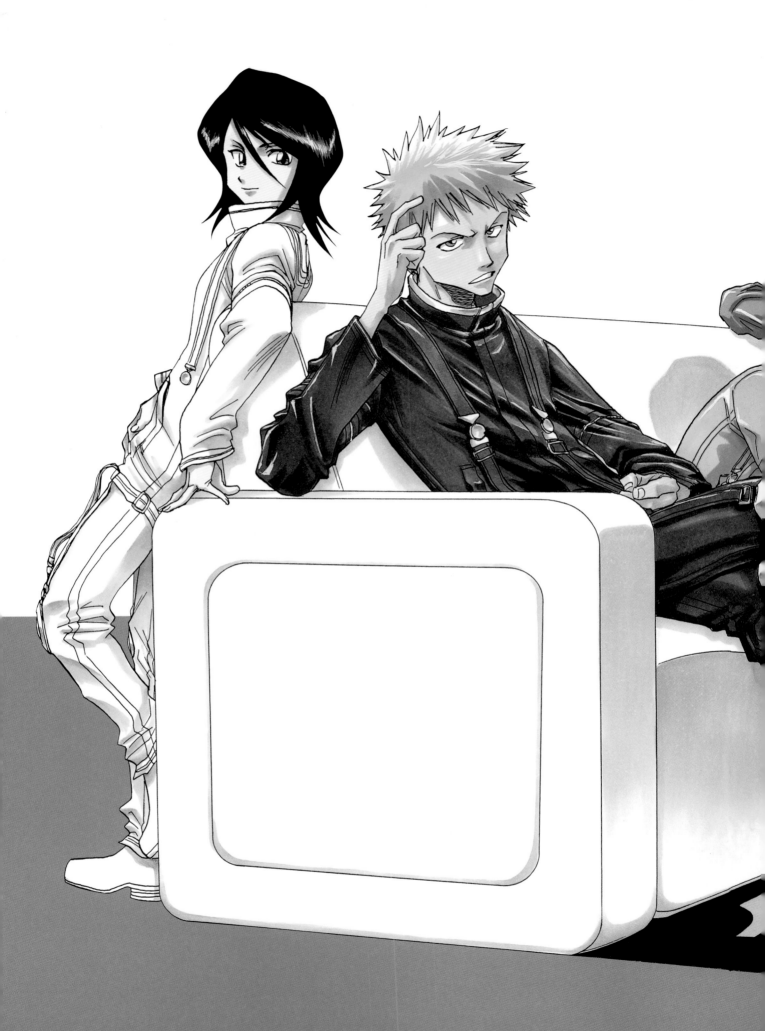

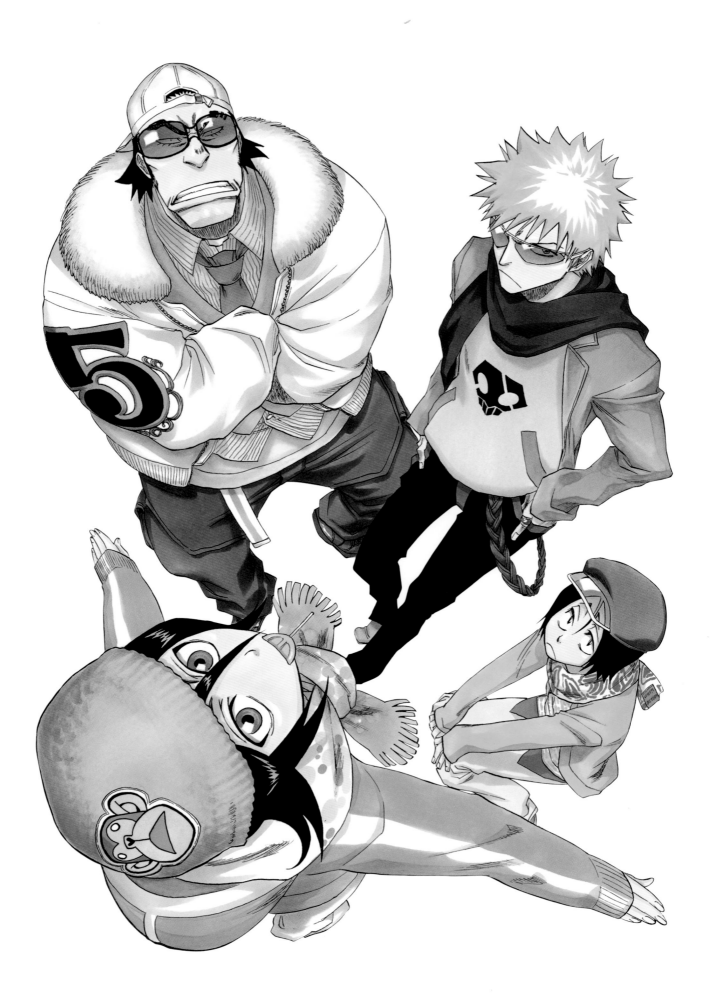

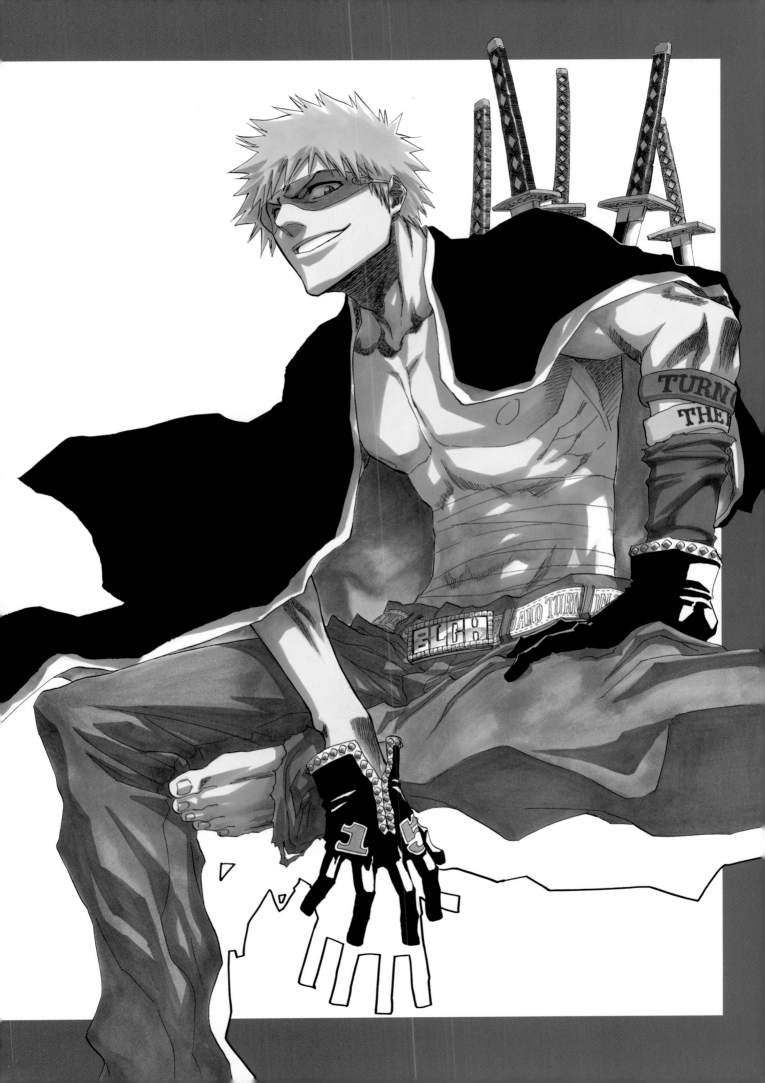

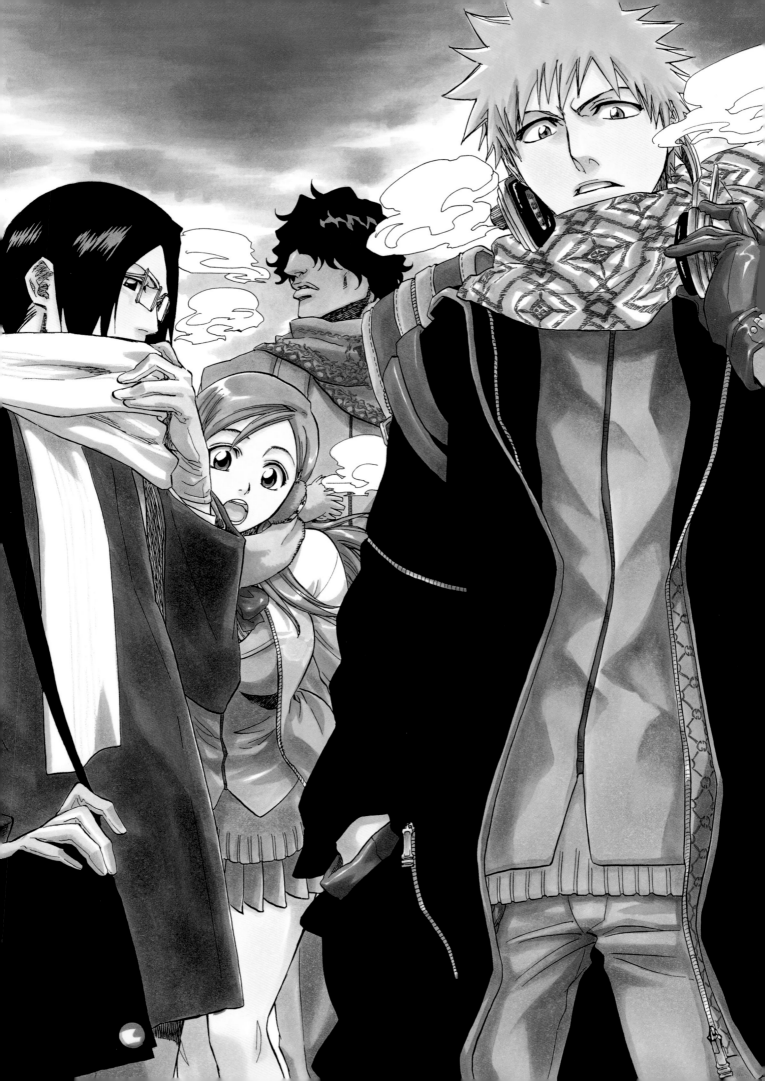

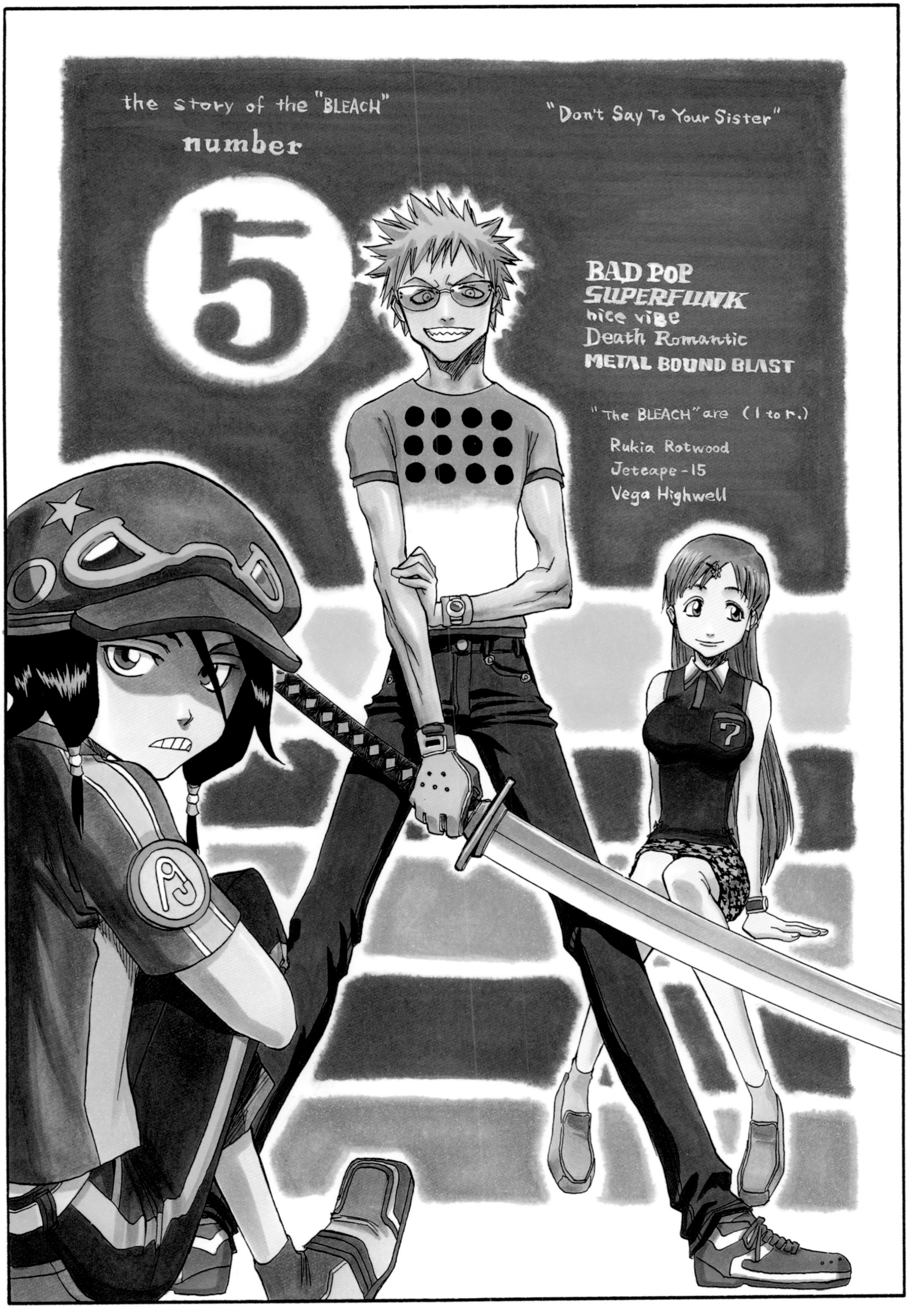
the story of the "BLEACH"
number
5
"Don't Say To Your Sister"
BAD POP
SUPERFUNK
nice vibe
Death Romantic
METAL BOUND BLAST
"The BLEACH" are (l to r.)
Rukia Rotwood
Jeteape-15
Vega Highwell

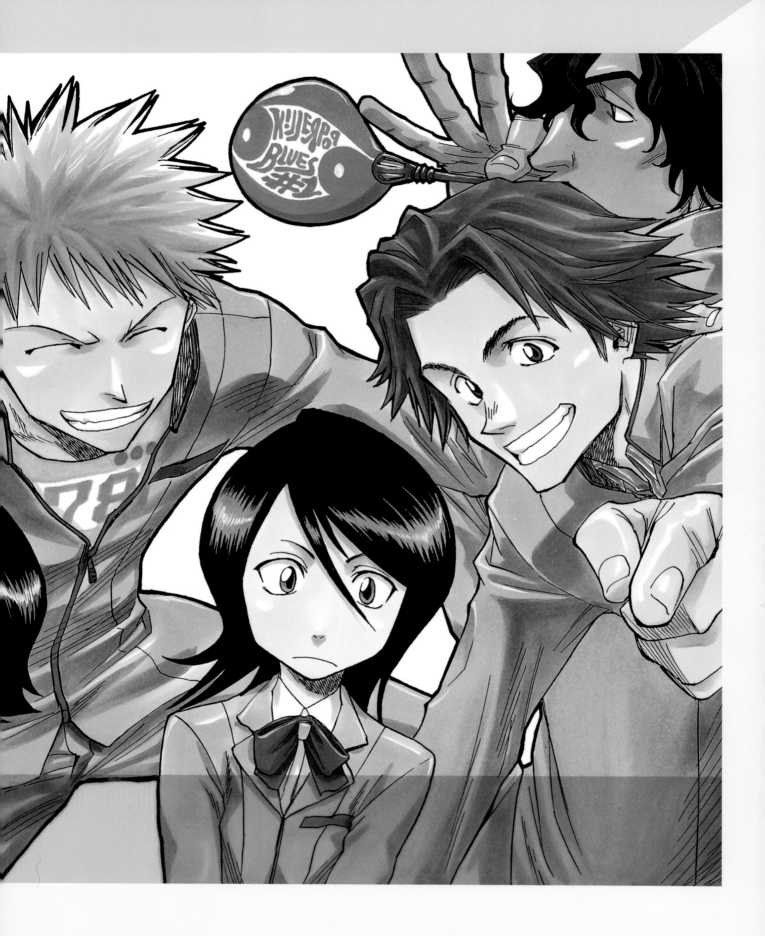

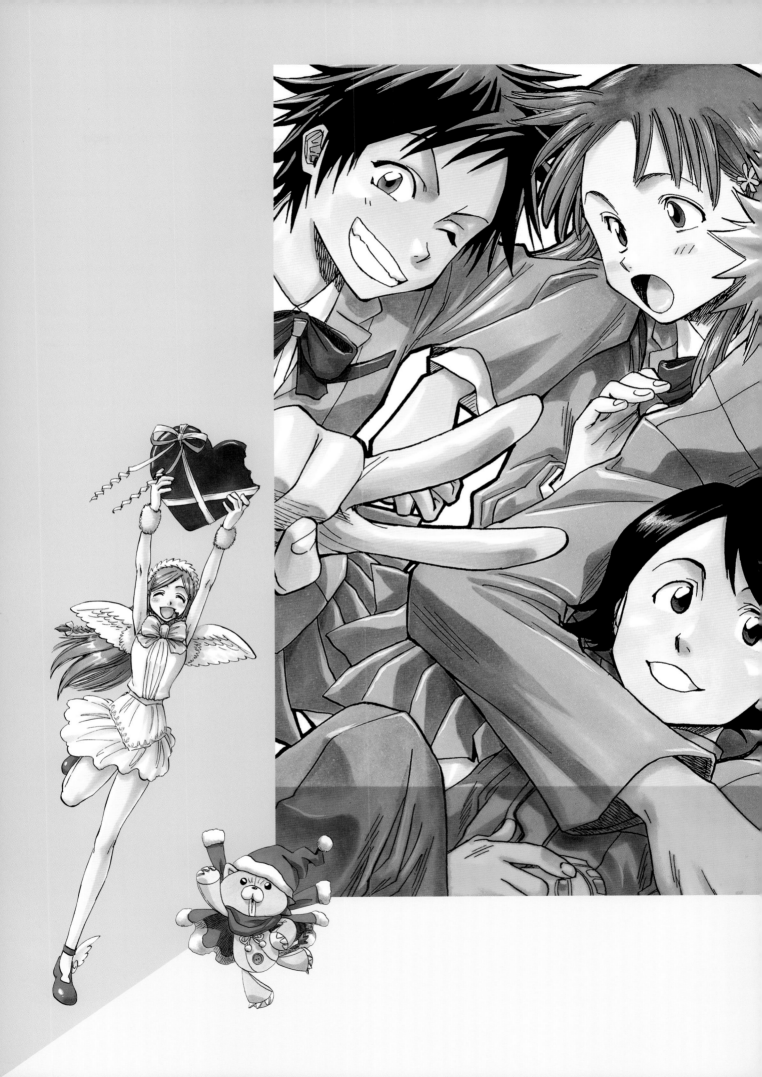

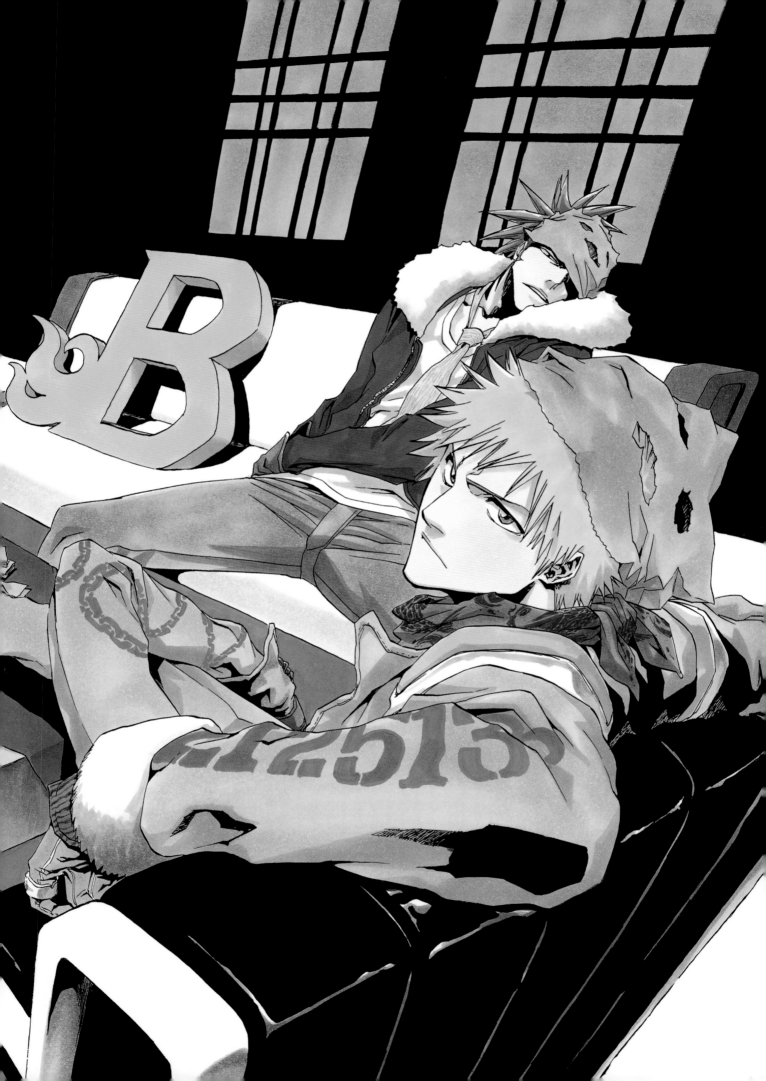

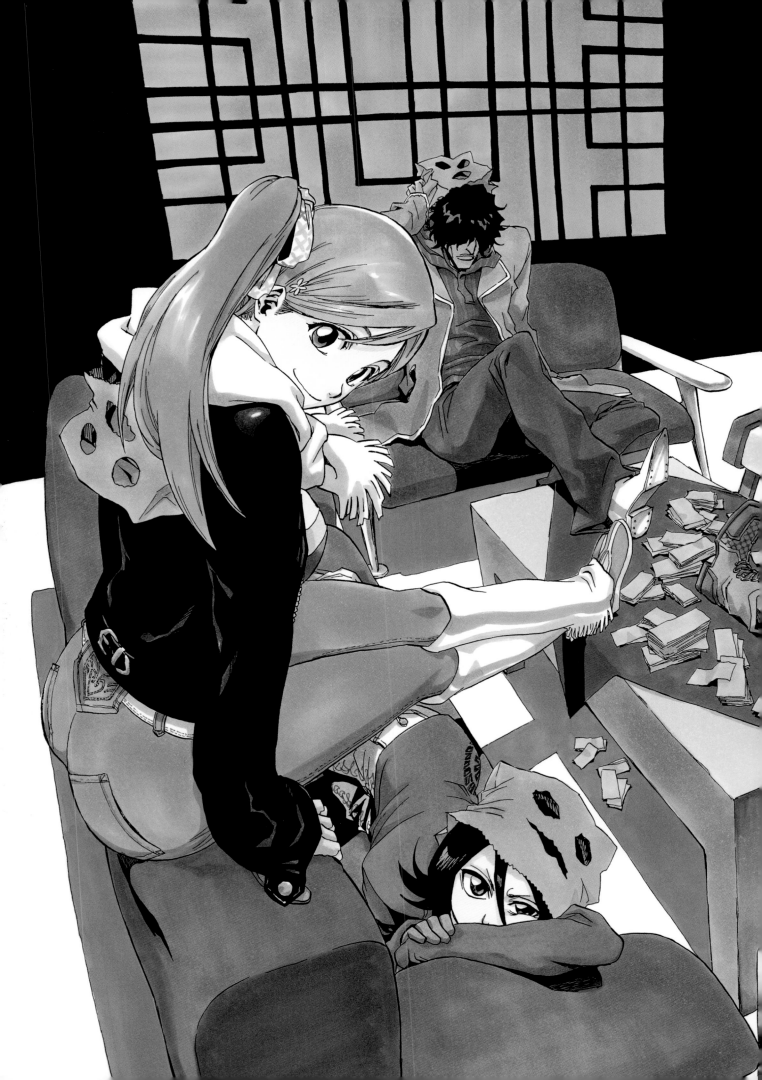

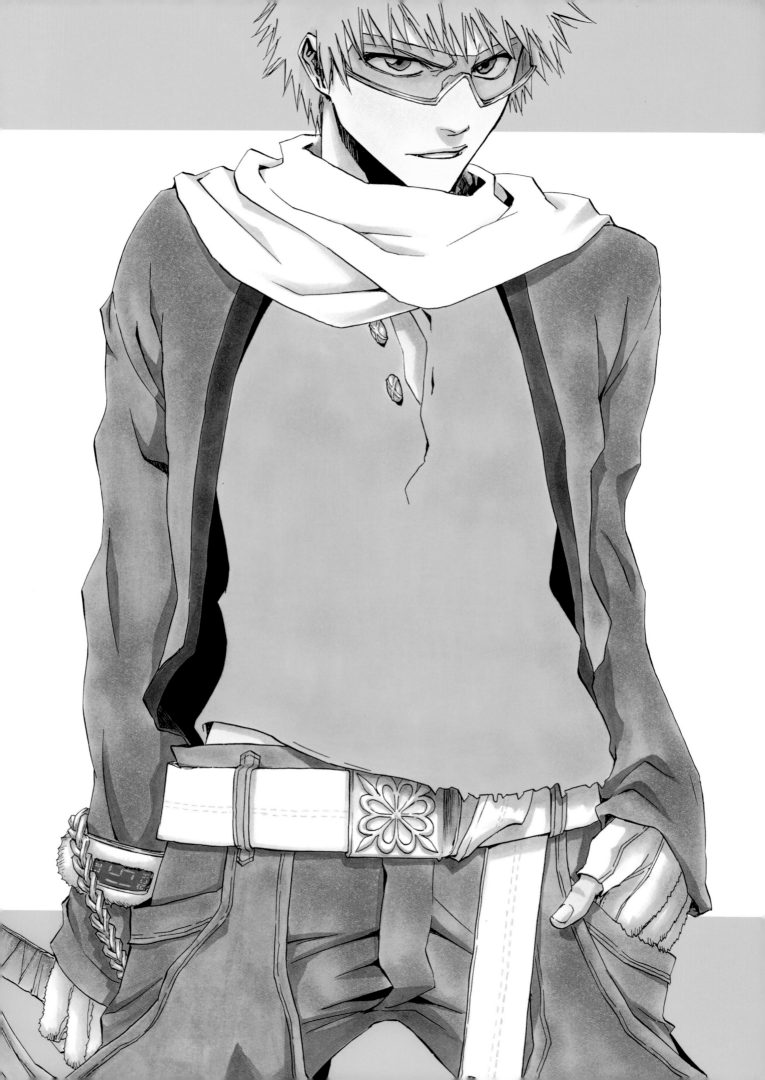

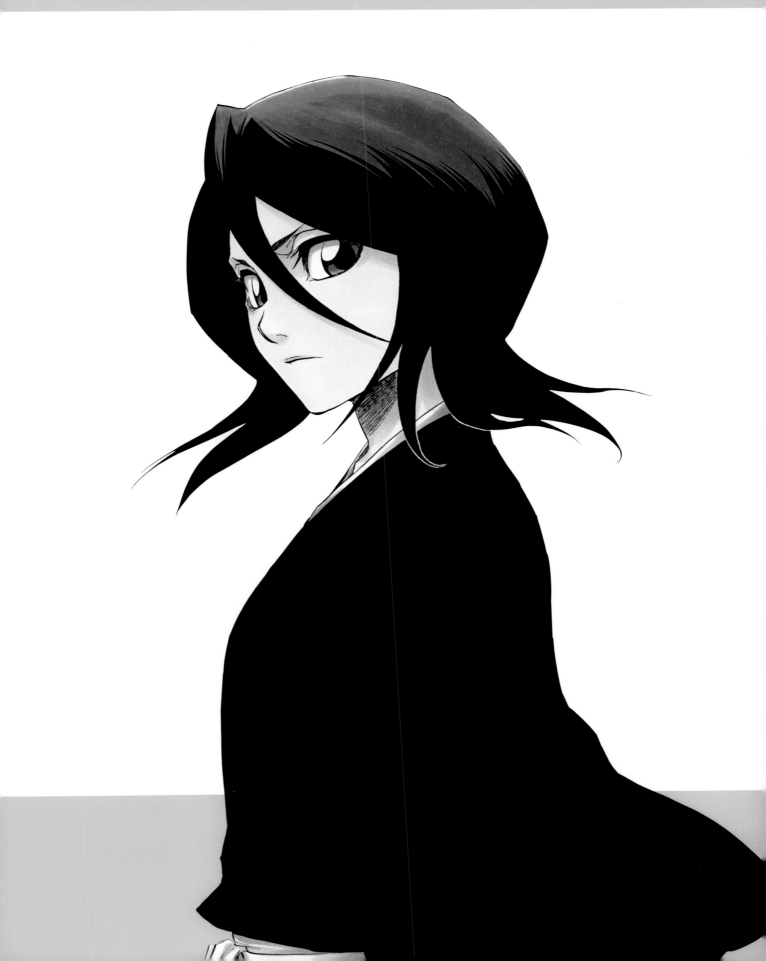

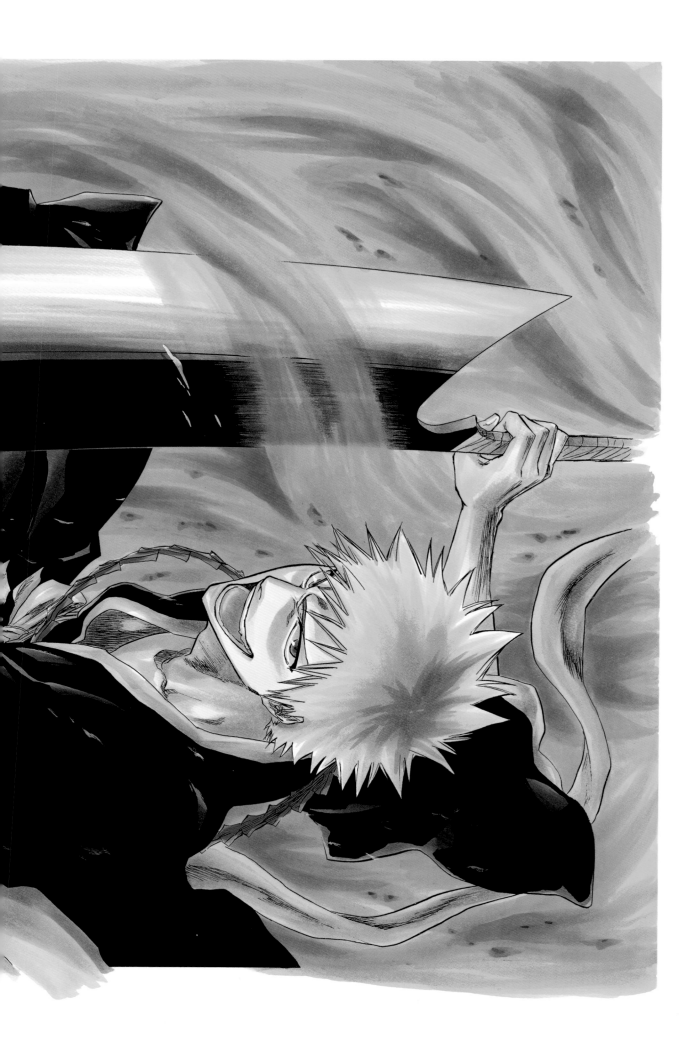

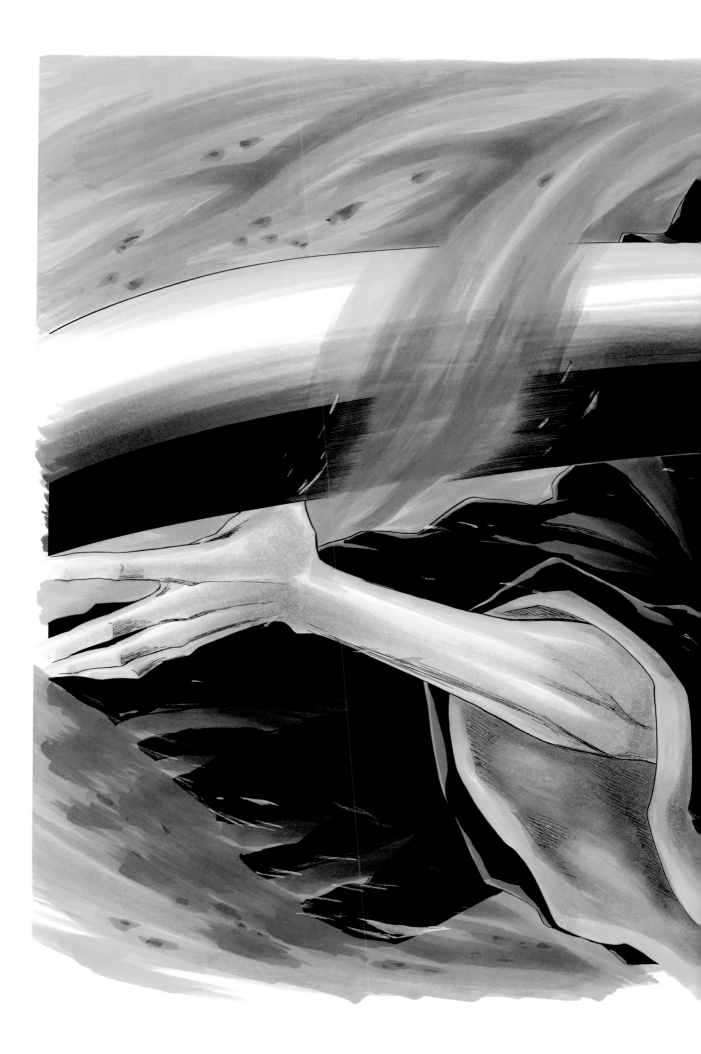

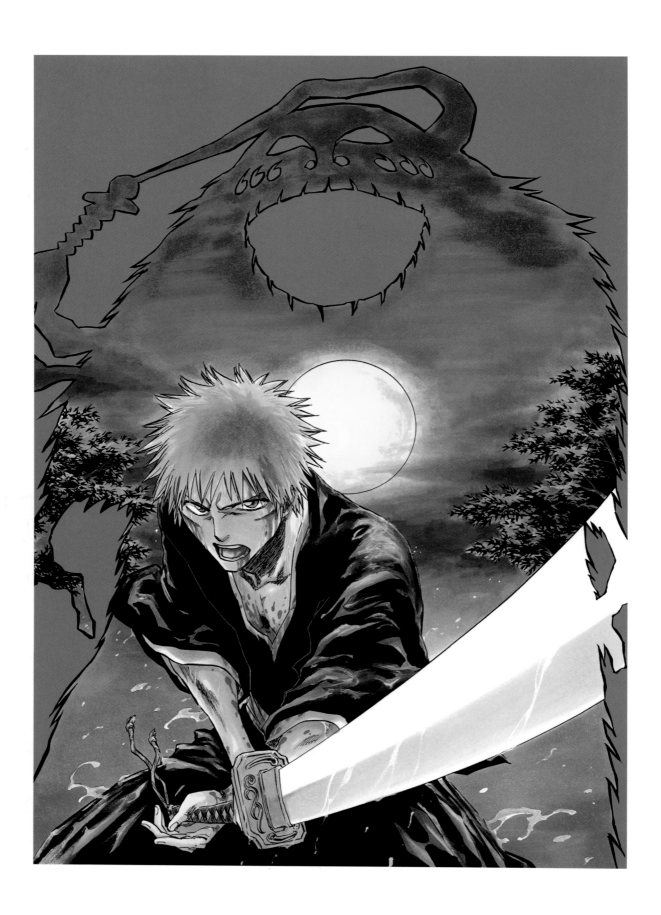

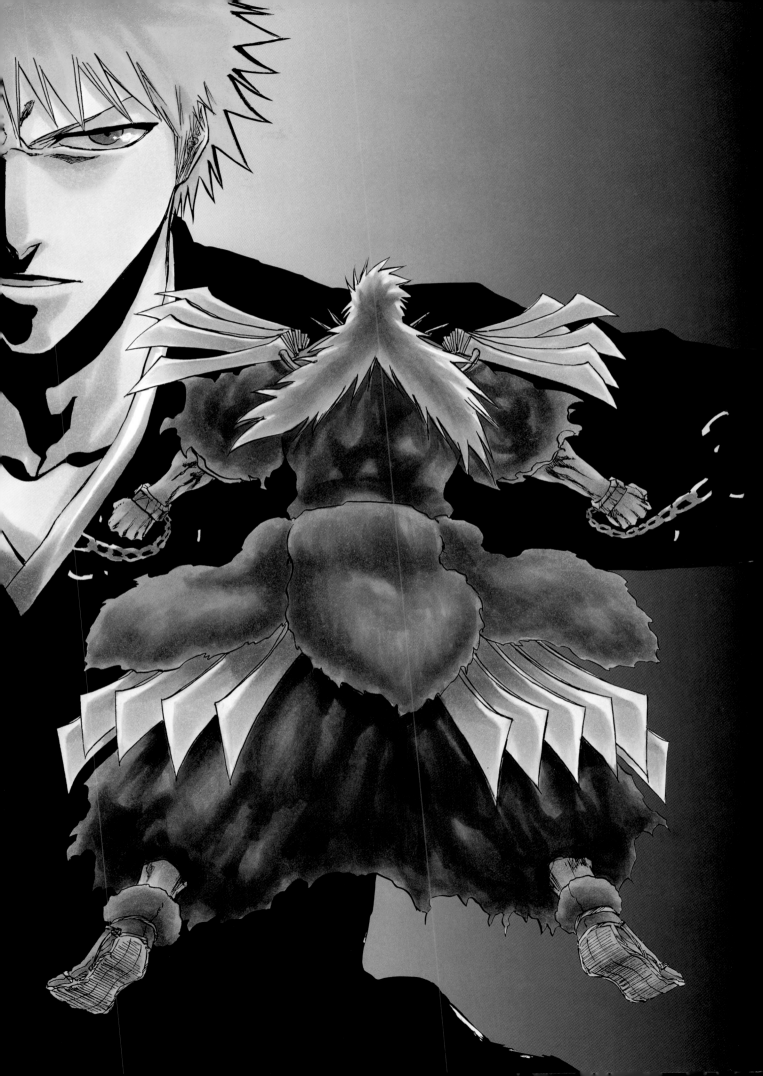

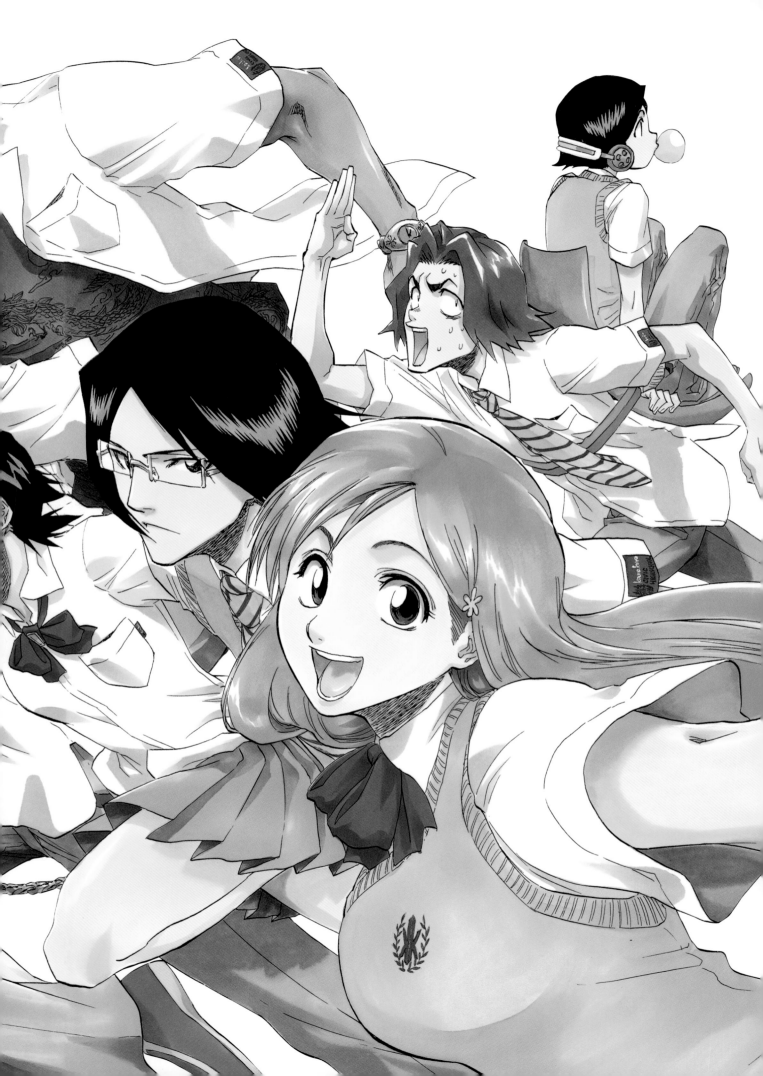

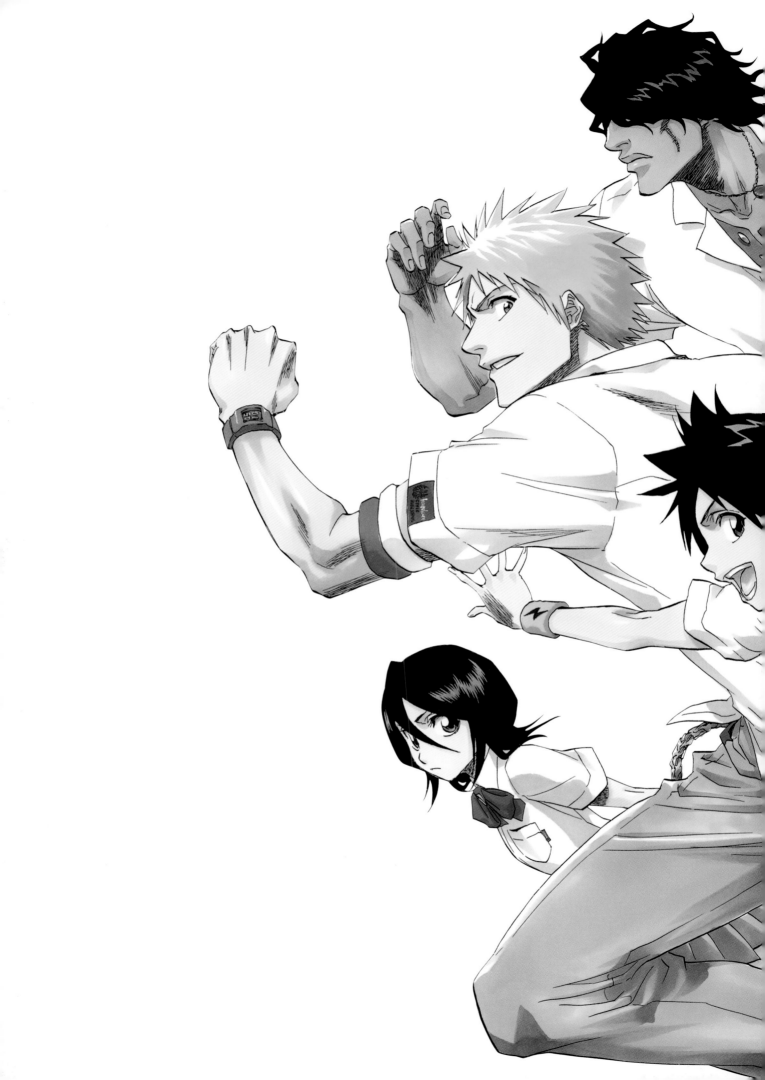

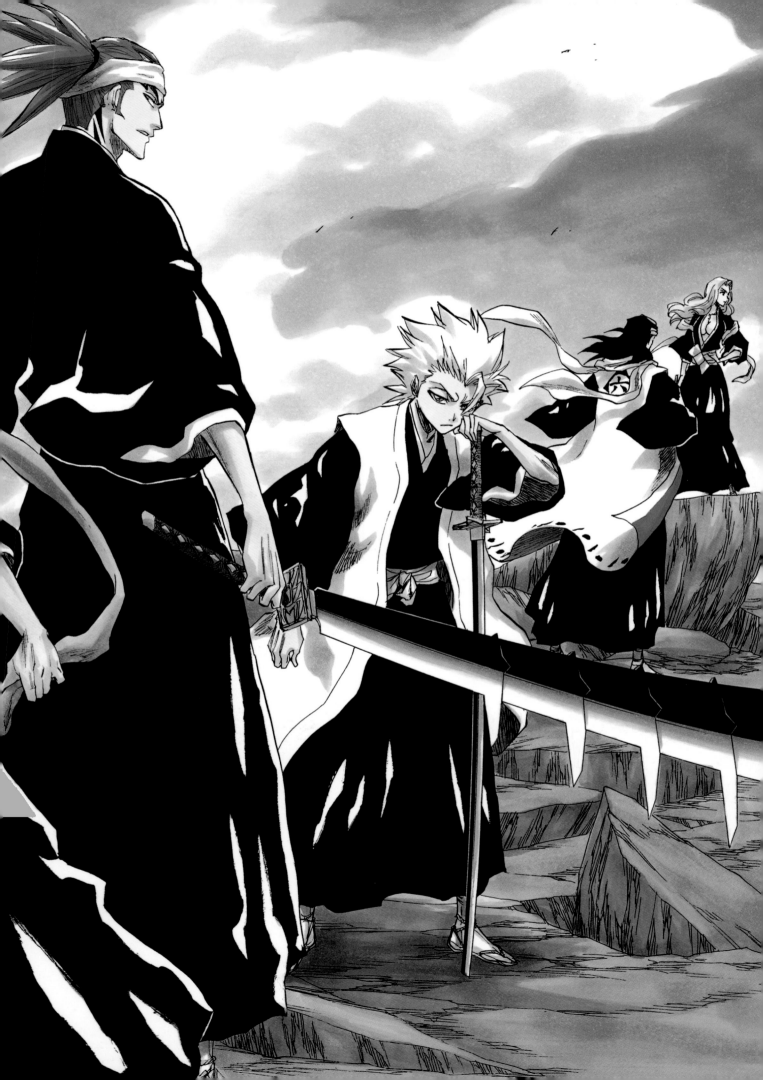

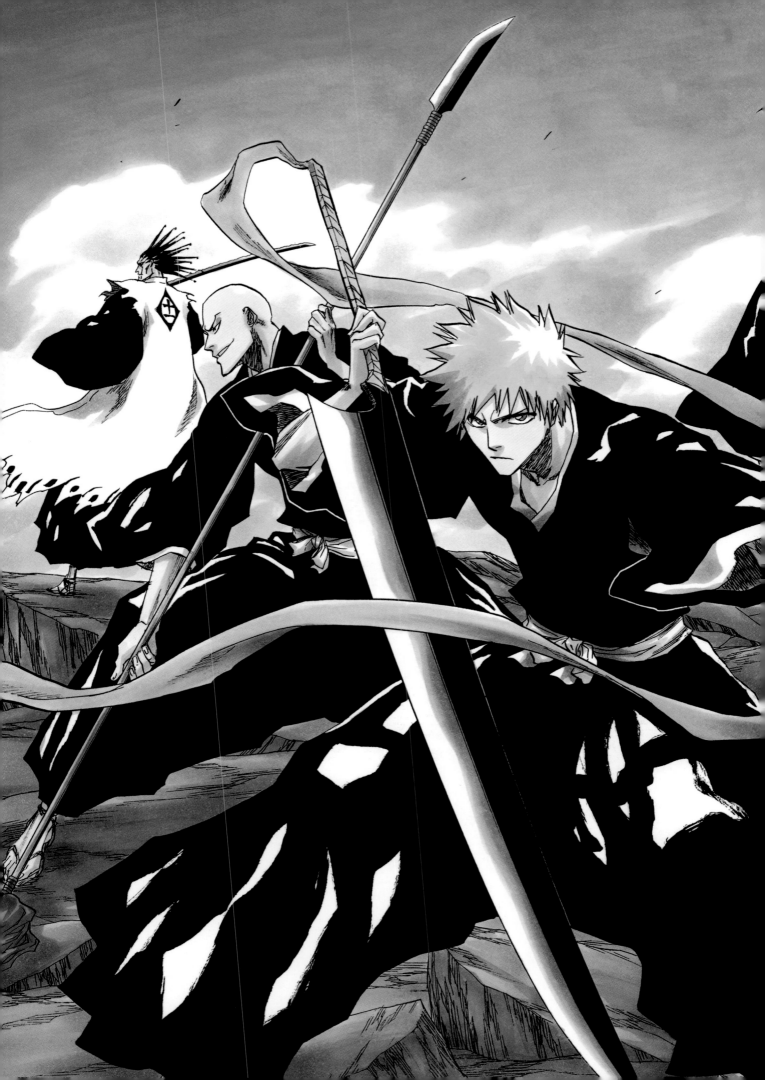

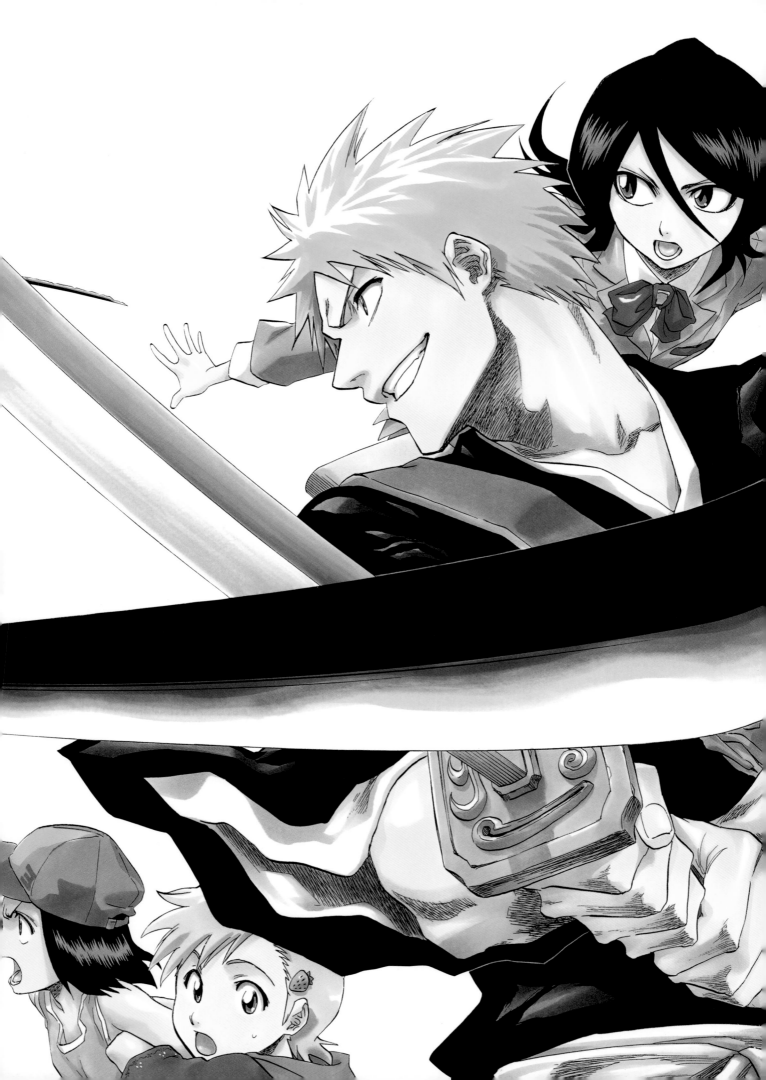

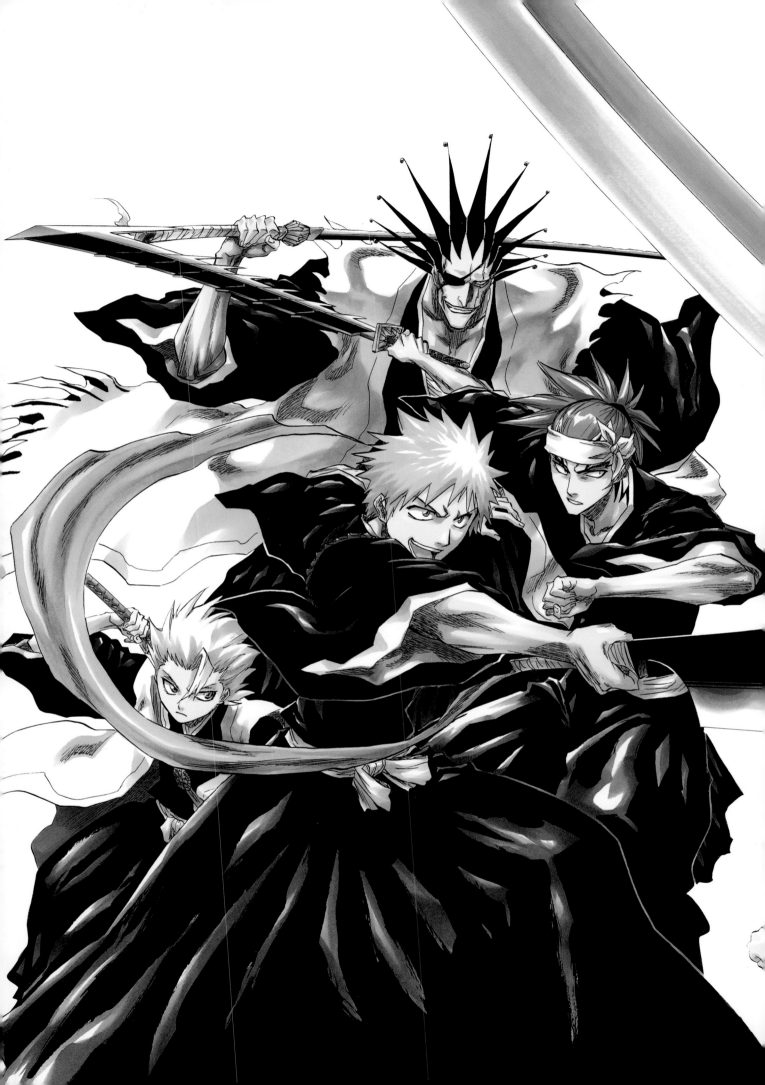

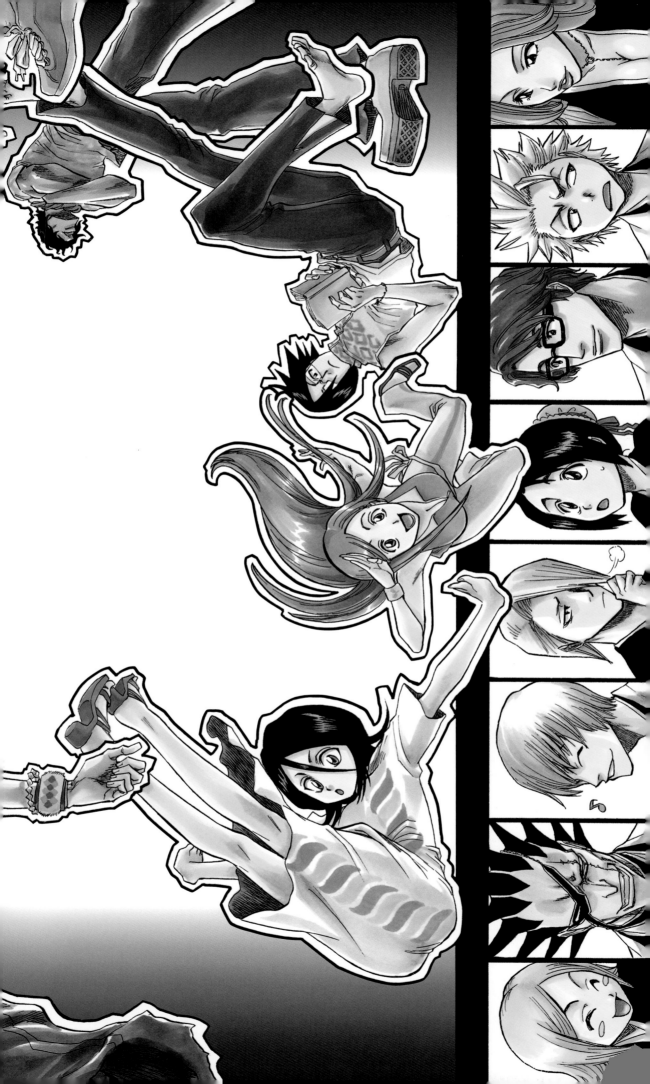

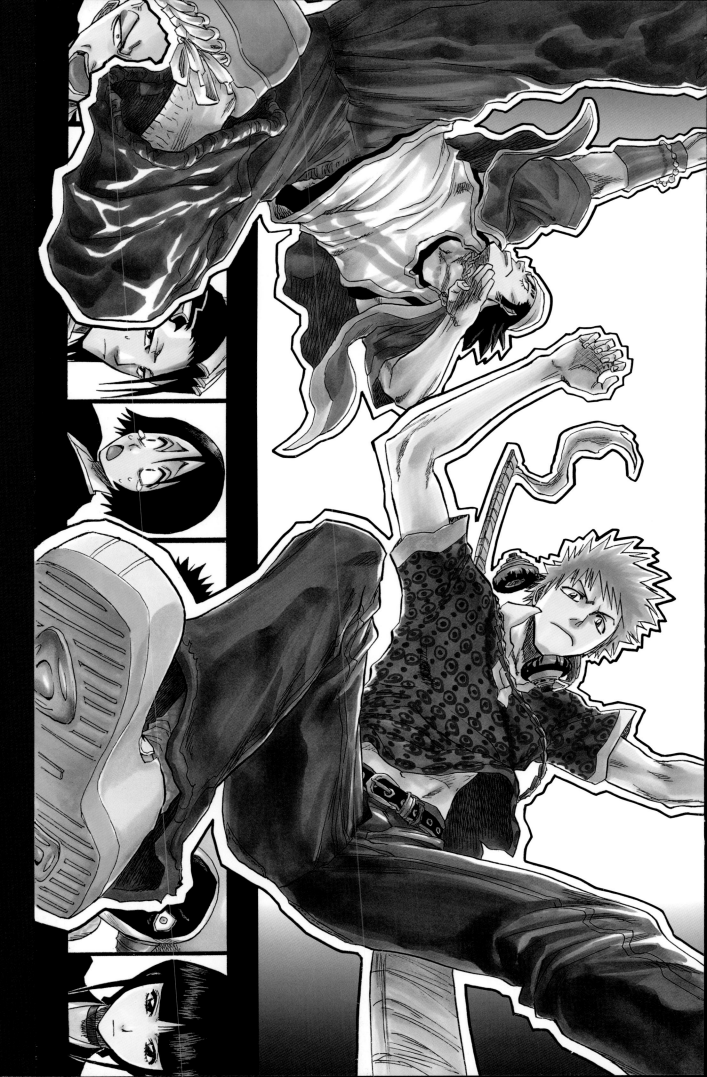

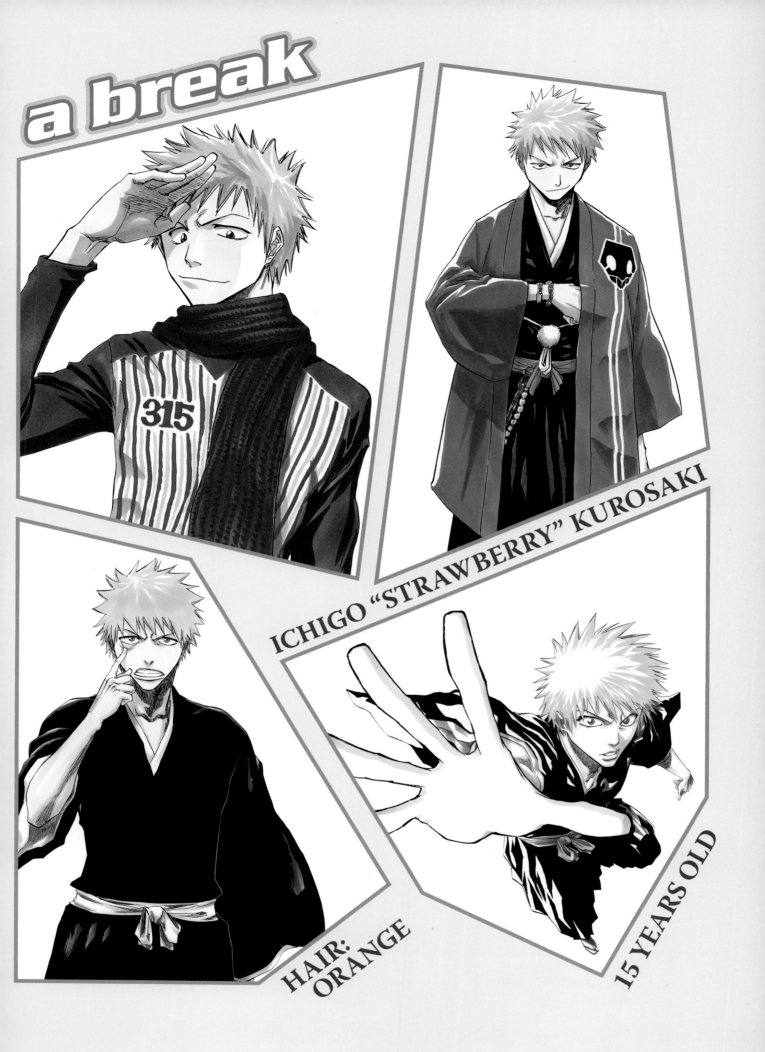

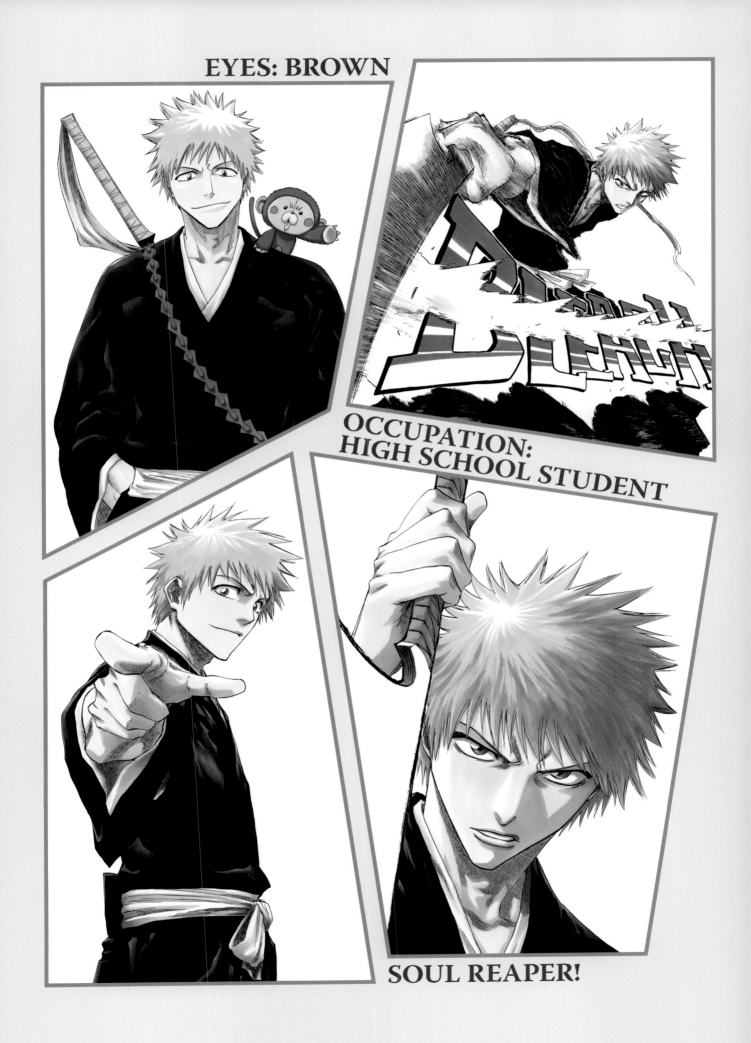

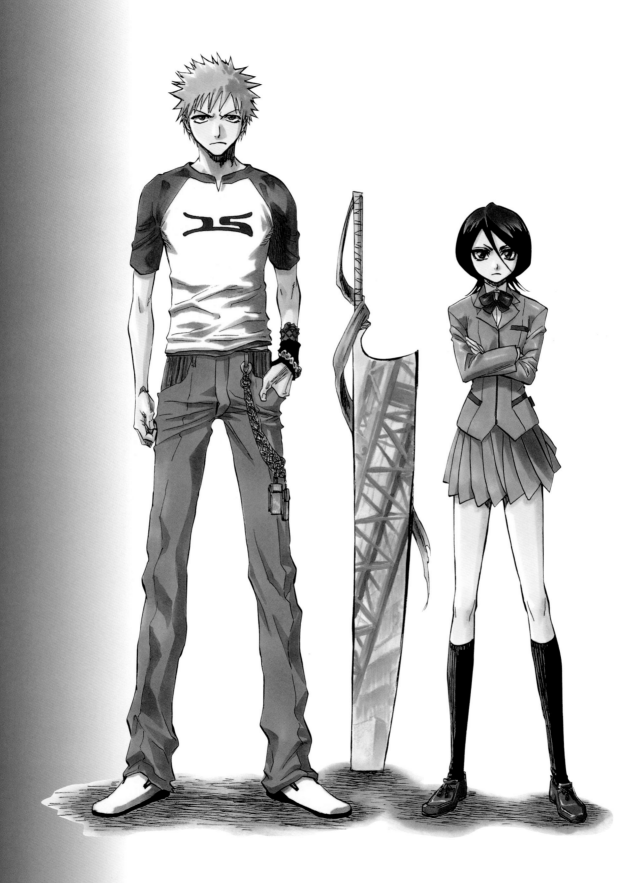

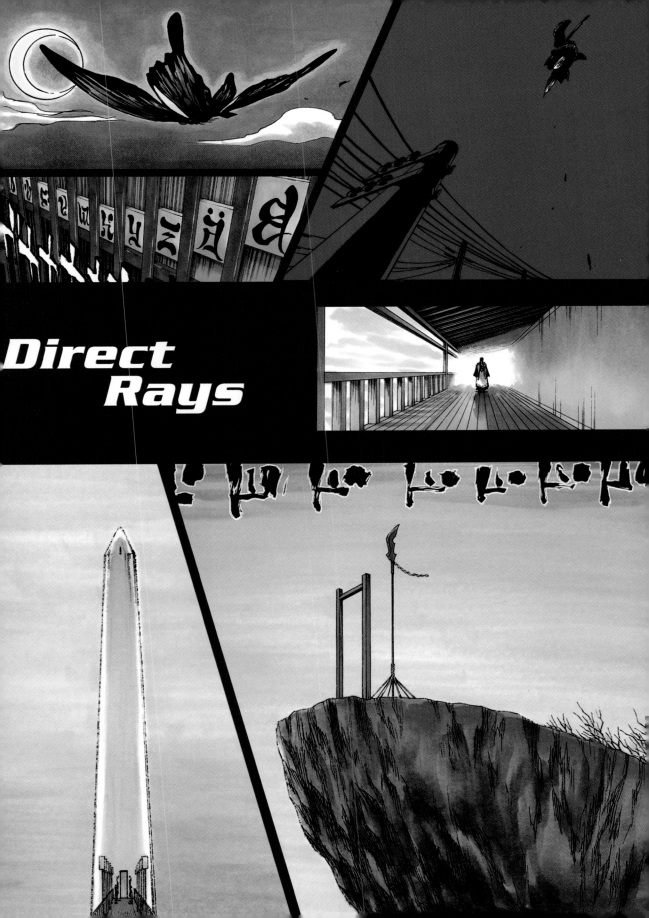

Direct
Rays

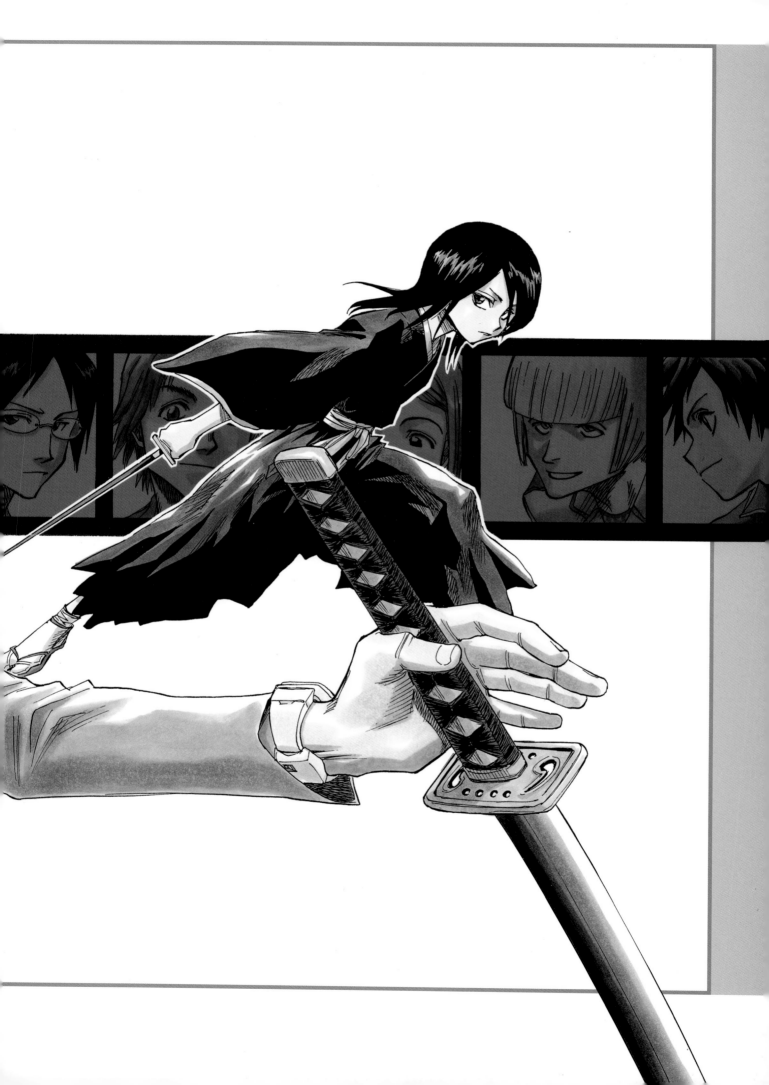

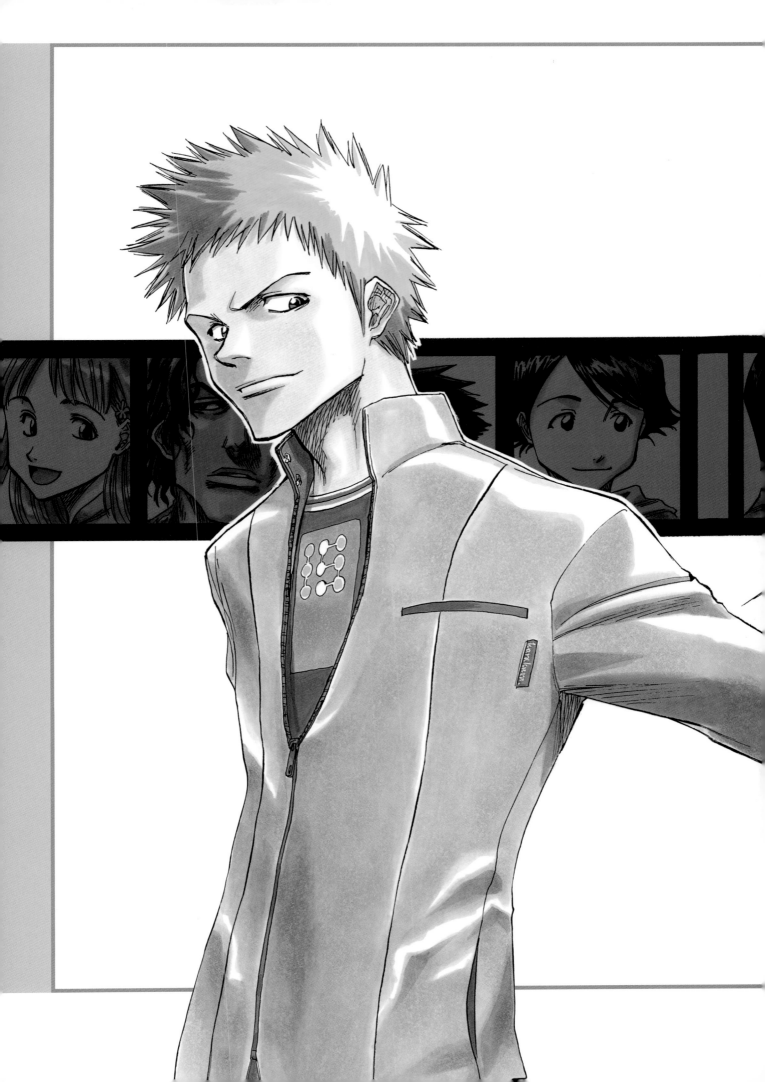

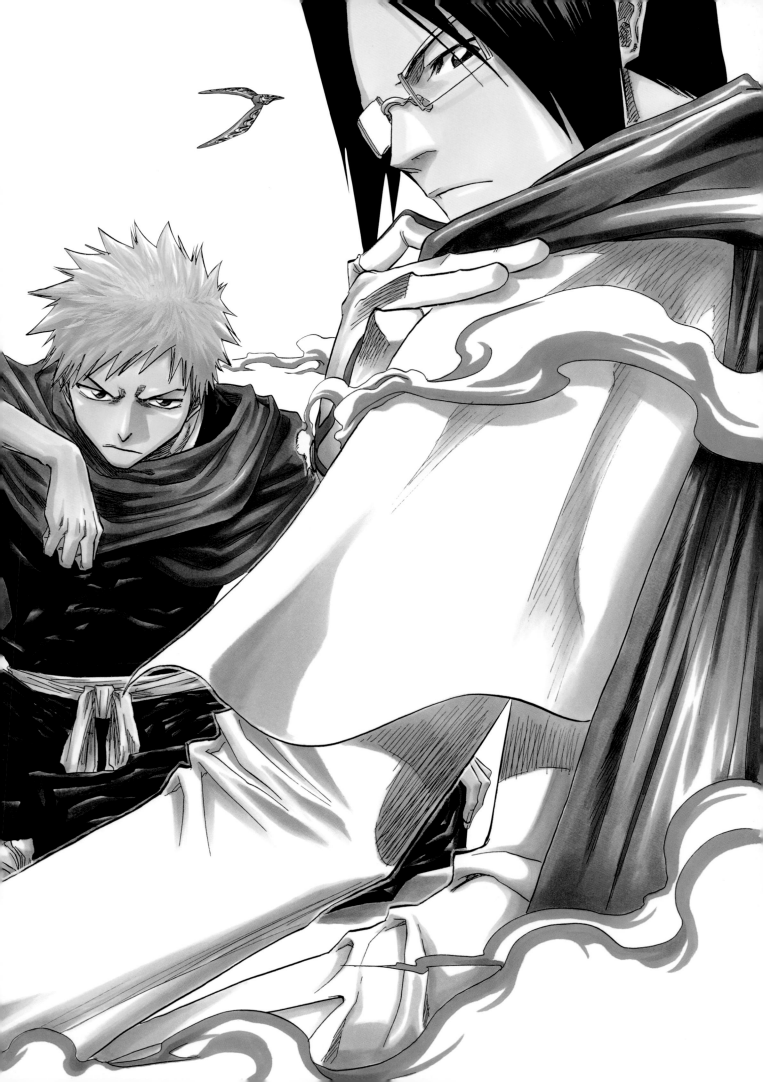

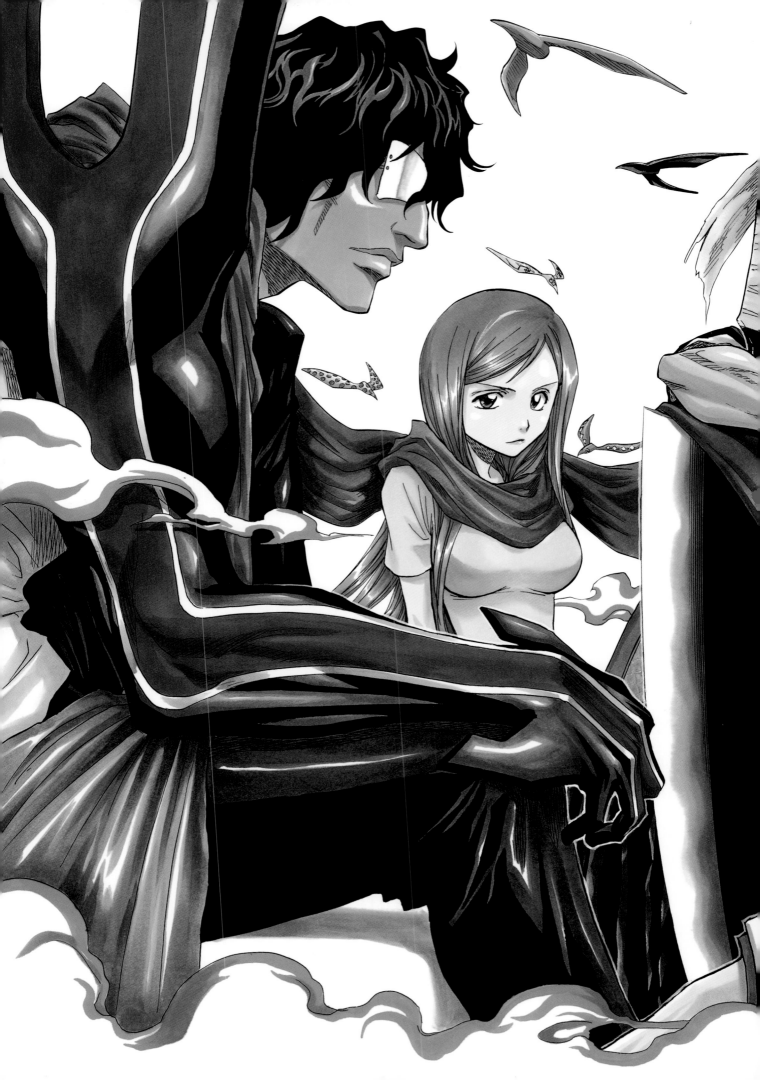

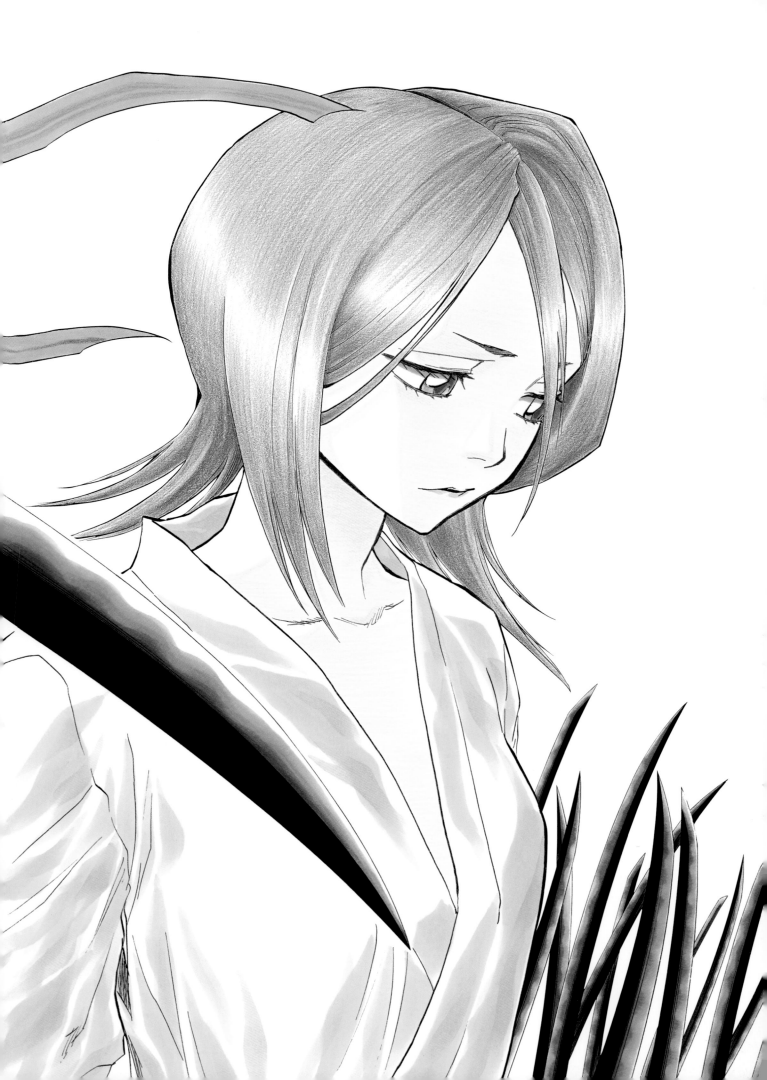

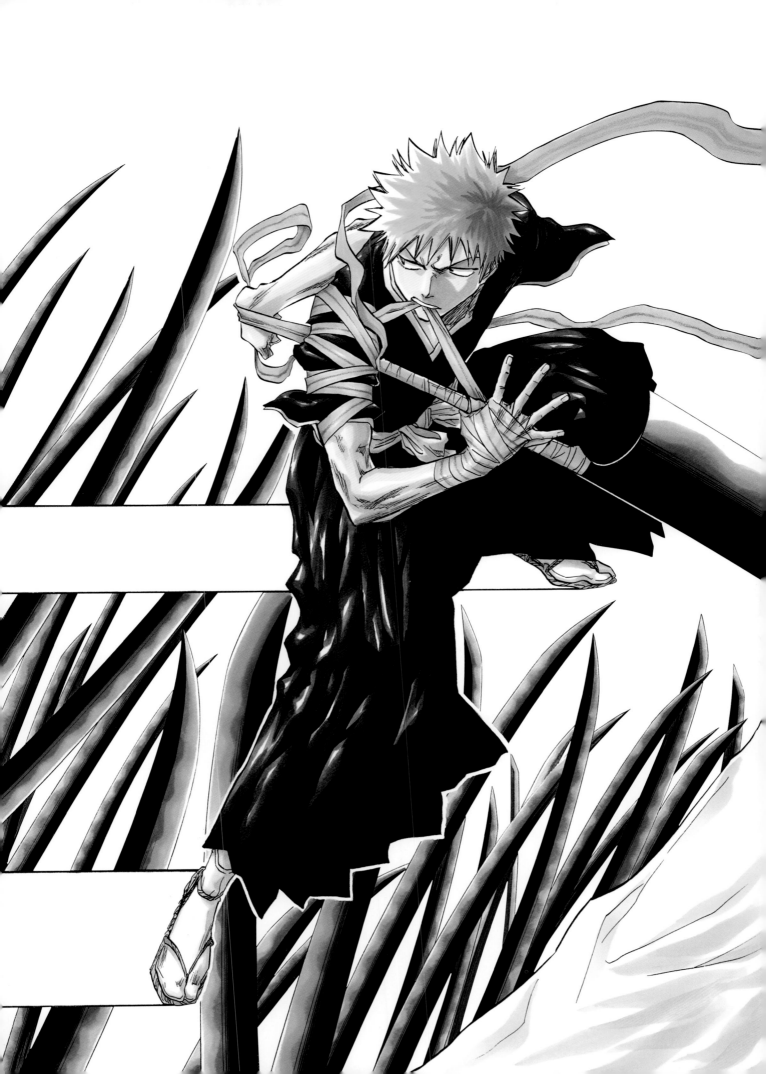

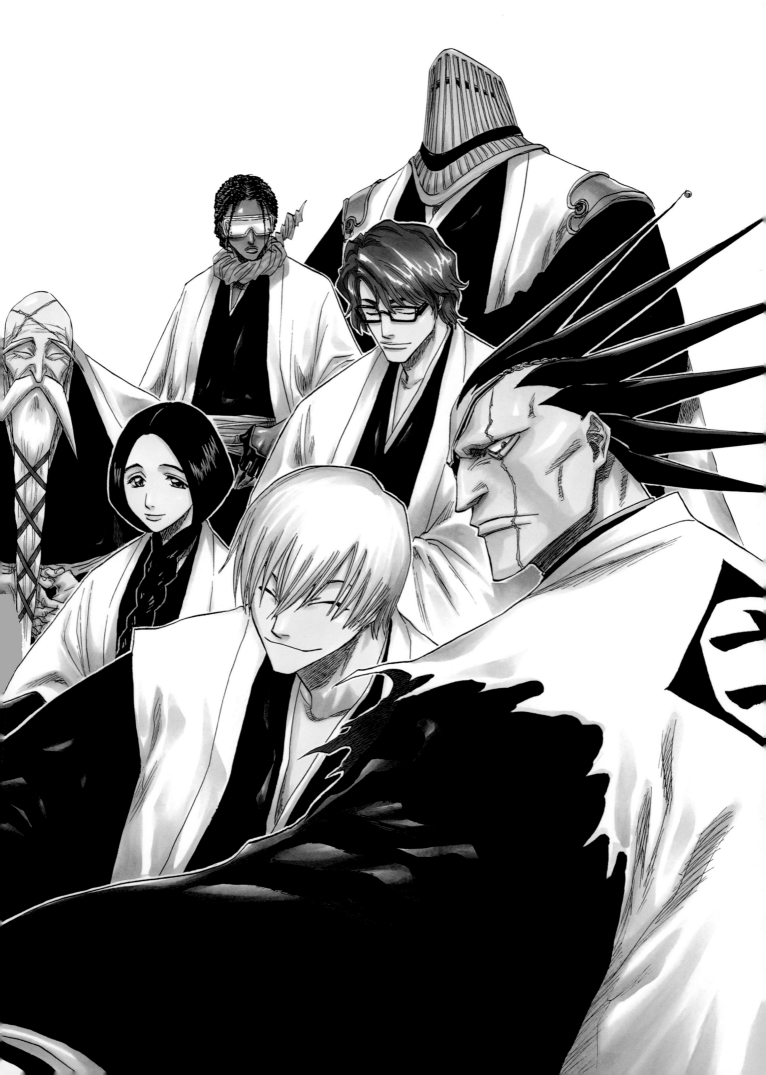

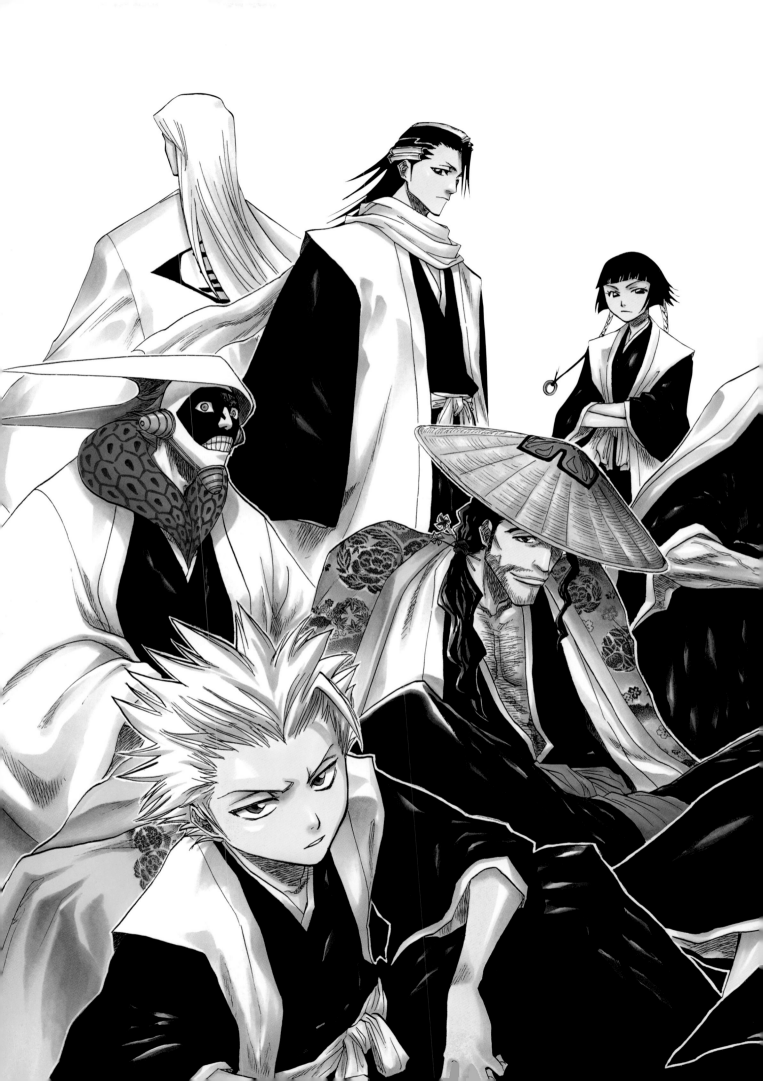

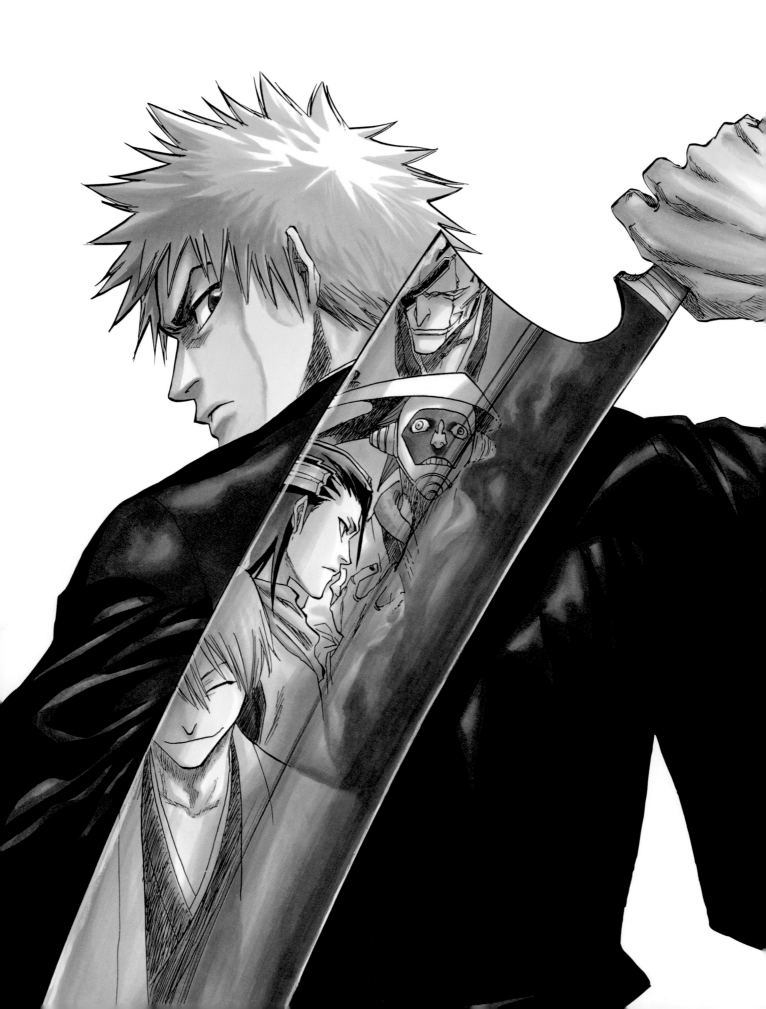

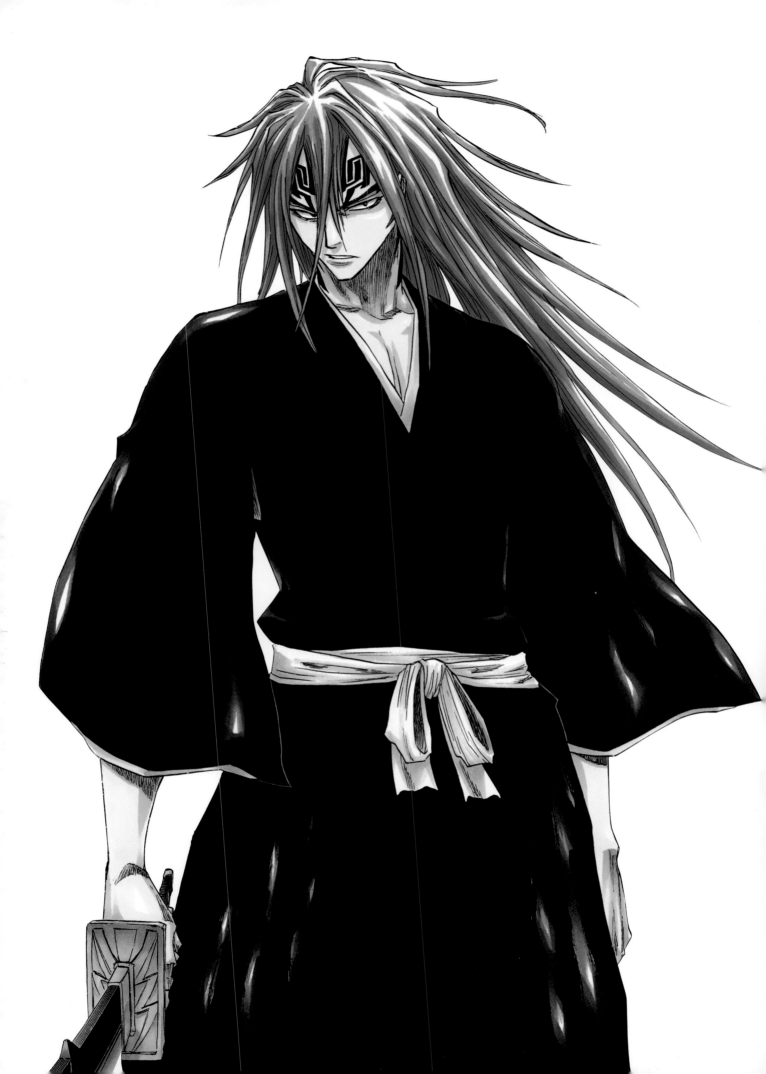

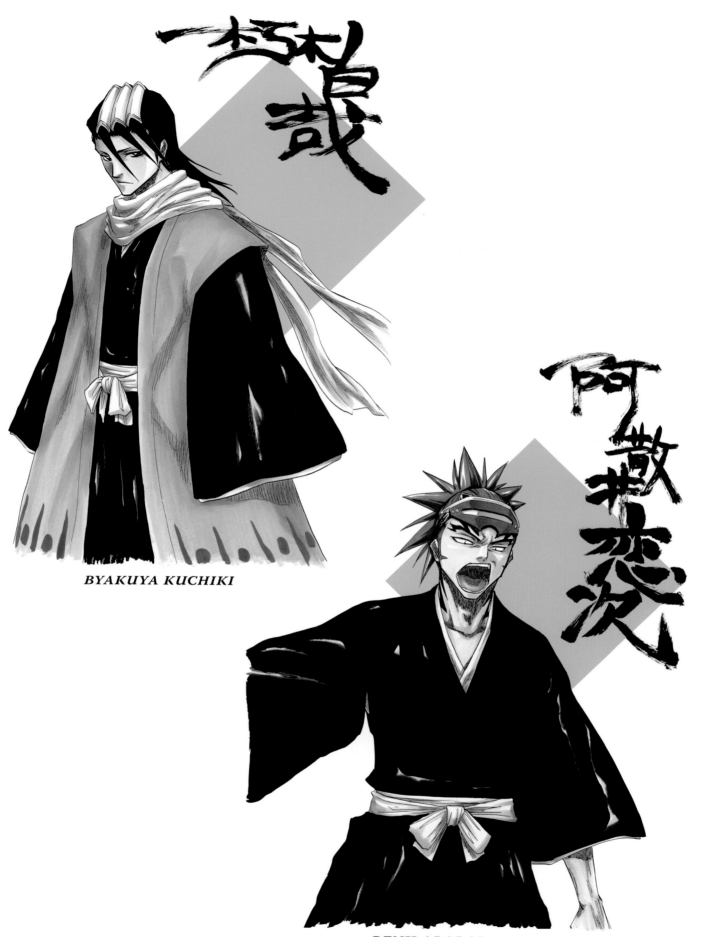

一五六心哉

阿散井恋次

BYAKUYA KUCHIKI

RENJI ABARAI

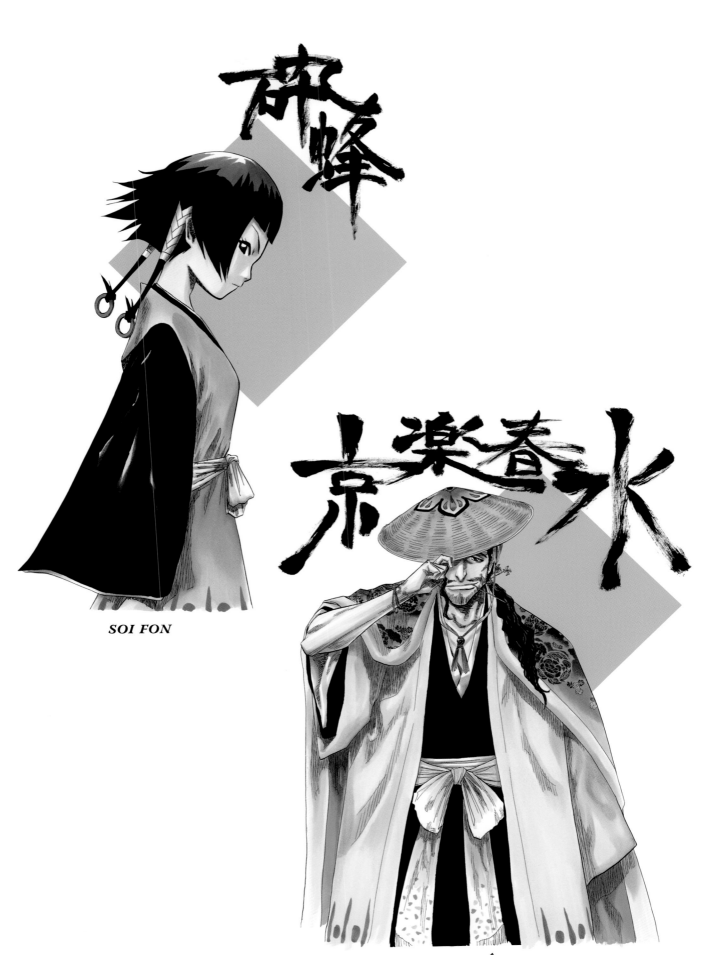

蜂梗

京楽春水

SOI FON

SHUNSUI KYÔRAKU

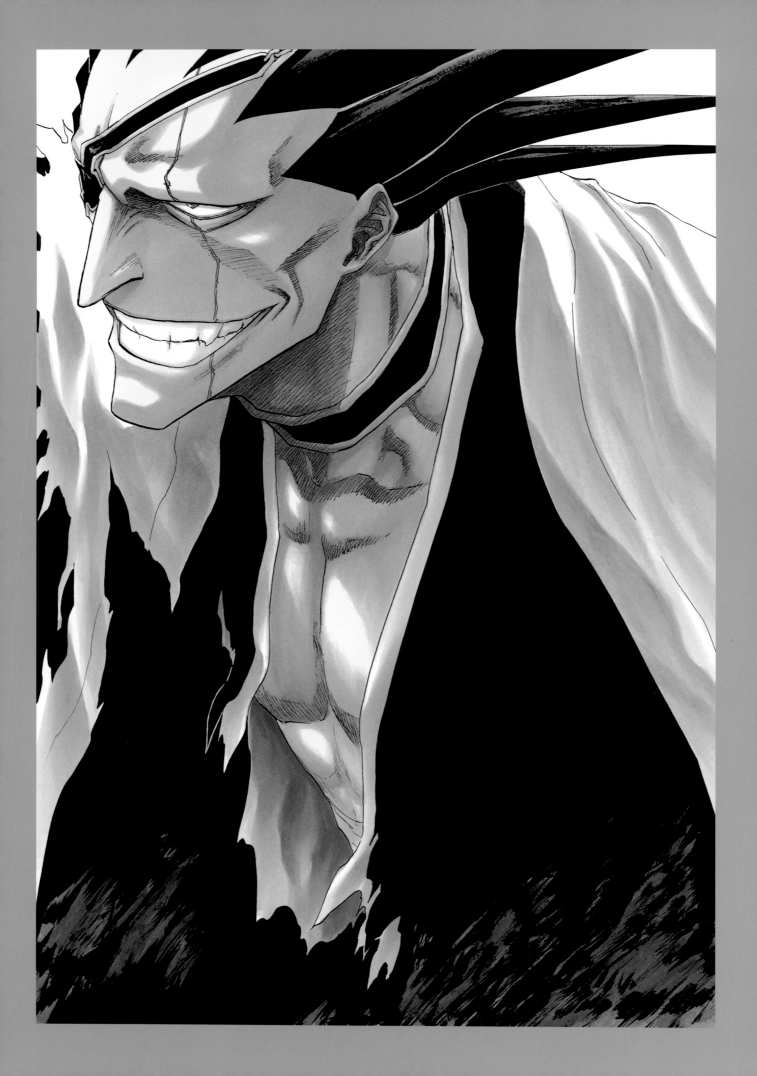

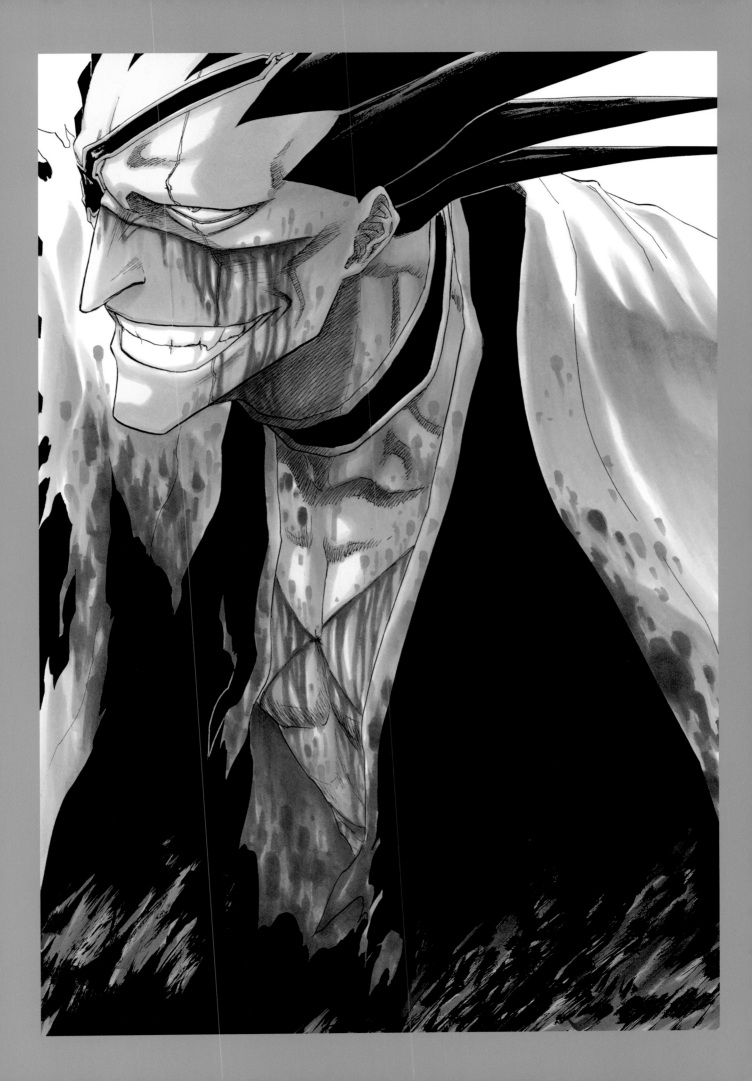

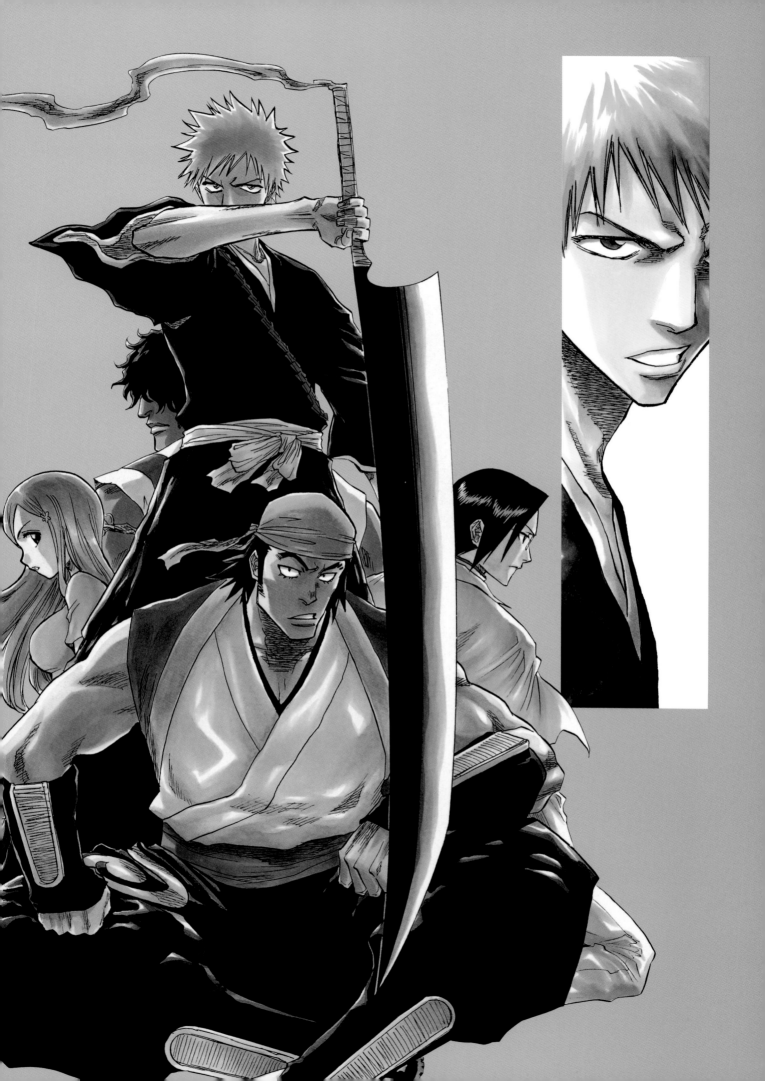

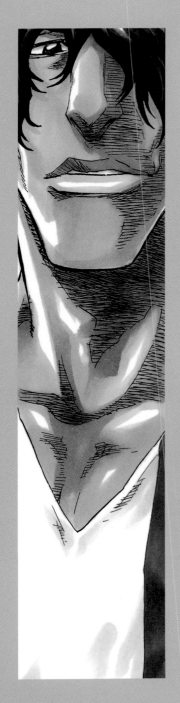
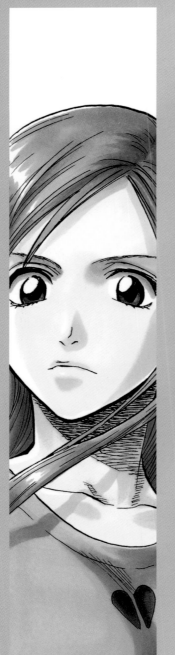
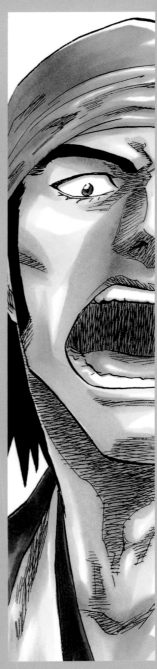
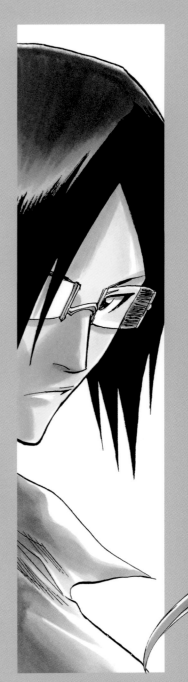
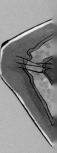

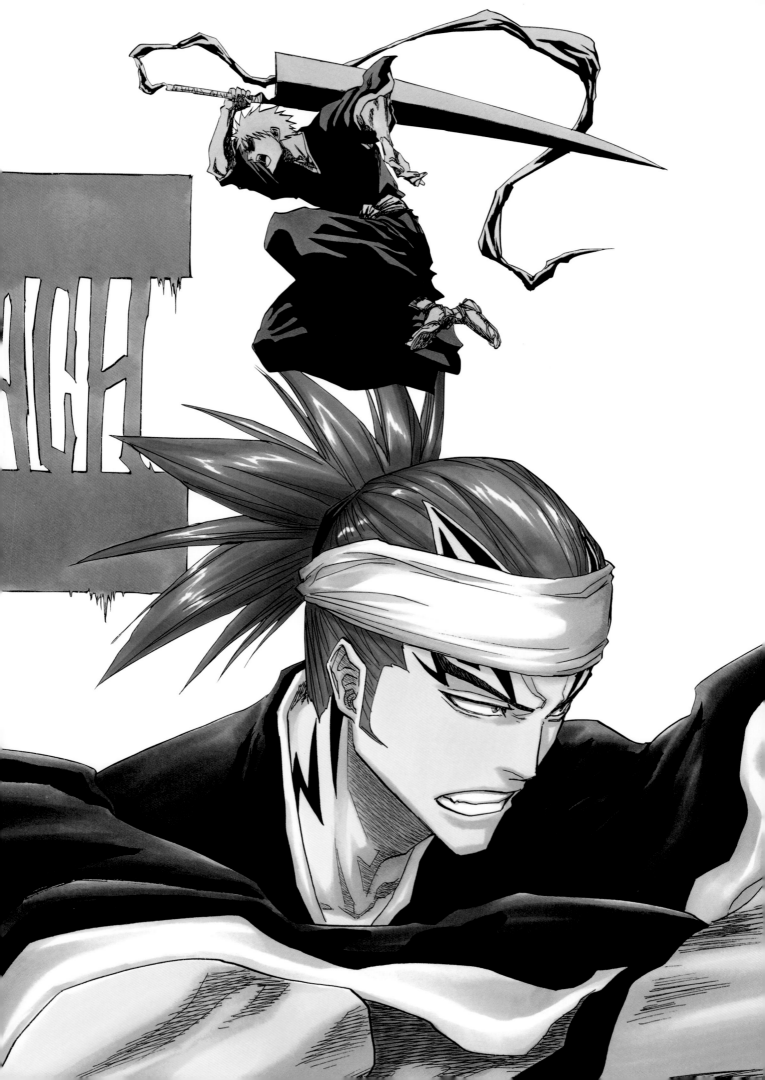

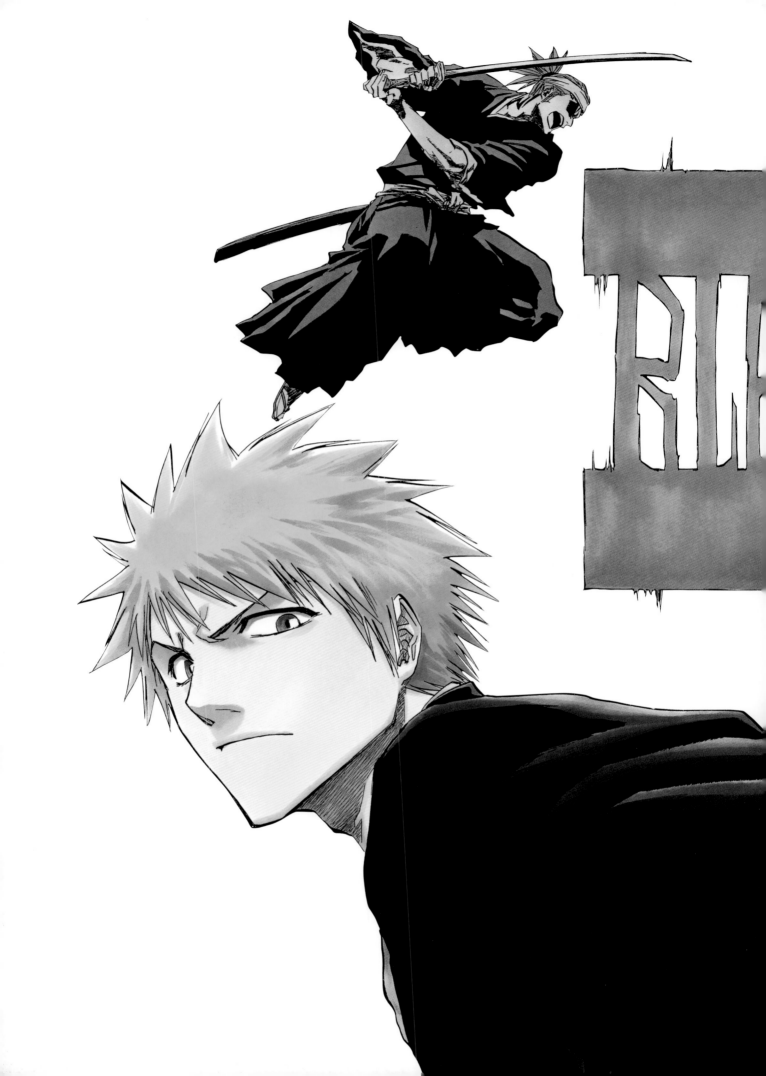

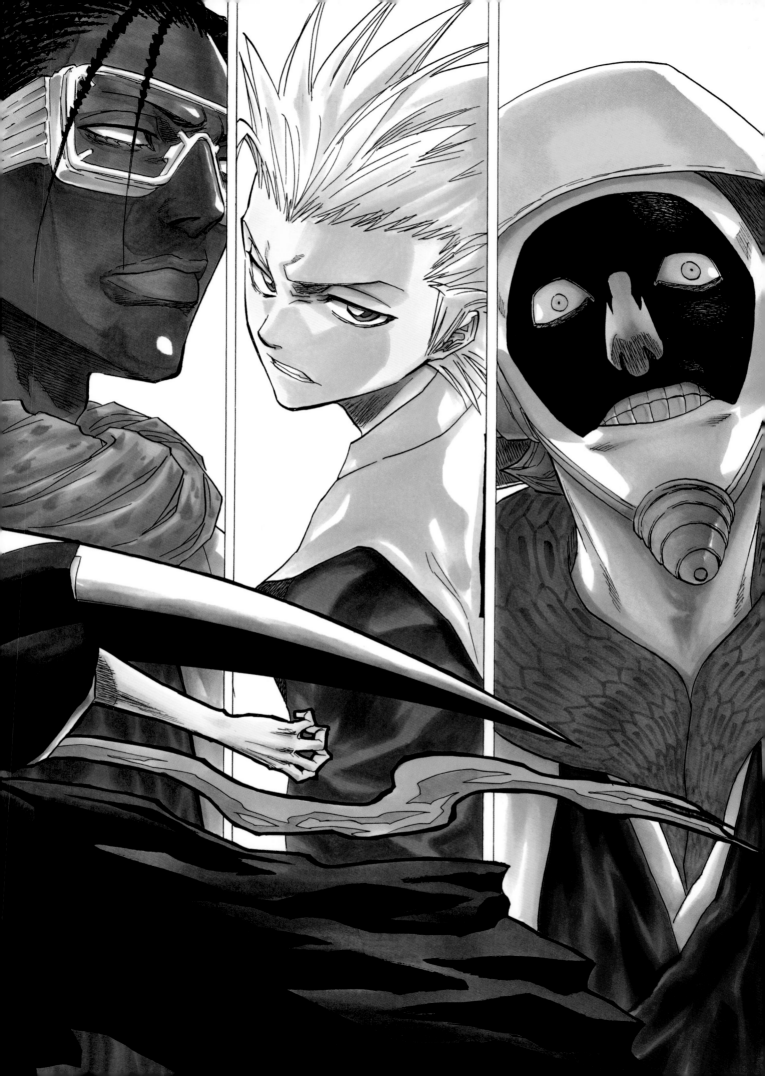

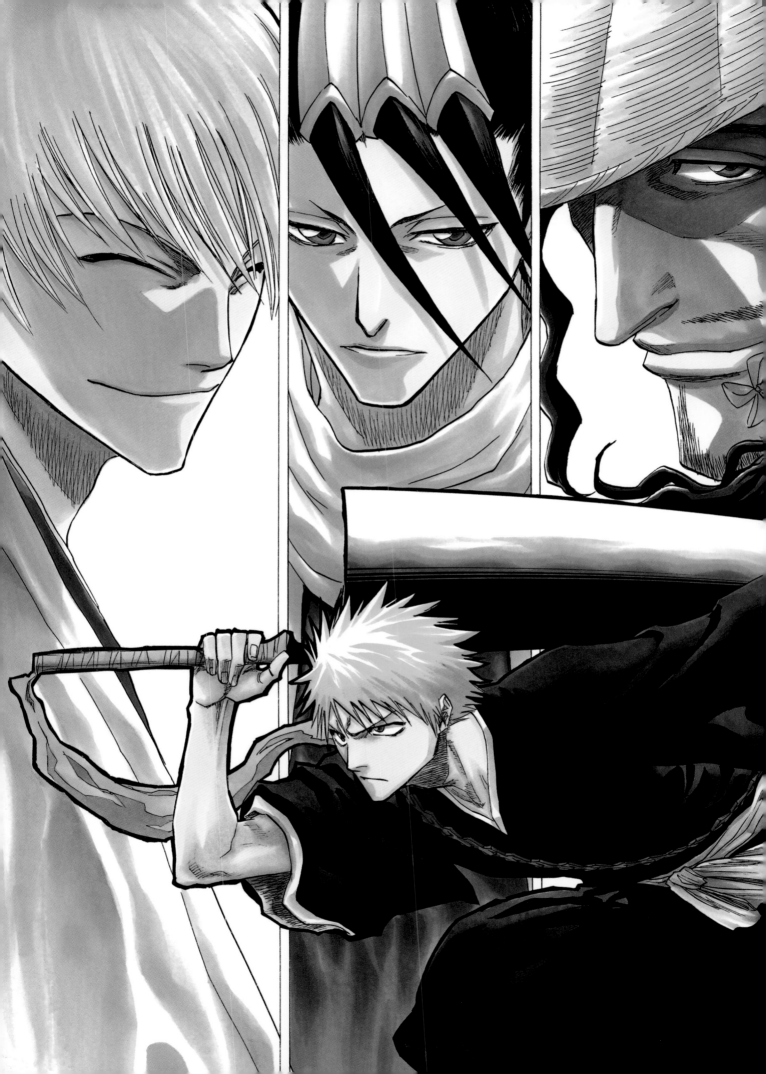

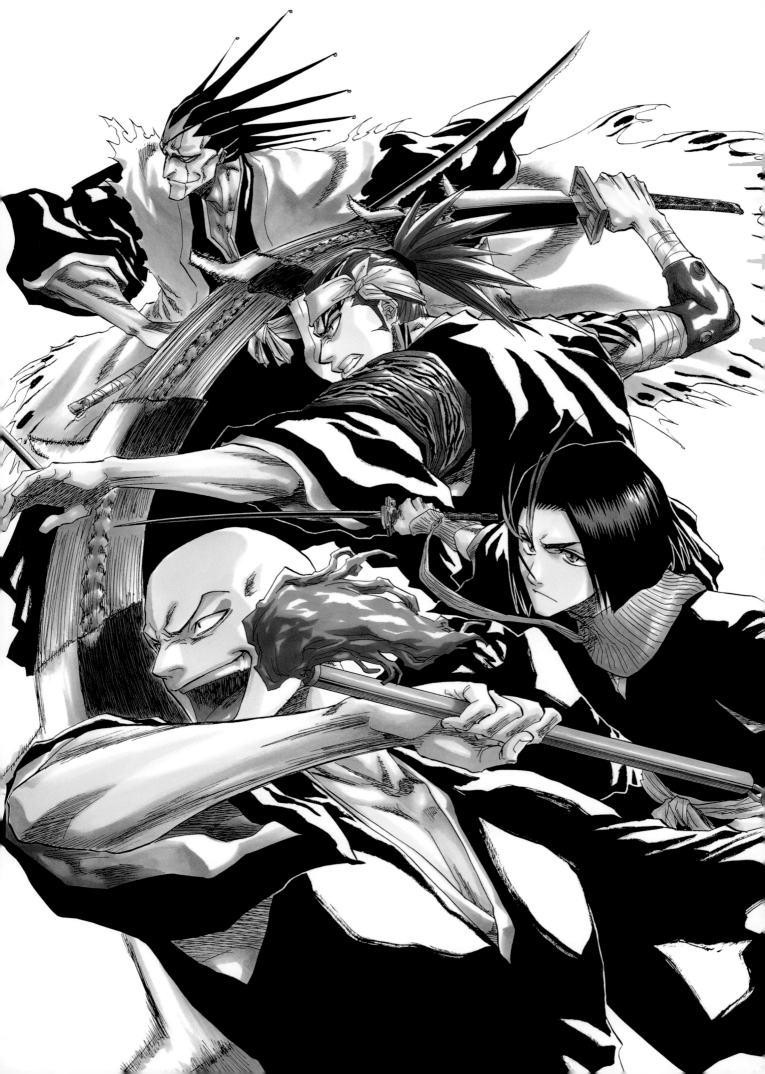

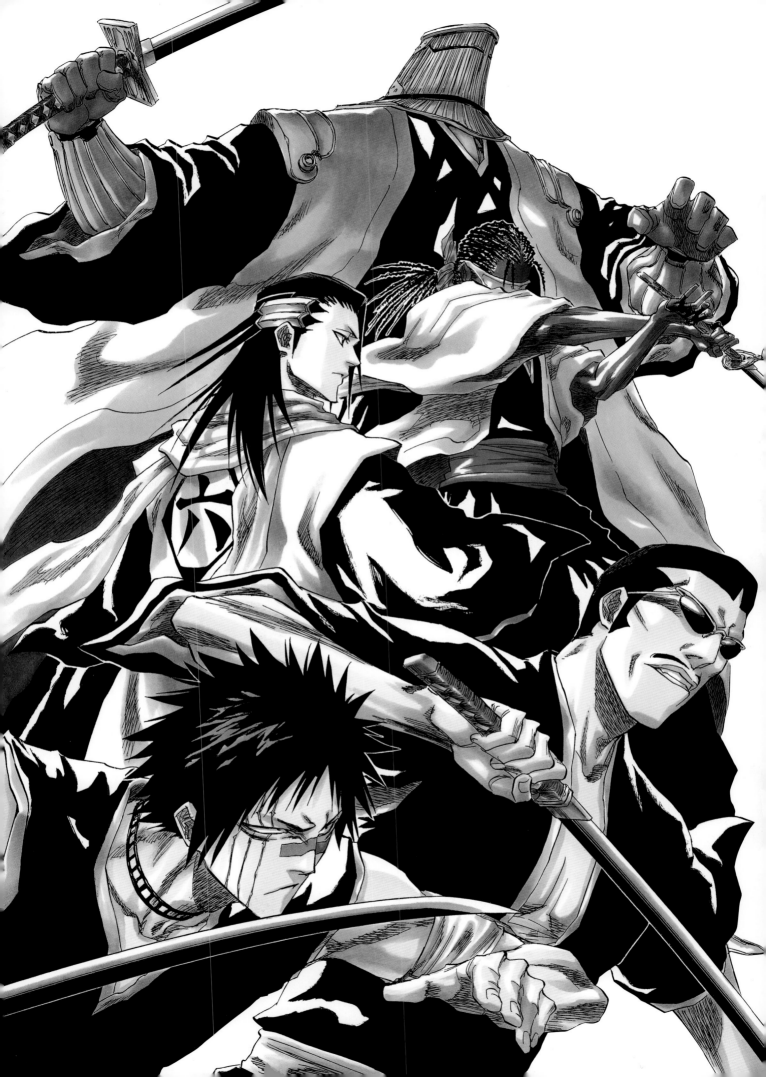

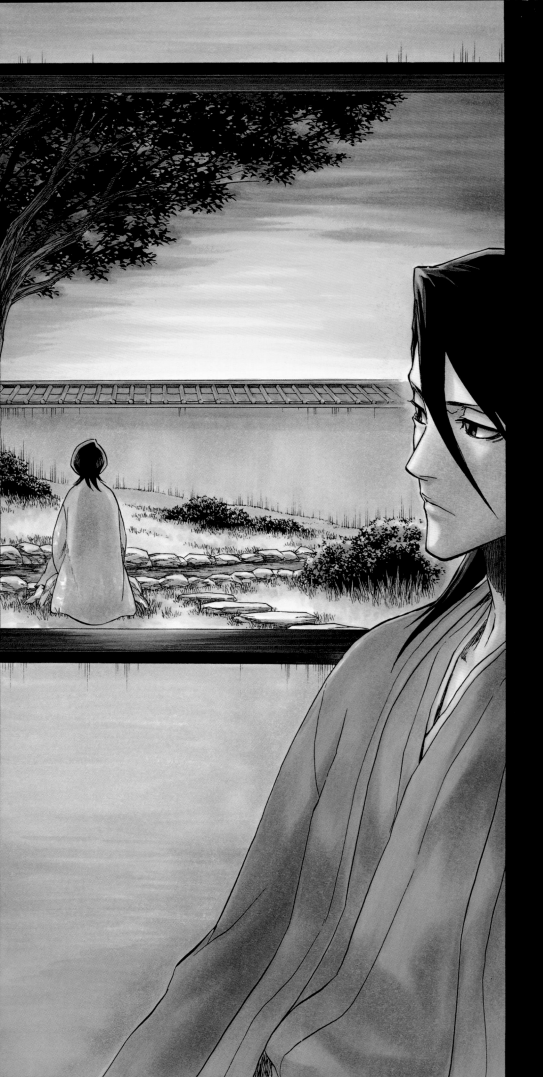

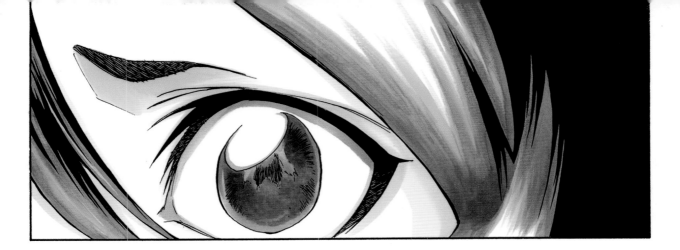

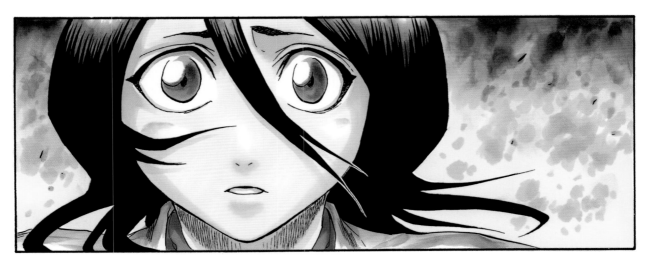

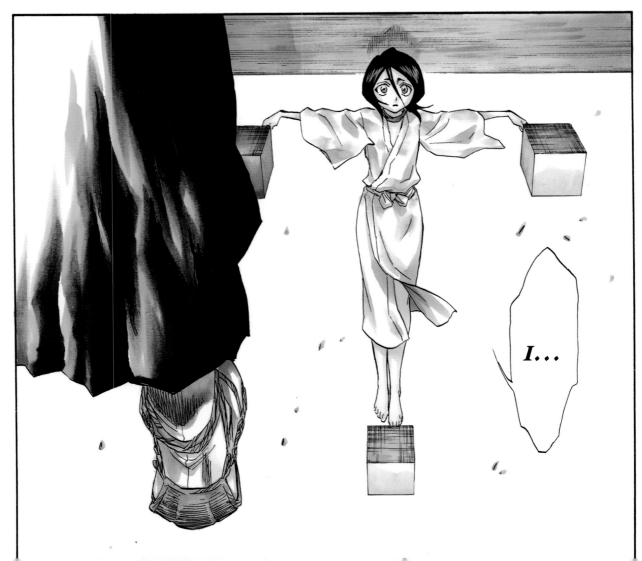

I...

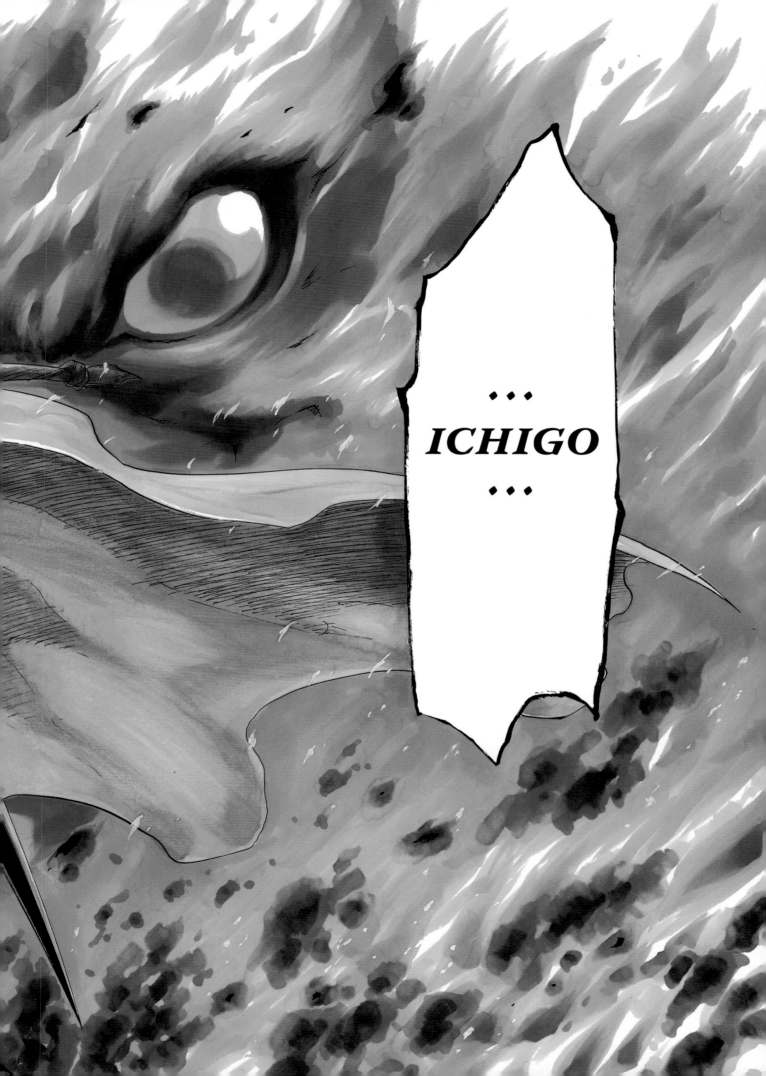

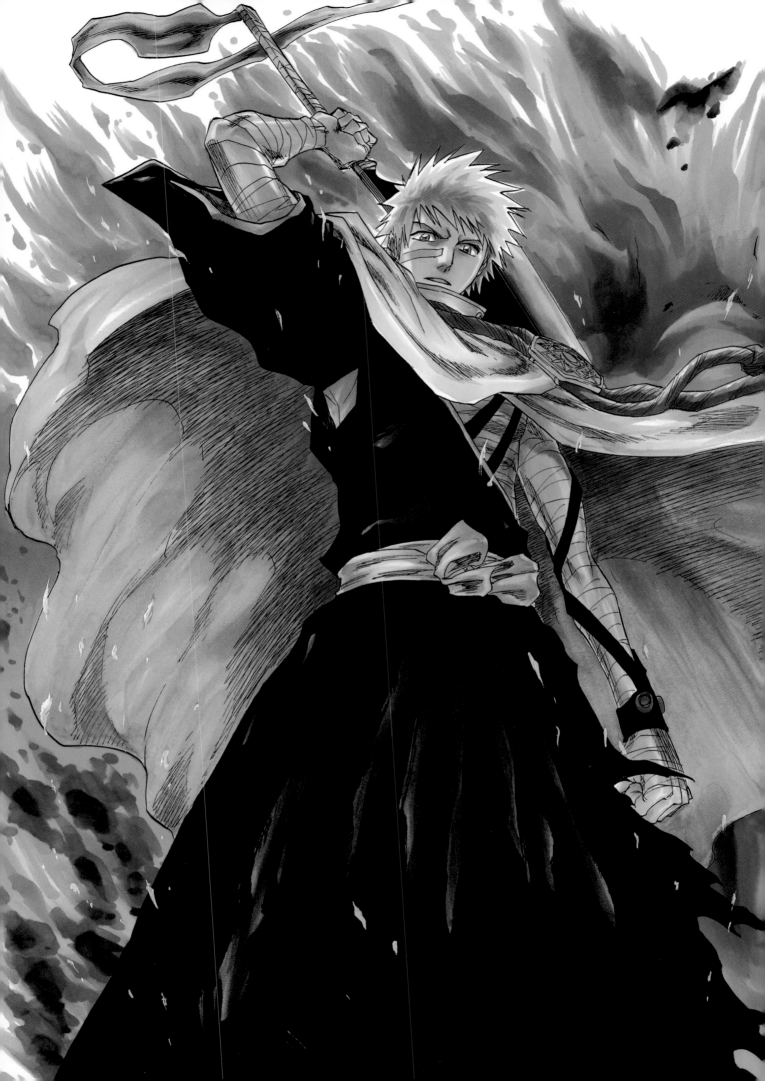

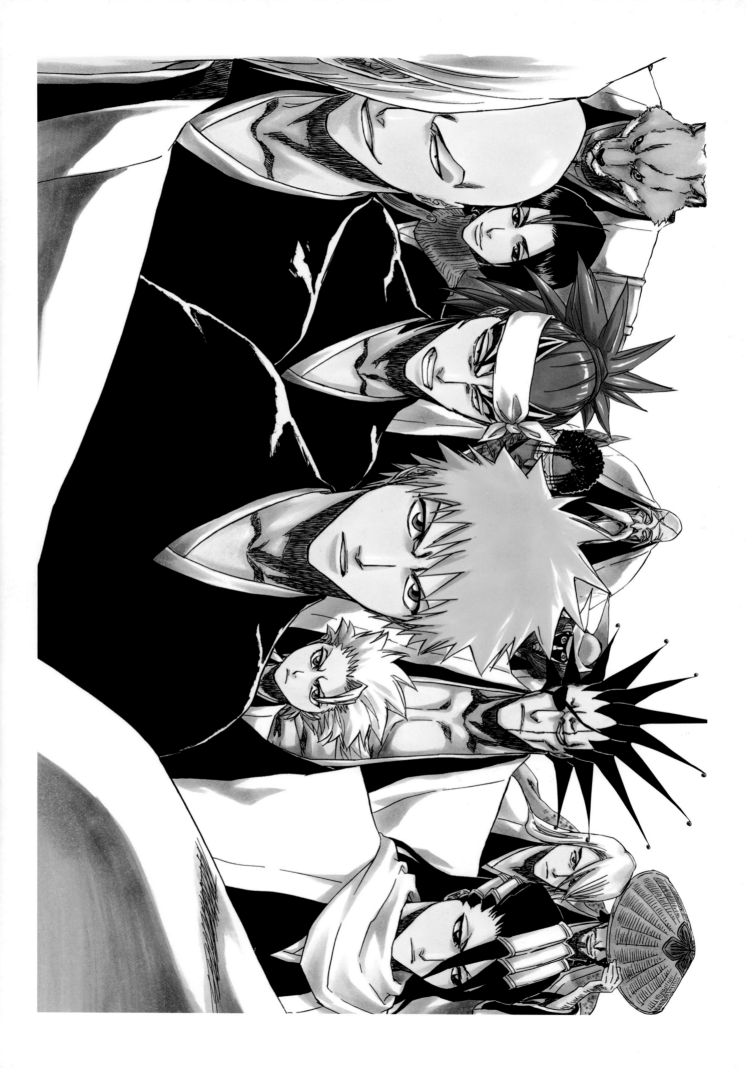

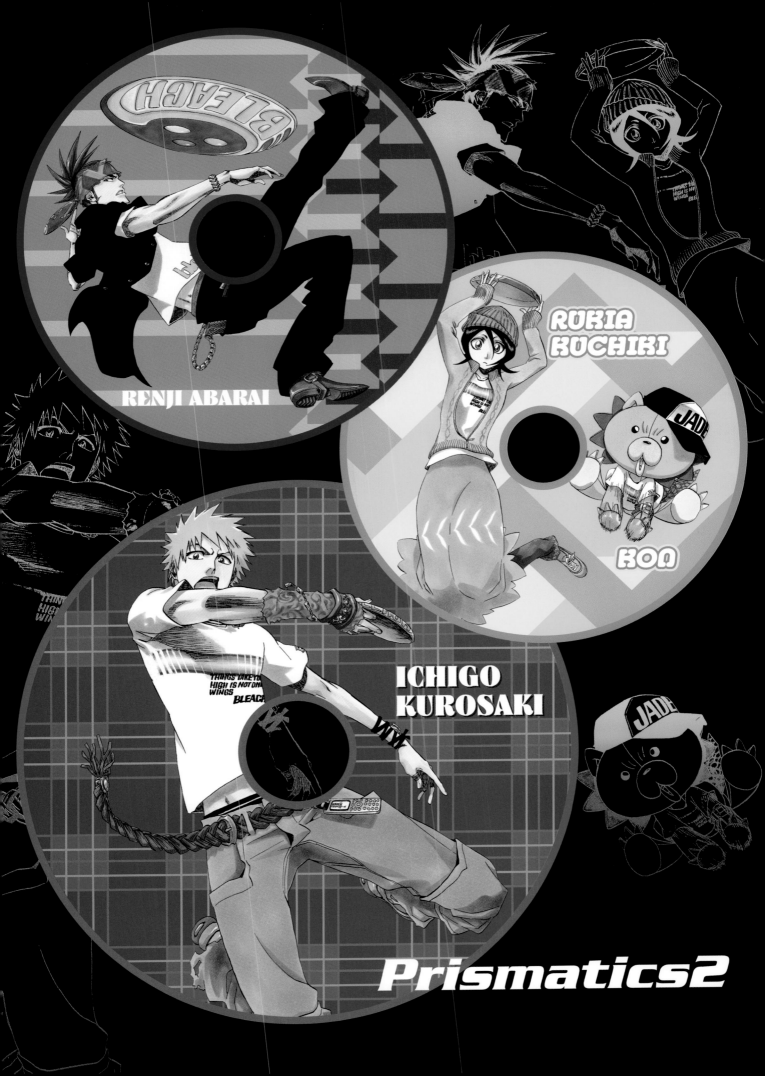

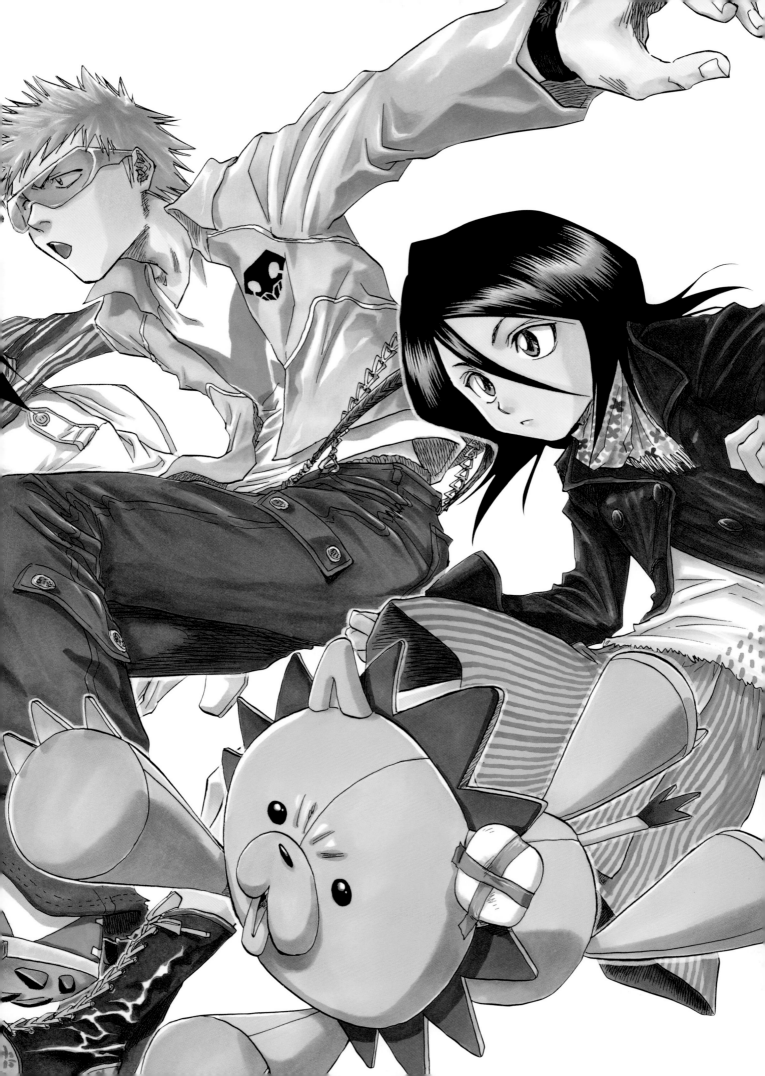

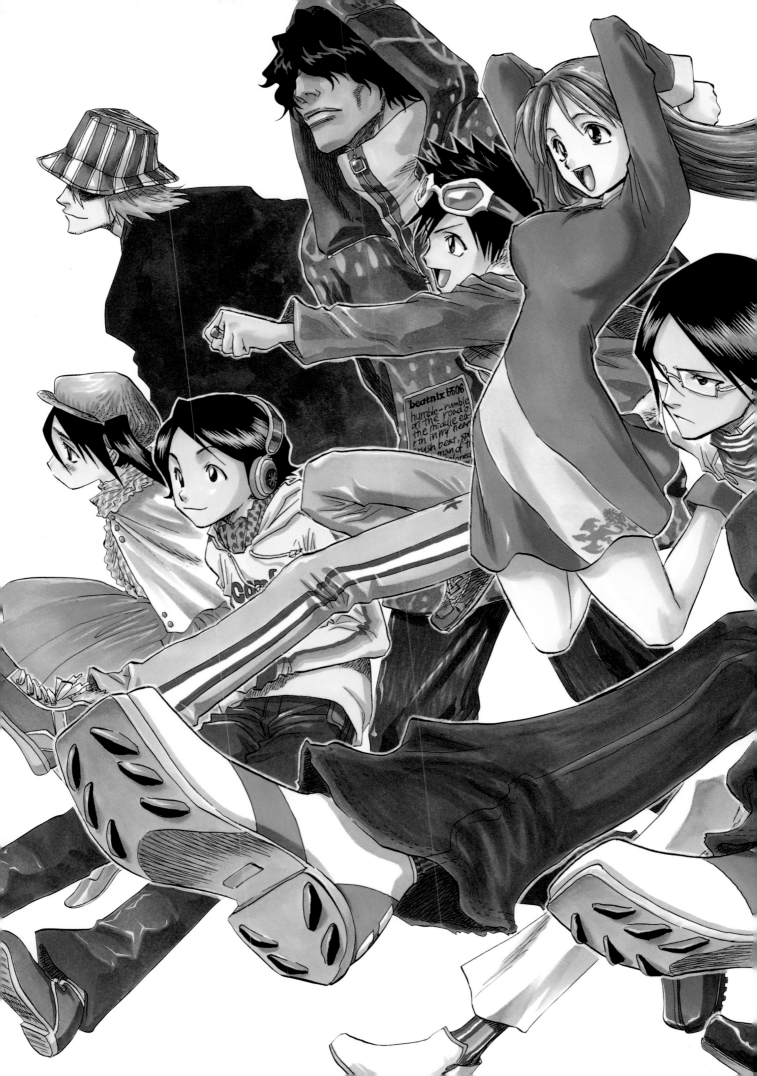

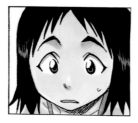
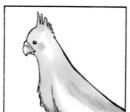
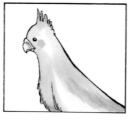
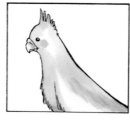
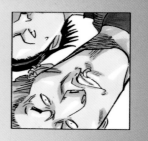
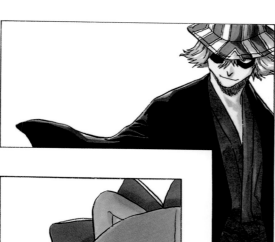
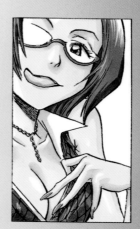
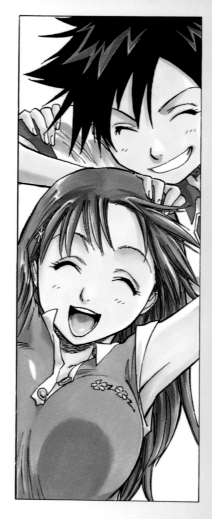
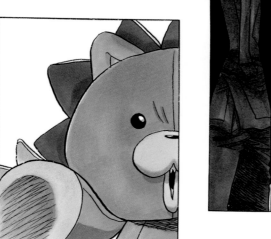
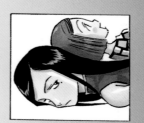
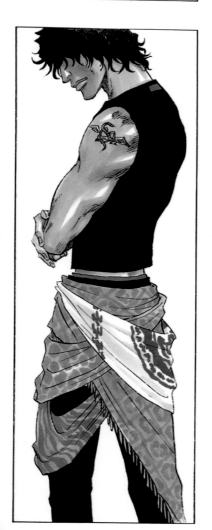
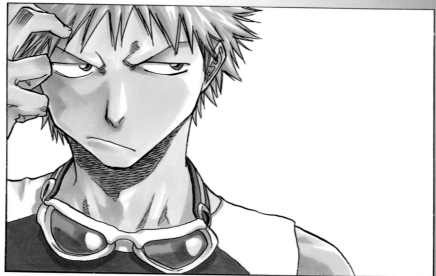
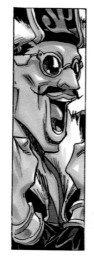

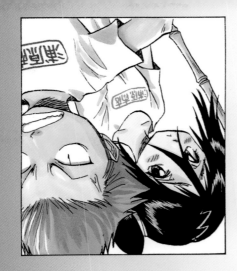
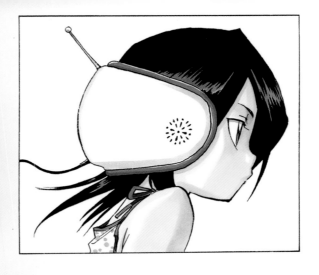
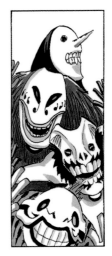
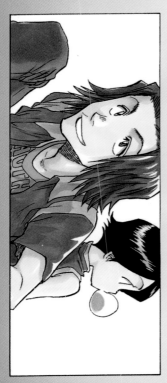
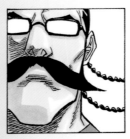
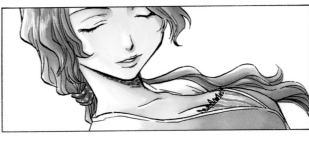
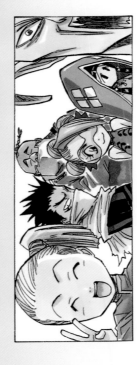
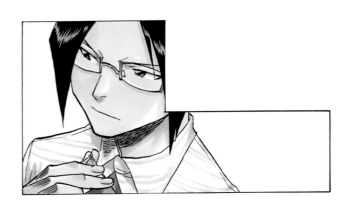
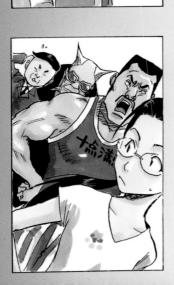
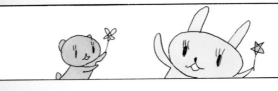
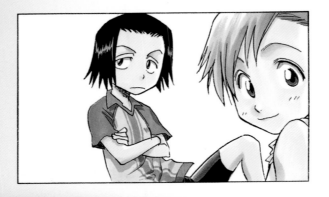
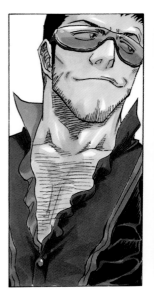

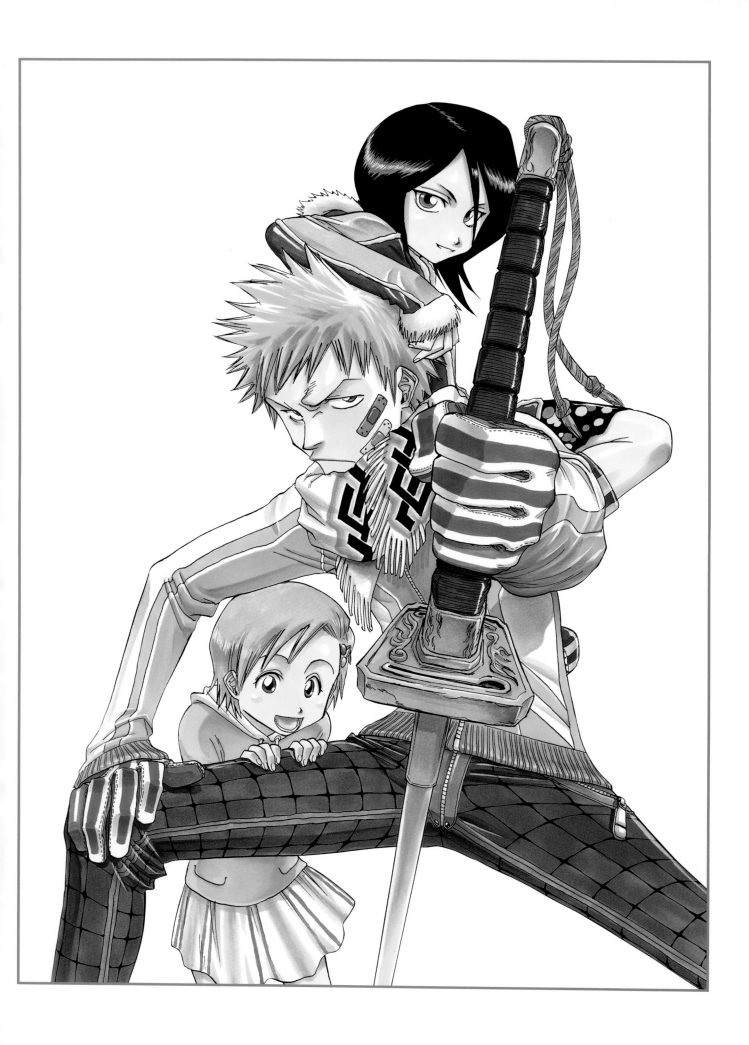

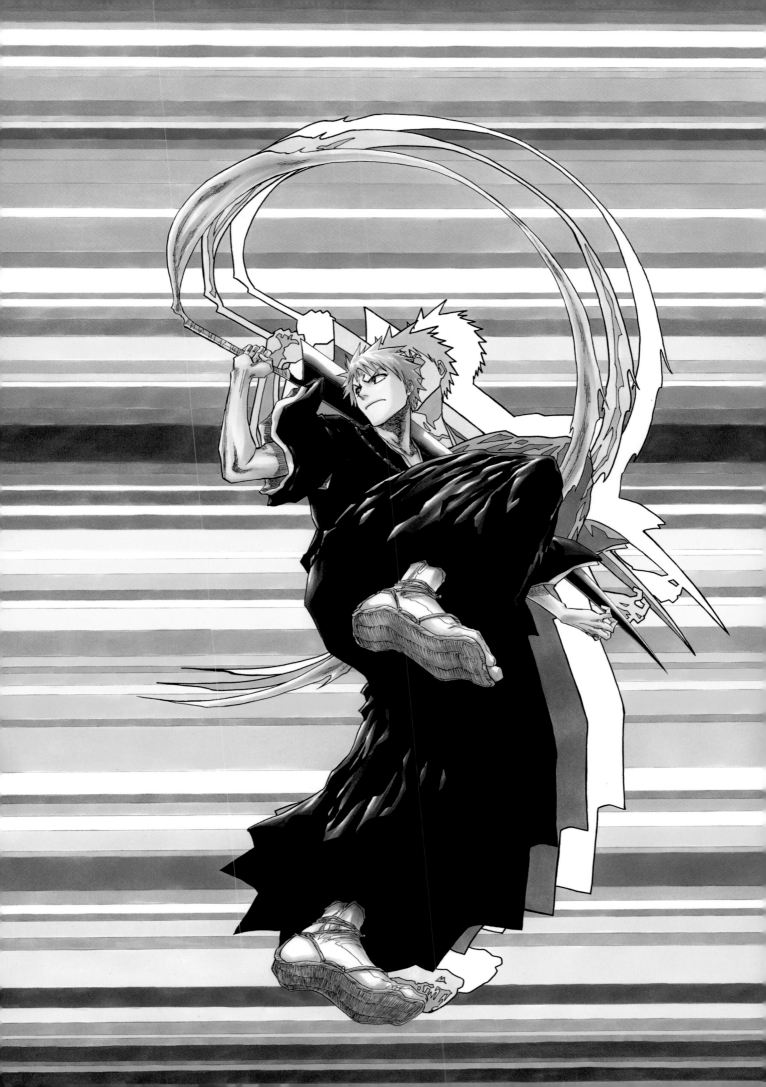

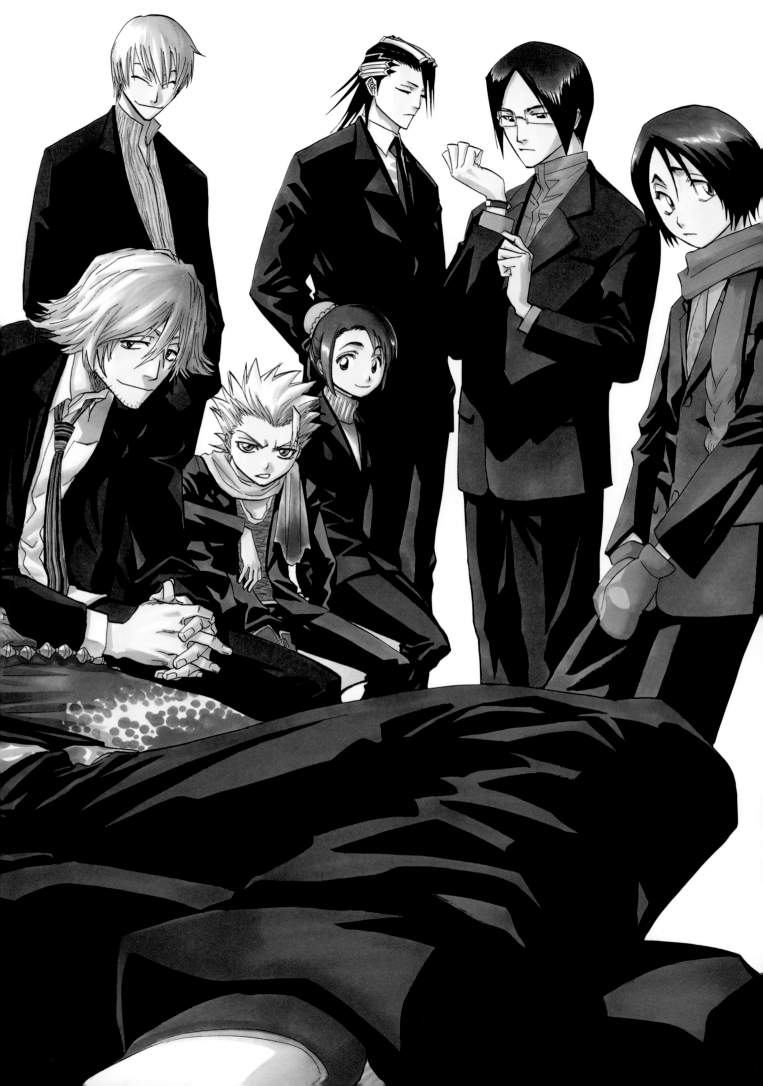

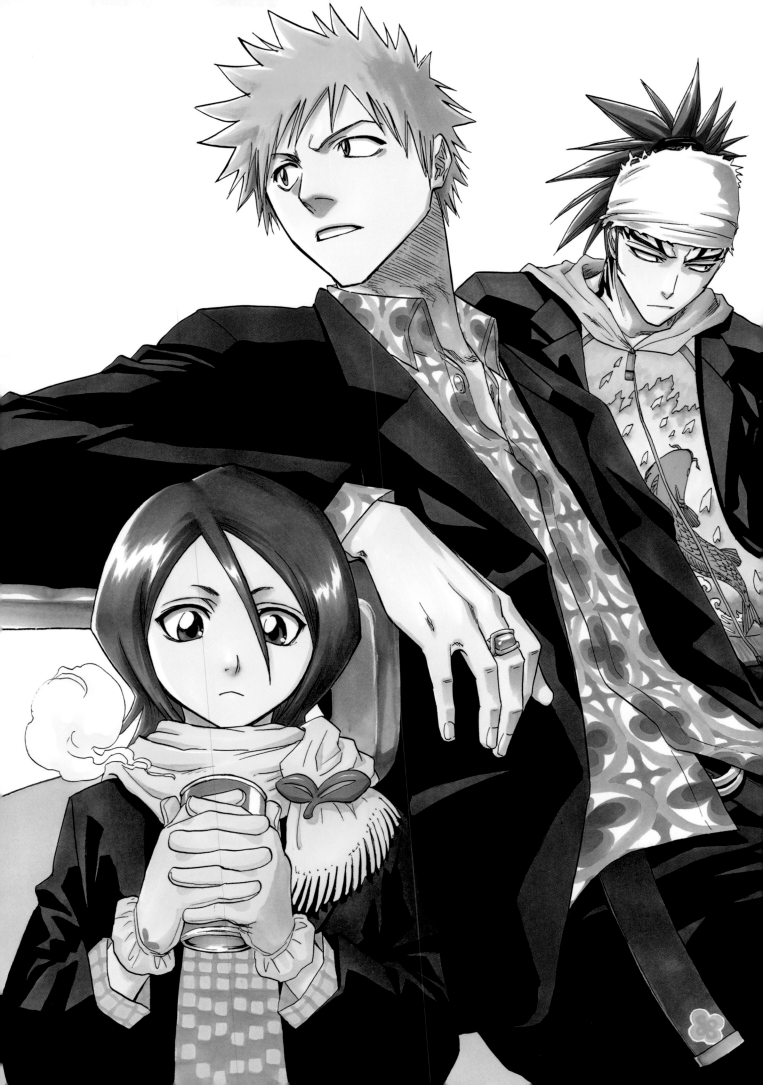

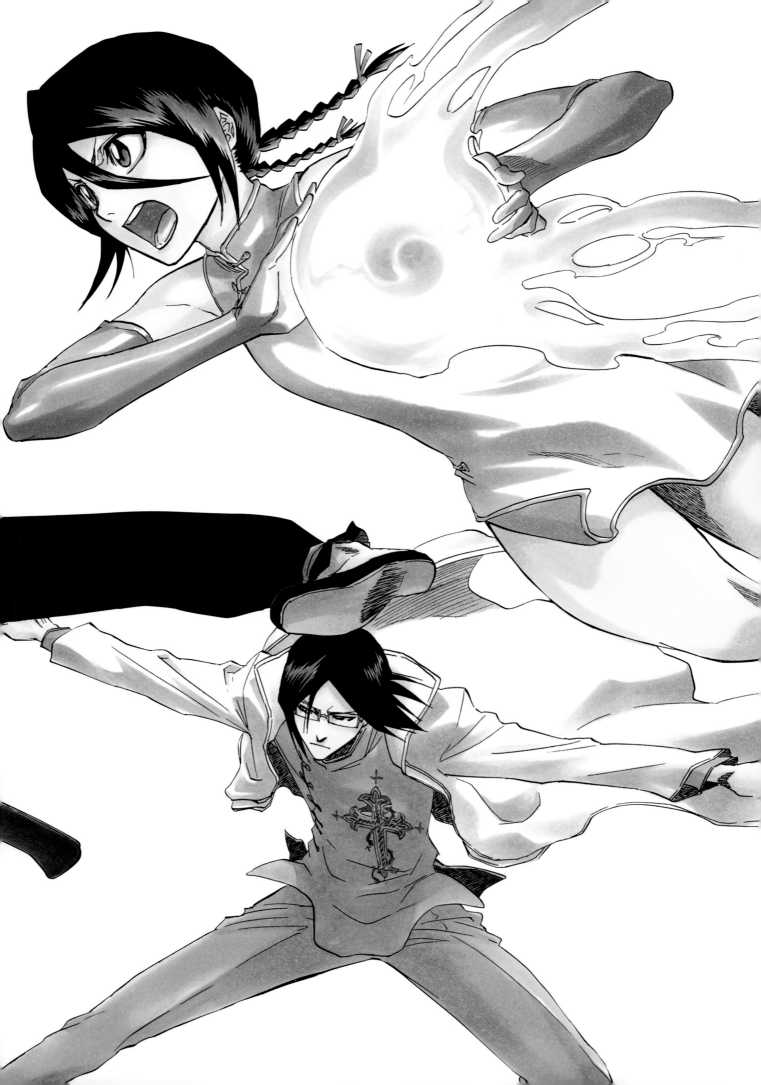

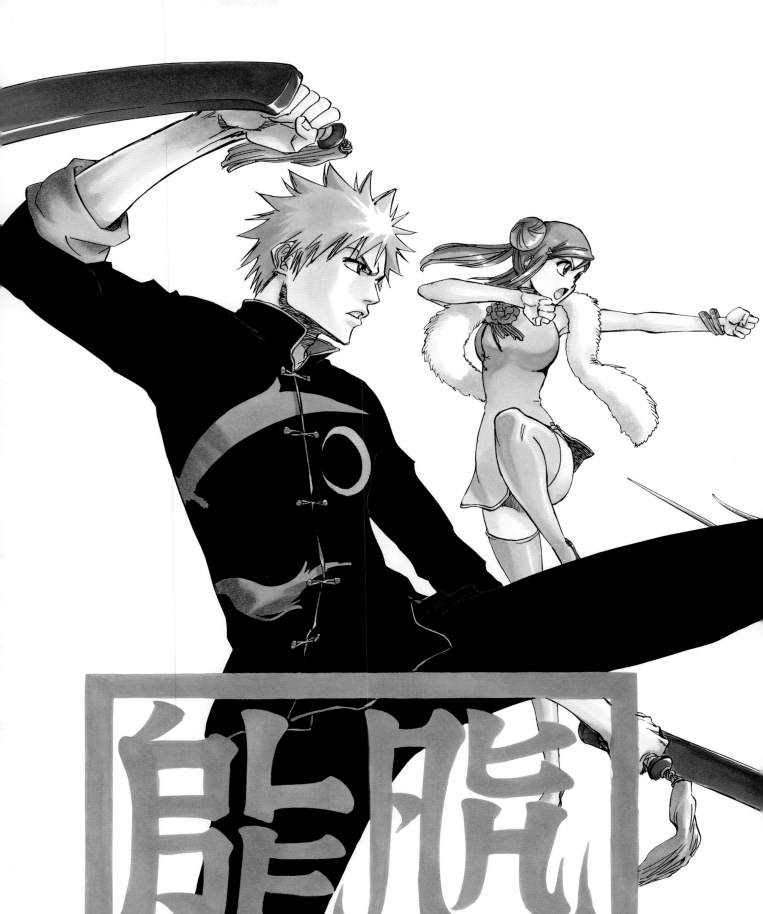

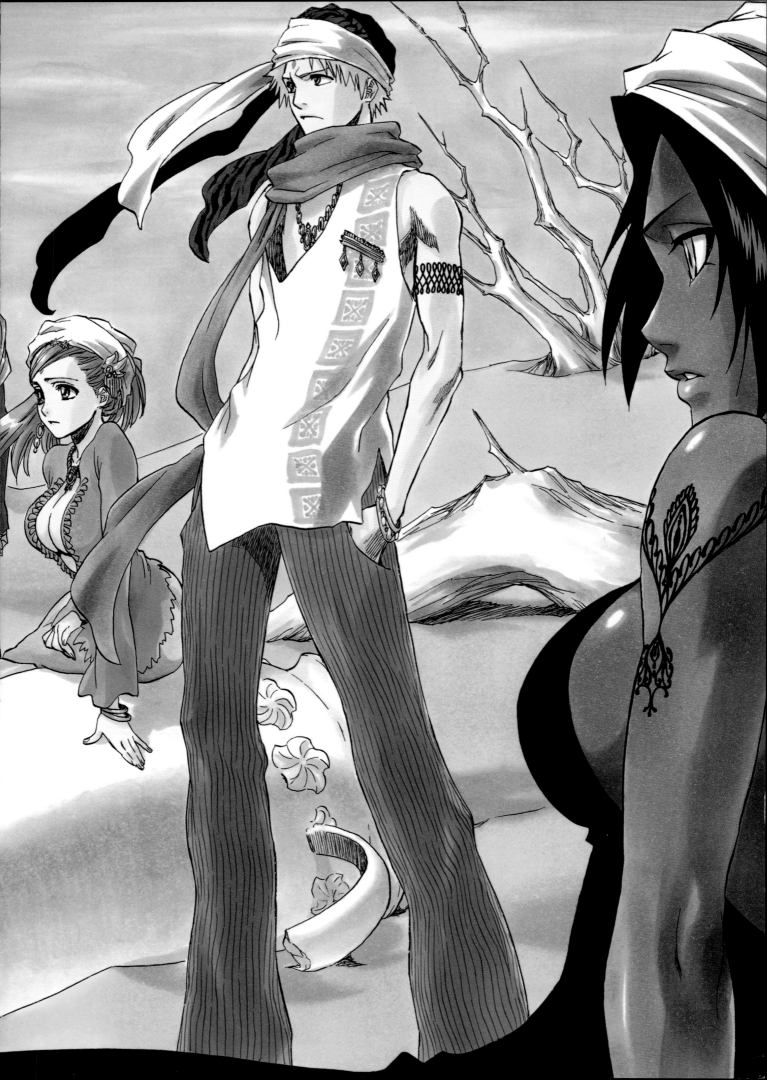

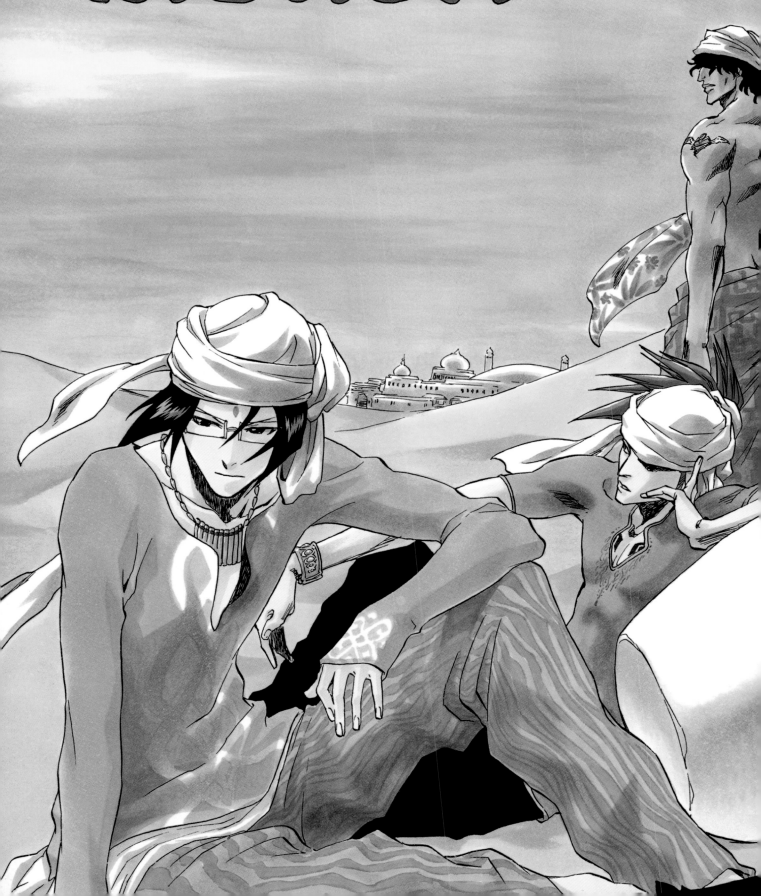

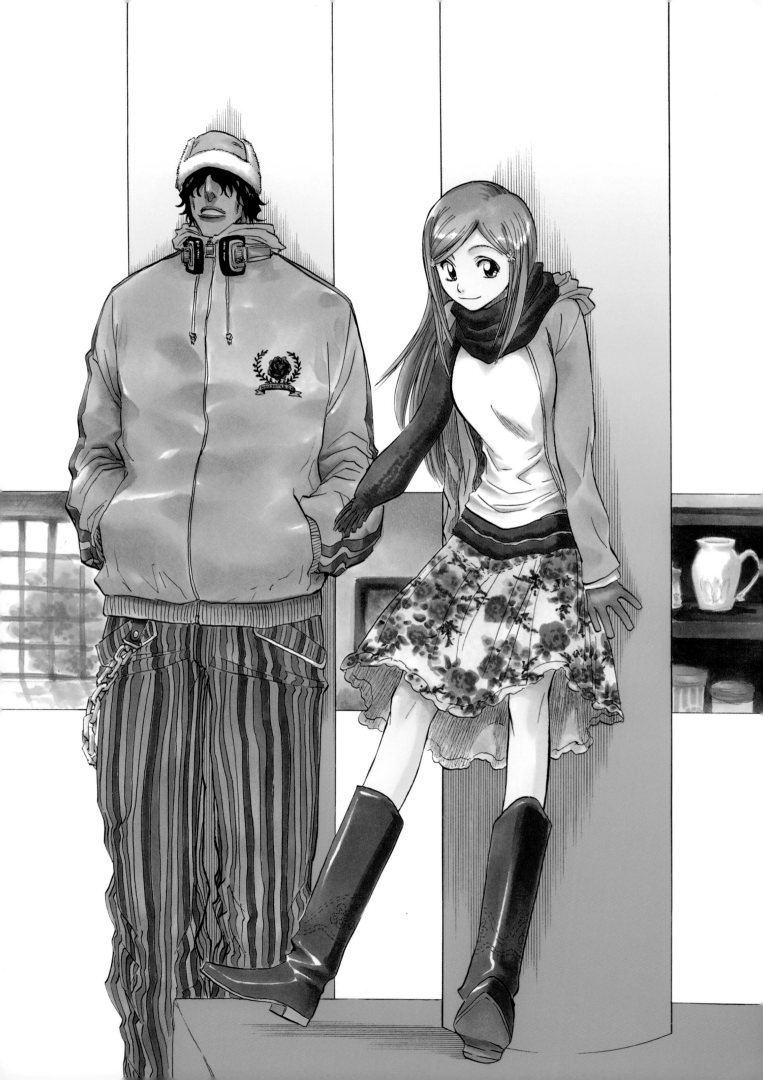

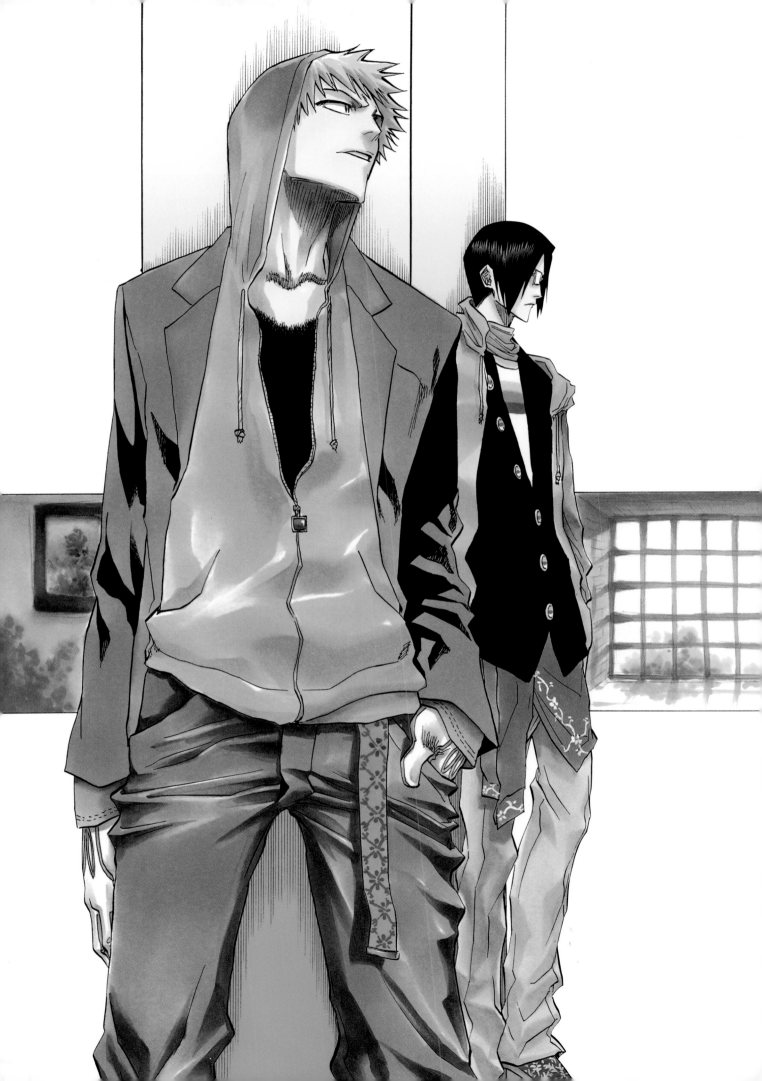

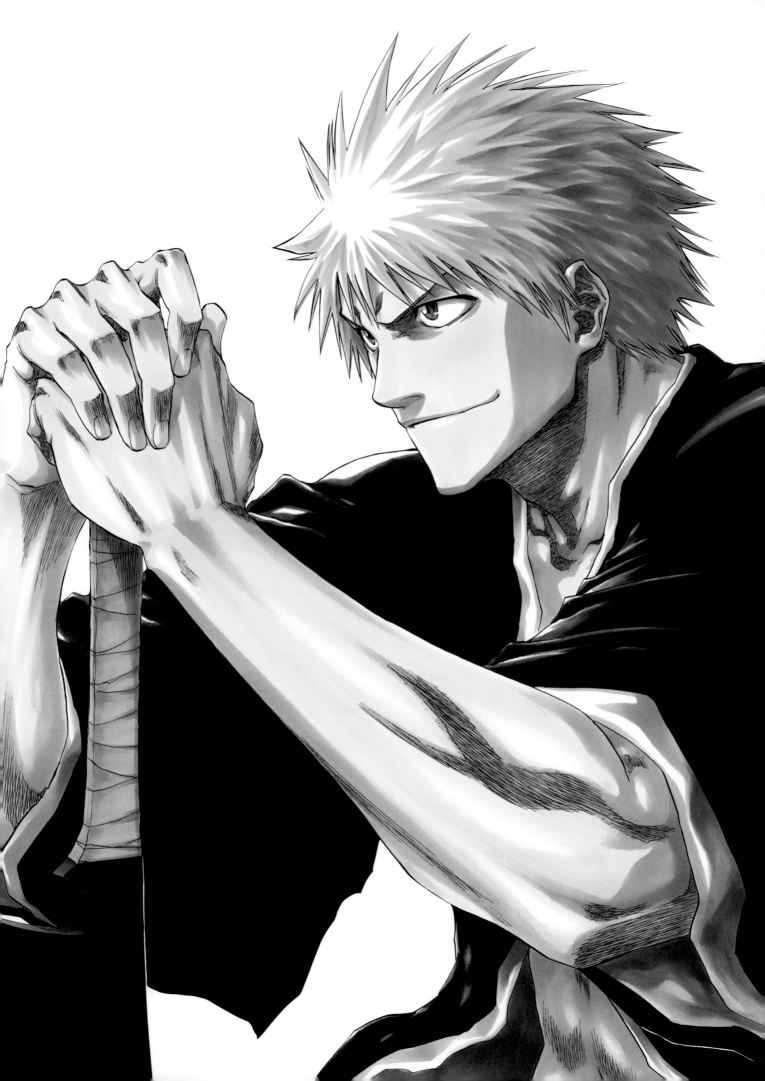

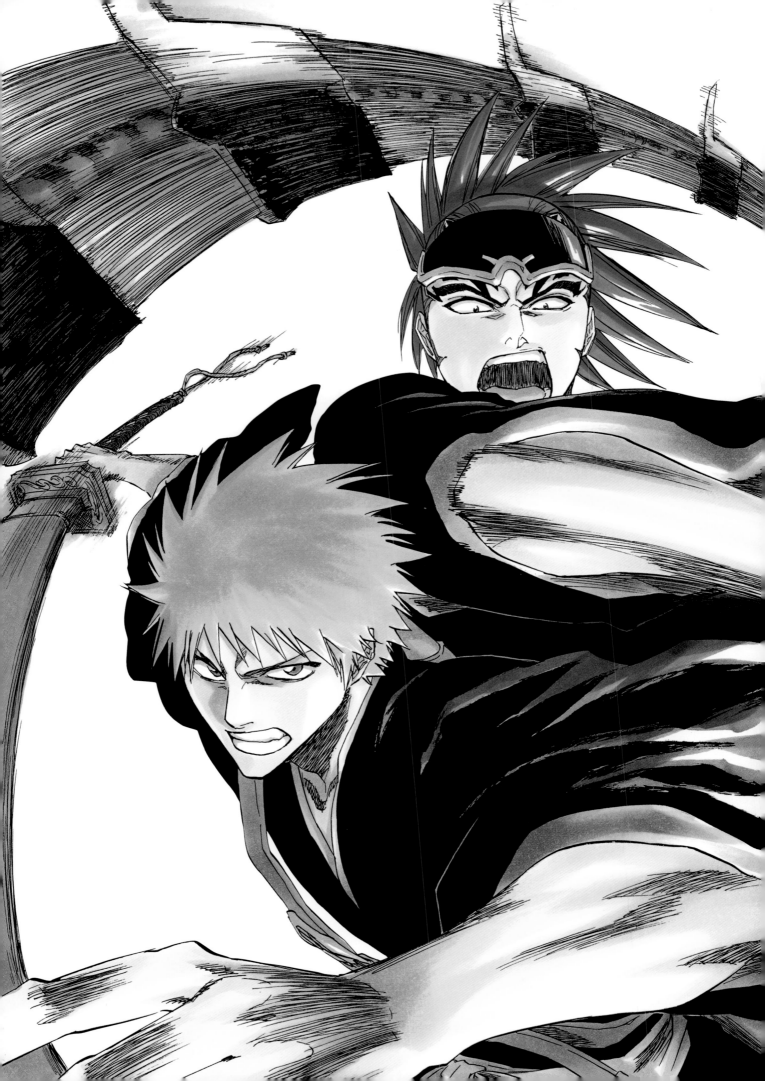

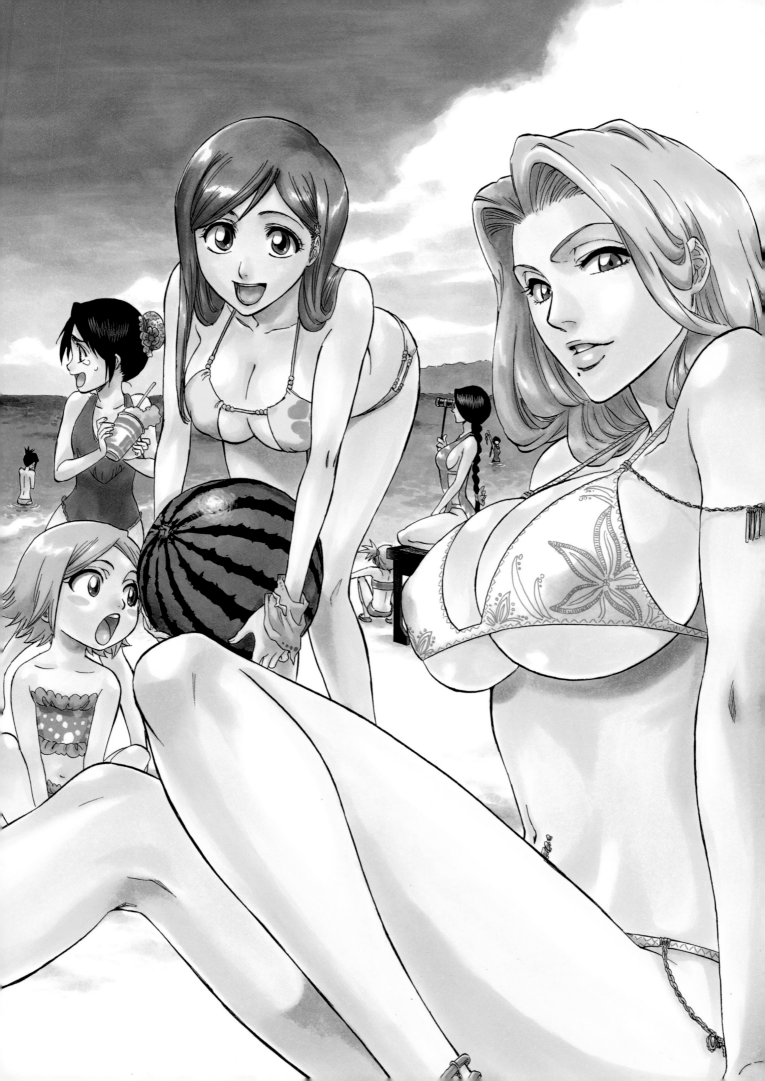

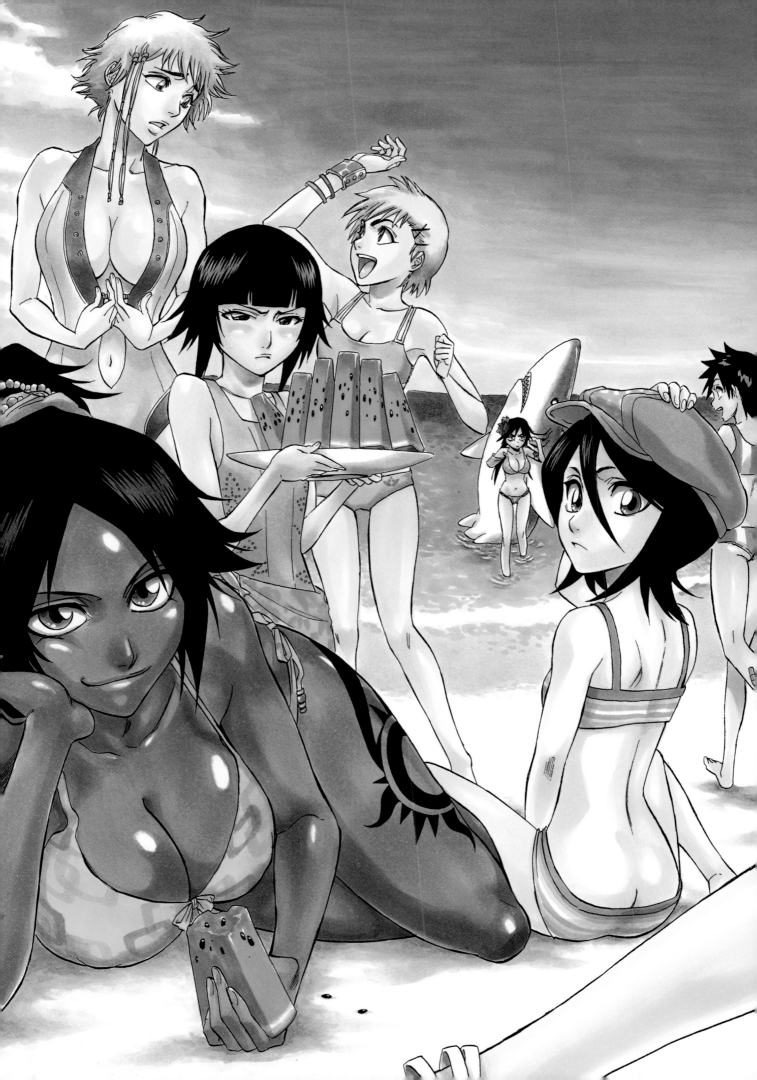

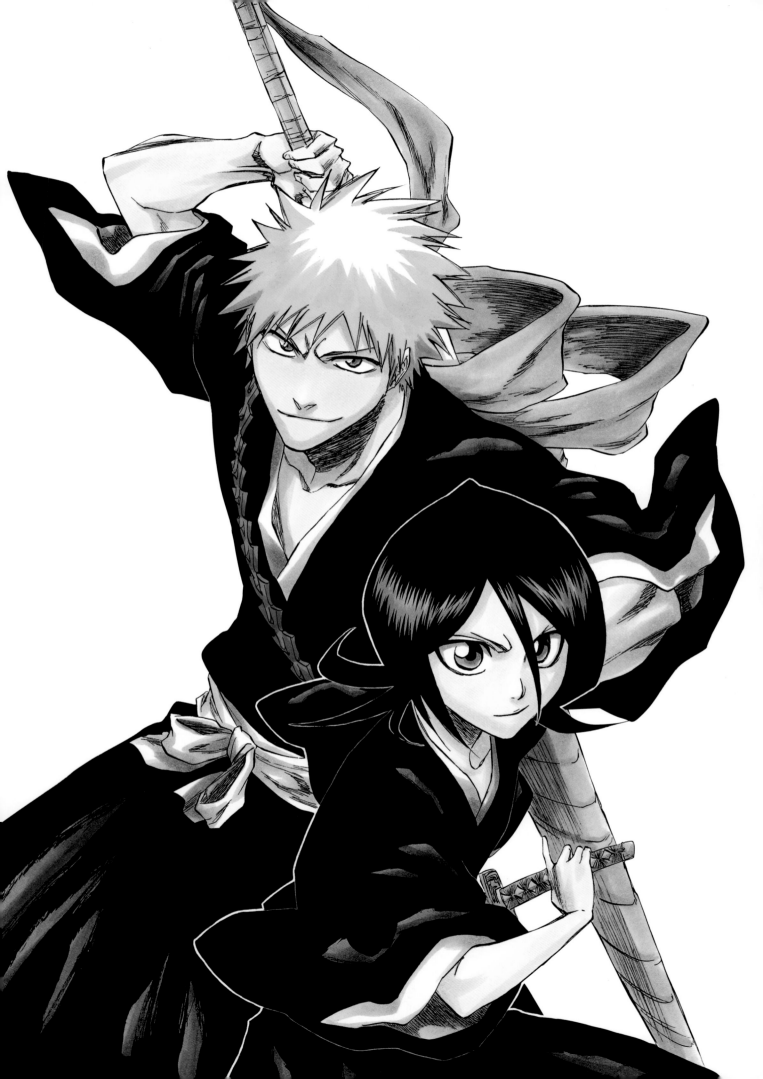

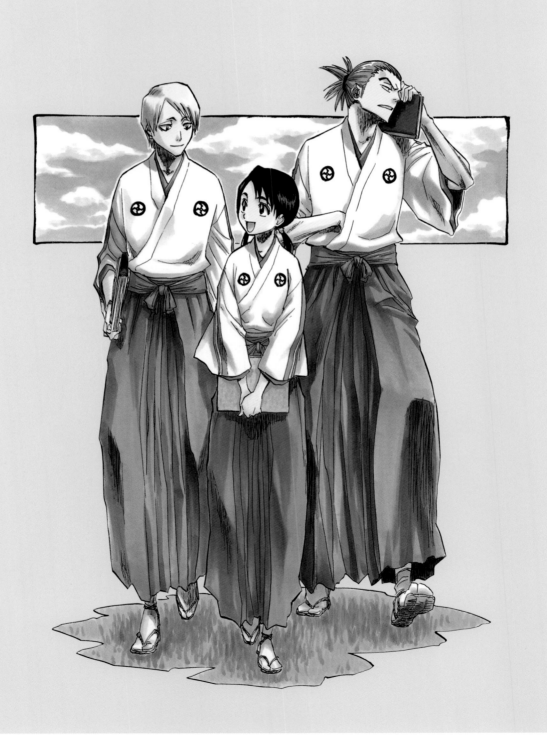

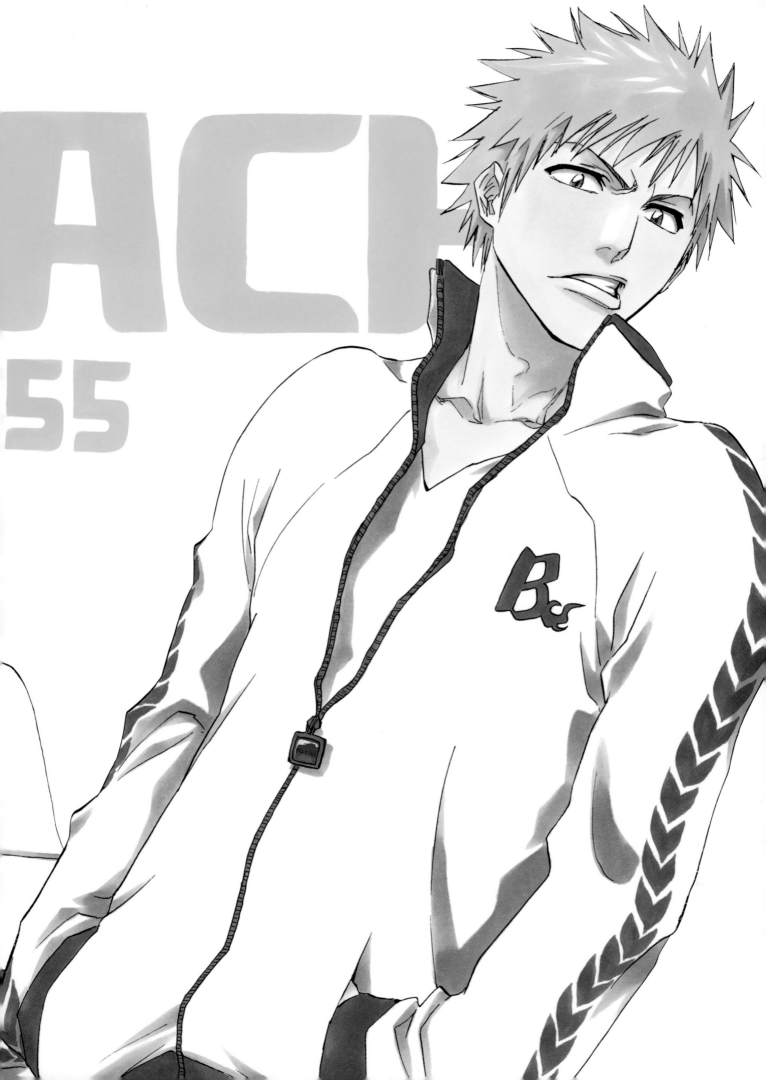

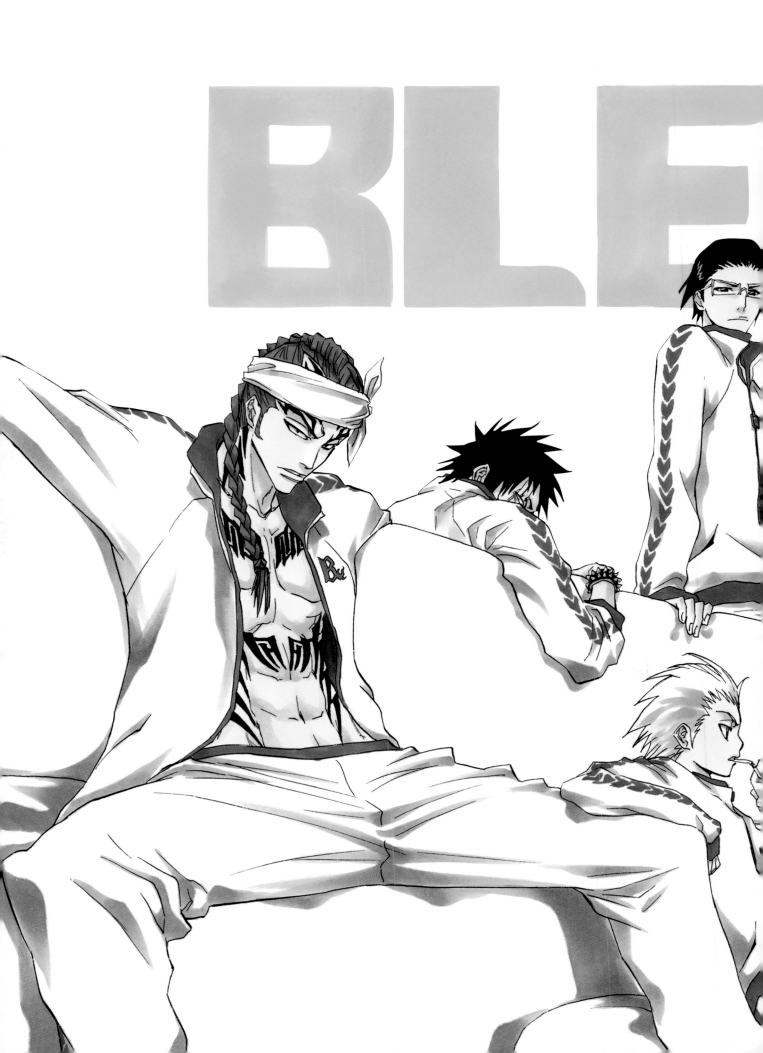

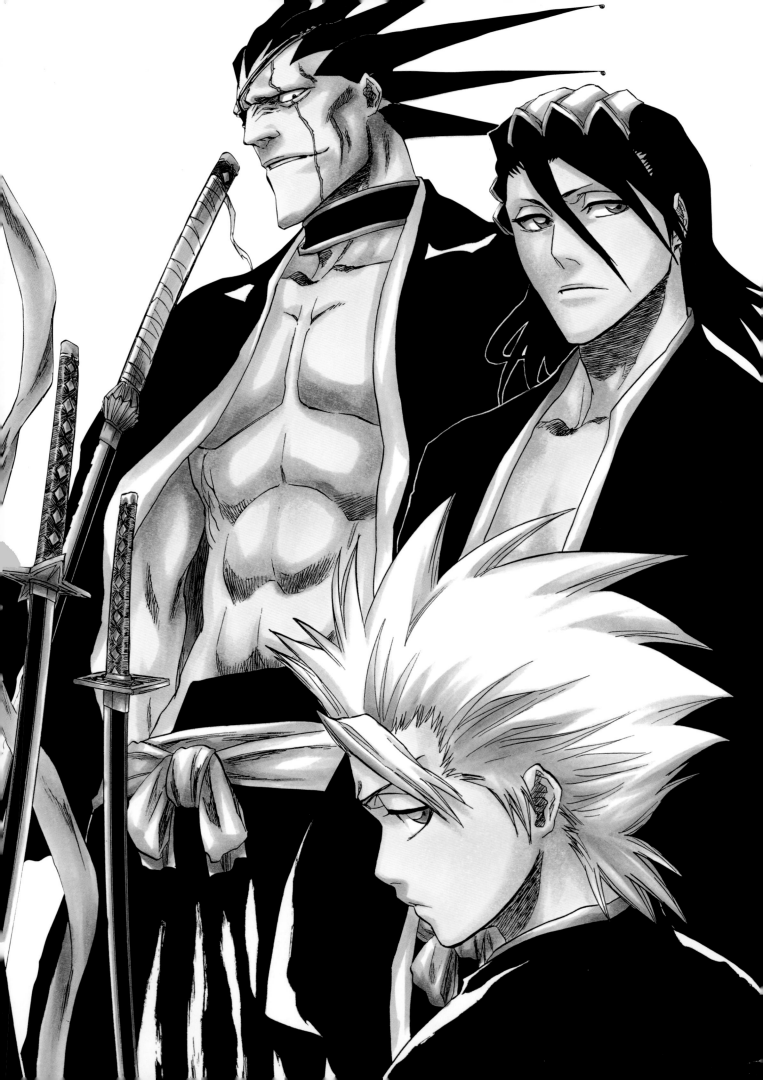

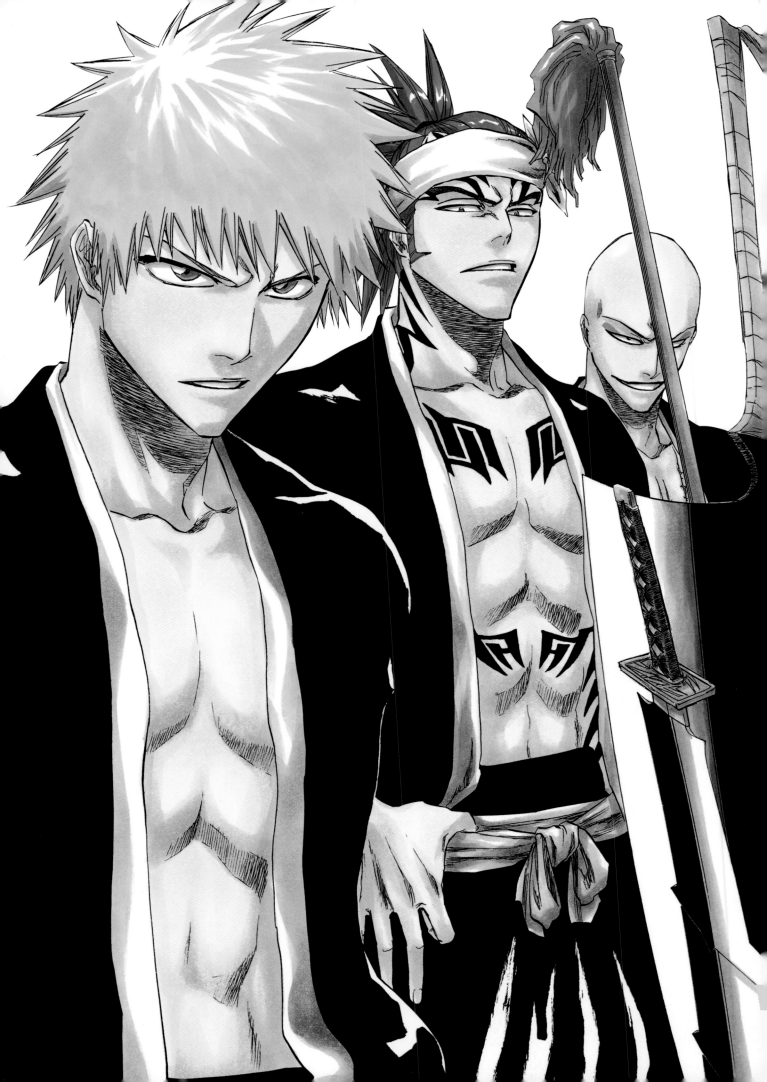

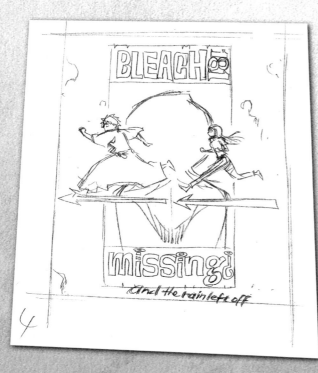
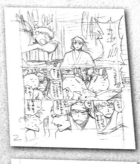
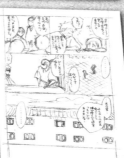
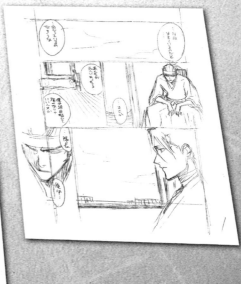
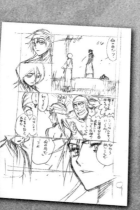
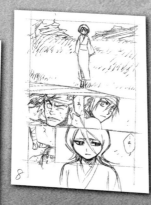
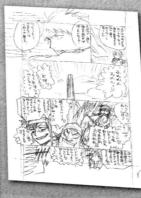
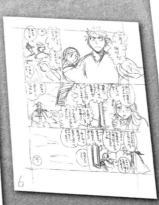
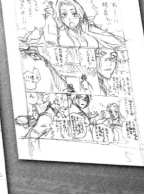
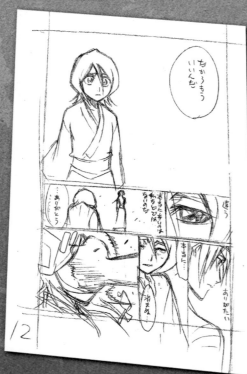
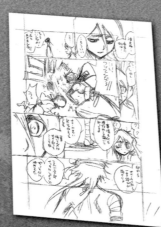
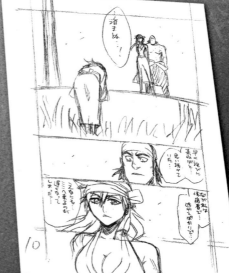

#181 *STORYBOARD*
AND THE RAIN LEFT OFF

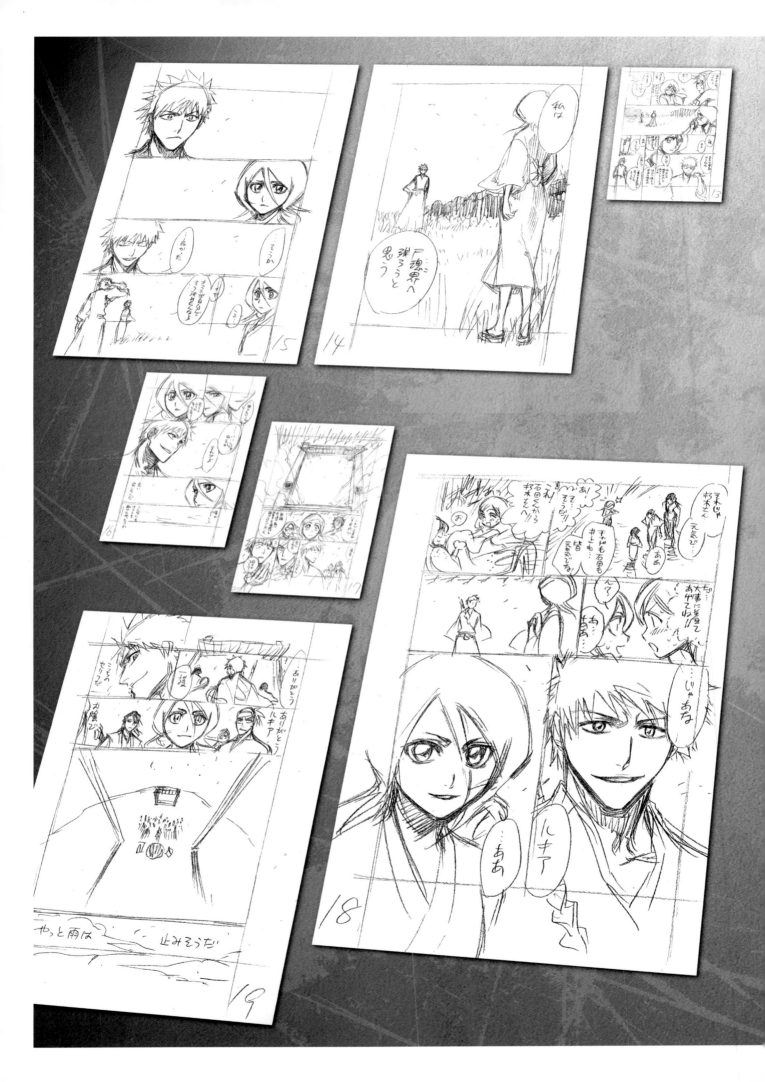

Good-bye 2005
                2006
Hallo 2007

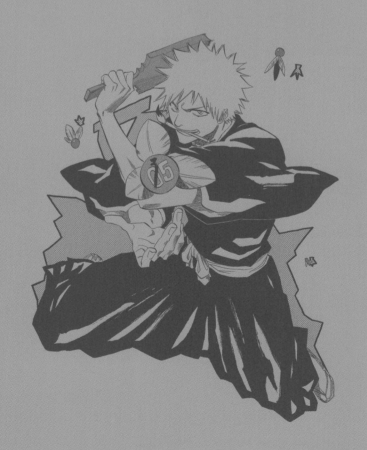

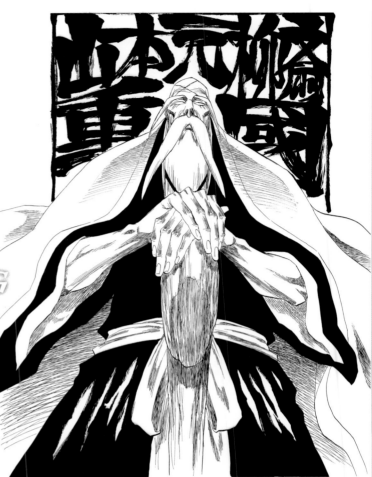

*THROUGH
YEARS OF LIFE
AND DEATH,
PURE AND IMPURE,
LOVE AND HATE—
AN UNWAVERING
TREE.*

GENRYÛSAI SHIGEKUNI YAMAMOTO

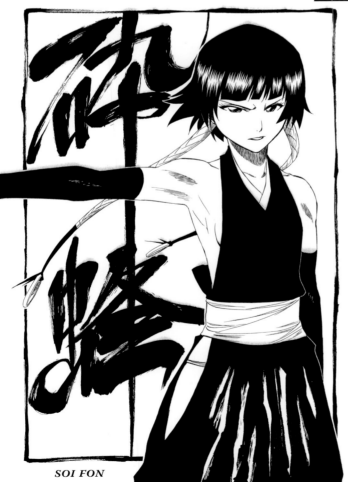

*THE
EYES
OF THE
QUEEN
STING
WITHOUT
HESITATION.*

SOI FON

GIN ICHIMARU

AN INTENTION TO KILL
BEAUTIFULLY, LIKE LOVE.

SUPREME HEALING.

A WHITE FLOWER SMILING QUIETLY.

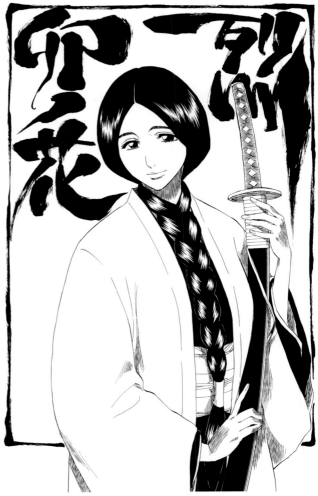

RETSU UNOHANA

FROM THE HEAVENS, FROM THE STARS, AND FROM EVEN HIGHER...

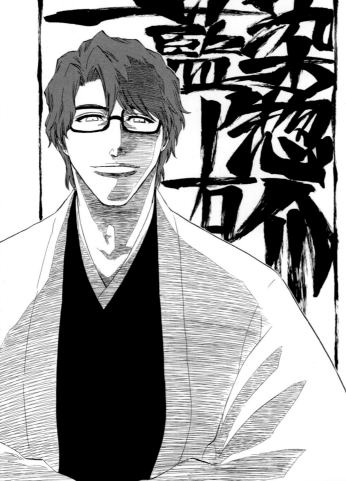

SÔSUKE AIZEN

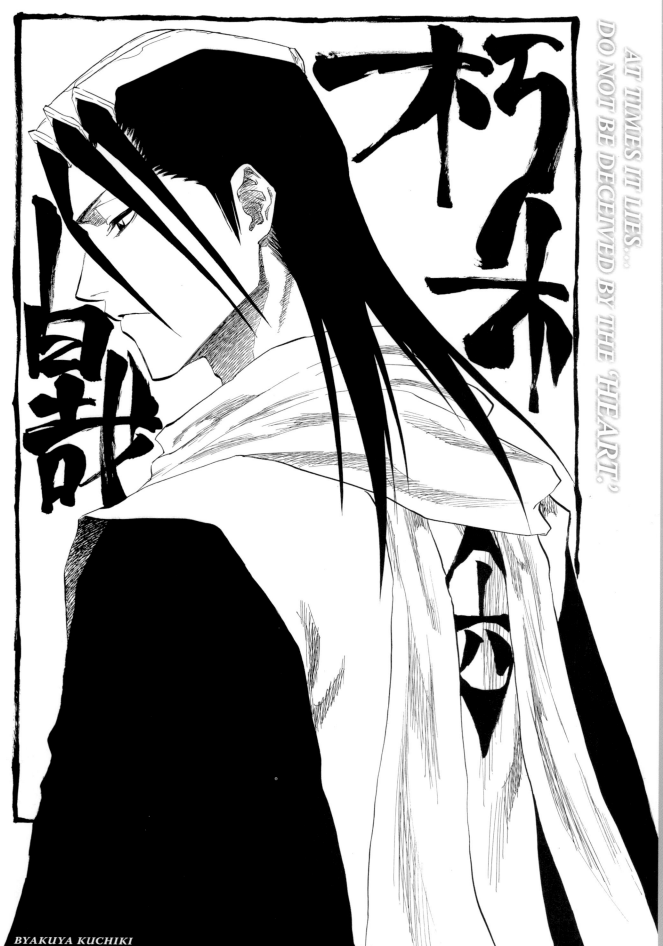

AT TIMES IT LIES...
DO NOT BE DECEIVED BY THE "HEART."

BYAKUYA KUCHIKI

THIS BODY MAY BE IMMENSE...
BUT NOT ENOUGH TO CONTAIN MY LOYALTY!

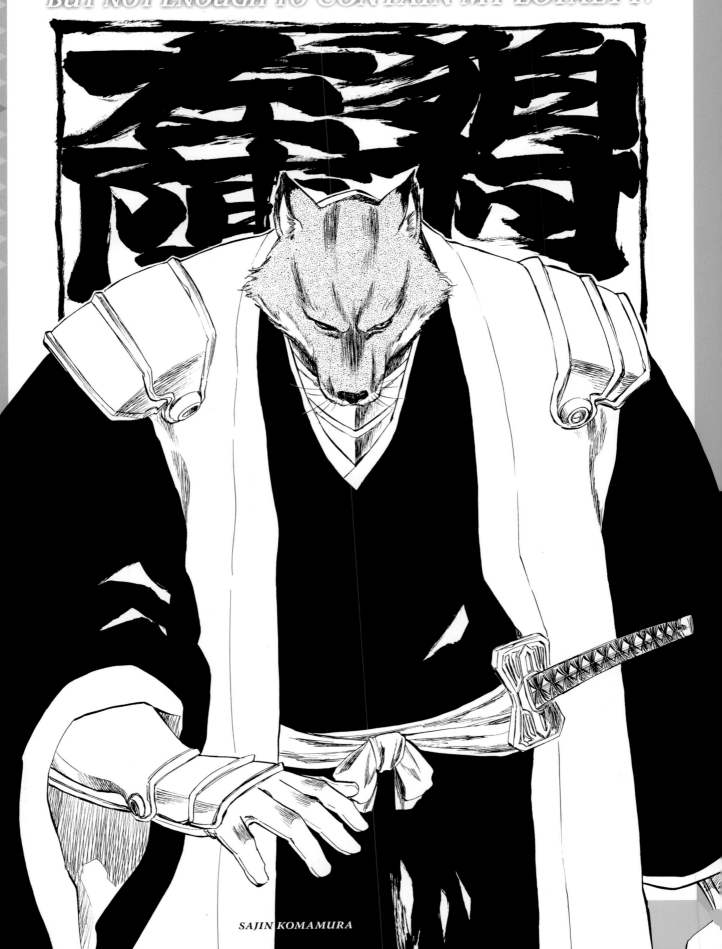

SAJIN KOMAMURA

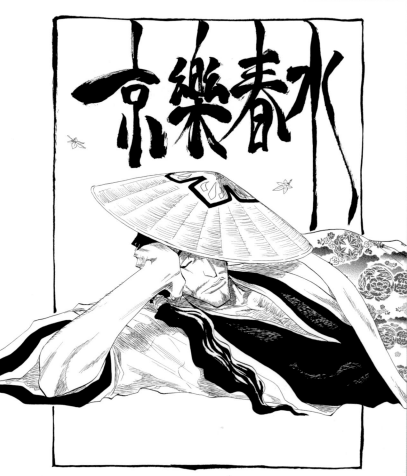

IDLY DRINK...
IDLY
DAYDREAM...

京樂春水

SHUNSUI KYÔRAKU

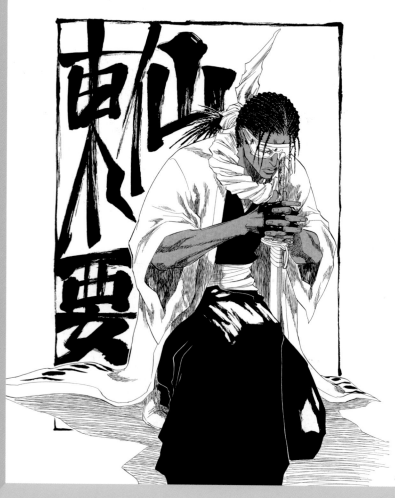

東仙要

KNOWING
IT IS AN IDEAL
NEVER TO BE
REACHED...
STRIVE TOWARD IT
AGAIN TODAY,
AS A MATTER
OF COURSE.

KANAME TÔSEN

TÔSHIRÔ HITSUGAYA

SWELLING CRYSTALS!

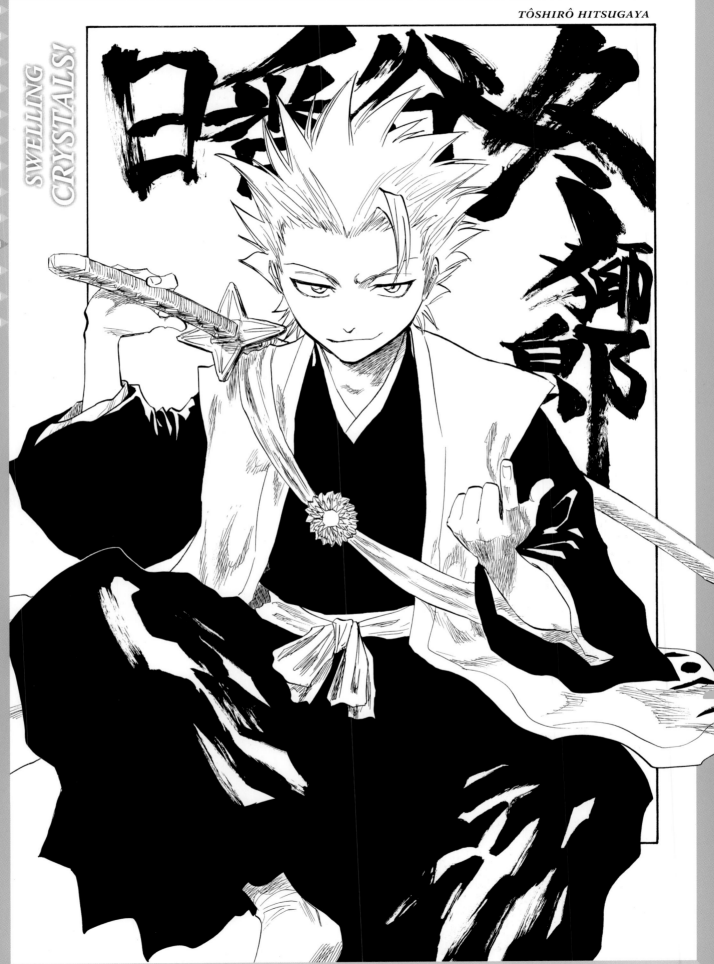

KENPACHI ZARAKI

DO NOT FEAR DEATH. TOY WITH IT INSTEAD. CARNAGE!!

FASCINATING.
THIS TOY
CALLED
LIFE.
PLAY WITH IT,
PLAY
WITH IT...
LAUGH,
LAUGH.

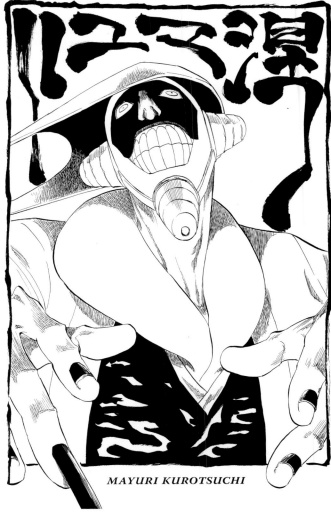

MAYURI KUROTSUCHI

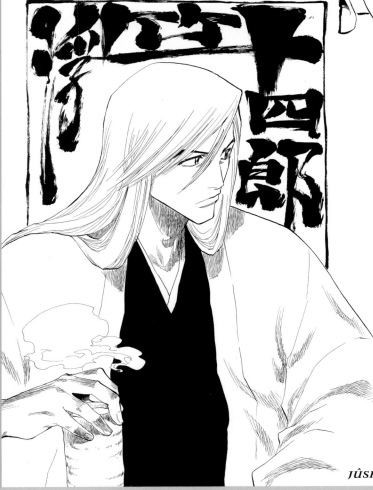

WHAT I
SHOULDER
MAY BE HEAVY.
STILL I HOPE
TO BE
THE ONE
WHO REMAINS
SMILING.

JÛSHIRÔ UKITAKE

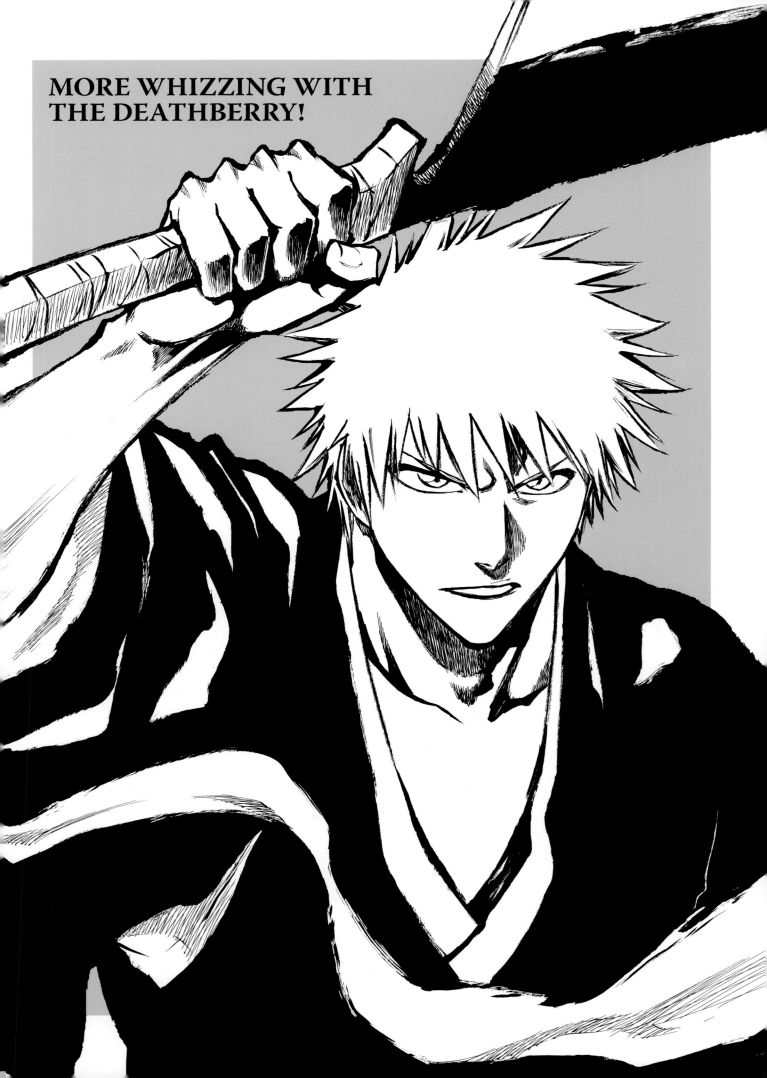

MORE WHIZZING WITH
THE DEATHBERRY!

Index

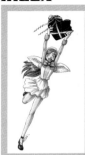

'04 WJ ISSUE 11 POSTER
A cut from the Valentine's Day poster illustration. They wanted an angel outfit, so I drew a super cheesy cosplay type outfit. I say "cheesy," but I don't know much about cosplay so it's based purely on my imagination. I didn't think Rukia would look good as an angel, so I chose Orihime, but I heard a lot of female readers saying, "I wanted to see a Rukia version too!!" But I think Rukia would probably refuse an angel cosplay (laugh).

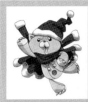

'05 WJ 3/4 DOUBLE ISSUE COVER
A drawing of Kon I drew in place of Ichigo from an issue around Christmas time. I like Kon cuz he always ends up being a little funny no matter what you dress him in.

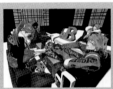

'05 WJ 5/6 DOUBLE ISSUE COVER
The concept here is them as a gang. They were wearing ski masks at first, but there were so many terrorist incidents around the world back then (though there still are) my editor asked if they could be without masks. I thought hard about it and settled on paper bags. But I think it ended up looking kind of cheap. Renji looks cool here. The series of numbers on Ichigo's sleeves is something I use in other places—"BLEACH" written out in numbers according to the order of letters in the alphabet.

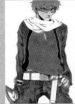

'05 WJ 3/4 DOUBLE ISSUE SUPPLEMENT JC COVER
A different version of volume 15's cover for the magazine. I like the watch covered with fur. I wish somebody would make something like that. When it made the cover, it had the volume number and logo outlined in white, and I'm personally uncomfortable without it.

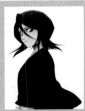

'05 WJ 3/4 DOUBLE ISSUE SUPPLEMENT JC COVER
I designed this one of Rukia with letters printed on her body (volume 15's subtitle "BEGINNING OF THE DEATH OF TOMORROW") so again, I personally feel better with that included. But she looks good here, so I still like it.

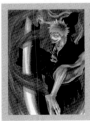

'05 CATCHPHRASE GP POSTER
A poster for the Catchphrase Grand Prix. I like it cuz Ichigo's eyes are lively.

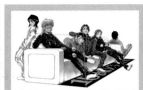

'01 WJ ISSUE 49
The title page after my first editor pushed for a weird concept like "Soul Reaper Five!!" (laugh) I like Tatsuki's pose and Chad wearing a pink jumpsuit cuz Orihime took the blue one. The writing at their feet is the names of the characters on the couch. From the front, 15 for Ichigo, a water drop with the letter C meaning "Water Color" for Mizuiro, K-V for Keigo, 7/7 = Tanabata for Orihime, and T2K for Tatsuki.

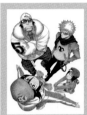

'03 WJ ISSUE 51 COVER
I like Ganju's outfit and Rukia's pose in this one. They wanted something like everybody's looking up into an elevator security camera, so I drew square-shaped lights on the bill of the casket hat, but then I realized security cameras aren't square and aren't that big. But I still left it in.

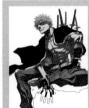

'04 AKAMARU JUMP SUMMER POSTER
A poster I drew for the anime's anniversary. It says "TURN OFF THE RADIO AND TURN ON TV" on the wristband and belt.

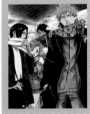

'05 WJ ISSUE 16
A scene of everybody going to school on a winter morning. Uryû and Orihime look cute. I like Orihime's velour jacket in this one.

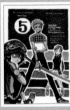

'01 WJ ISSUE 41
Title page for chapter 5. It's supposed to be like a band photo, so that's why there's the (l to r). I received letters saying "Isn't 'Highwell' a little strange for Orihime? Shouldn't the name be 'Abovewell' instead?" But I never heard of anybody having the word "above" in their name, so I used "high." [The kanji in Inoue is *I* as in "well," and *ue* as "up/high/above." And Orihime-sei = Planet Vega.] The "Don't Say to Your Sister" was the subtitle for chapter 5, but I changed it to "Binda, blinda" later. Orihime's hair color is a bit different here than it is now. I think I was using light sepia back then. I'm using a color called caramel now.

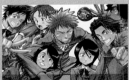

'01 WJ ISSUE 44
A rare picture of Ichigo laughing. One of my favorites from the early years. I stuck a strip of color tone at the bottom so they could print the subtitle on it. But I actually don't remember what they ended up doing with it.

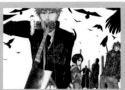

NEW ILLUSTRATION
My new place was right in front of a cemetery and crows would come flying down onto my balcony, so I drew crows. Renji's jacket was inspired by Dolce & Gabbana. Ichigo's belt was based on the belt I'm wearing now. Ichigo's bangs are my favorite part about this.

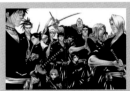

NEW ILLUSTRATION
I really liked everybody singing the title song for the second Rock Musical "The Dark of the Bleeding Moon" at the opening and ending of every performance, so I based this on a scene from that. This is the first appearance of Nanao and Nemu's zanpaku-tô.

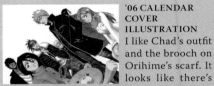

'06 CALENDAR COVER ILLUSTRATION
I like Chad's outfit and the brooch on Orihime's scarf. It looks like there's something like a tiger on Renji's bandana. I come up with the patterns for Renji's bandana on the spot, so I don't quite remember (laugh). That necklace that looks like a cow or devil's skull was based on a necklace I used to wear in high school. I still use it in the comics once in a while.

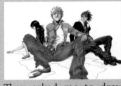

'05 CALENDAR COVER ILLUSTRATION
You can tell it's from the '05 calendar if you look at Ichigo's chest. They asked me to draw something where Renji's looking at Rukia and Rukia at Ichigo, but Ichigo's facing forward and Kon is looking at Rukia, so their line of sight crisscrosses each other. I usually dress Renji in rock 'n' roll type clothing in the comics, so I was surprised when I saw him wearing that outrageous outfit in the anime (Kisuke's prank).

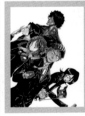

'02 WJ ISSUE 39 COVER
The one-year anniversary cover art for the magazine. I like Rukia and Kon in this one. I also like Uryû taking a peek at Orihime.

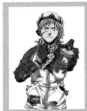

'04 WJ 22/23 DOUBLE ISSUE COVER
This is a cut from the magazine cover where the concept was everybody doing graffiti. The color of the spray can he's holding is grayish blue. The "Sasquatch" on the spray can and the "Beatnix" on the jumpsuit are brand names within the comic. Sasquatch is a mythical creature said to exist in the American northwest. The animal on the can is not a gorilla. It's a Sasquatch.

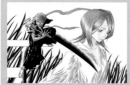

'03 WJ ISSUE 24
My first drawing using colored pencils (Rukia's hair and skin). I felt like it was the first time since kindergarten that I used color pencils... It was kinda fun coloring with colored pencils.

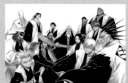

'03 WJ ISSUE 47 POSTER
A poster of all the captains. Ukitake, who hadn't made an appearance yet, has his back turned, and Aizen, who's about to die, has his eyes closed. Back then I had no idea Hitsugaya would become so popular... But then again, he and Aizen mix things up at the end of the Soul Society story arc, so if he didn't end up being popular, that would've been a problem too.

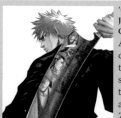

'03 AKAMARU JUMP SPRING COVER
An *Akamaru Jump* cover early on in the Soul Society story arc. The captains Ichigo fought are reflected on Zangetsu... but then there's Mayuri. I think I drew him in there cuz I liked Mayuri's looks.

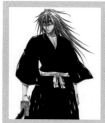

'04 AKAMARU JUMP WINTER SUPPLEMENT JC COVER
A different version of volume 11's cover for *Akamaru Jump*'s supplement. This is the only color version of Renji with his hair down, so it's rare.

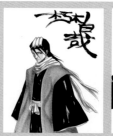 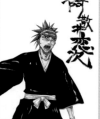

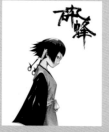 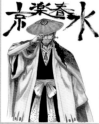

'03 WJ ISSUE 20 COVER
Illustrations that were used in Ichigo's background for the magazine cover. You may think "Why Soi Fon?!", but what surprised me the most is everybody's haori is a different color. (Currently the color of the lining is different for everybody.)

 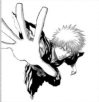

'03 WJ ISSUE 20 COVER   **'04 AKAMARU JUMP SUMMER COVER**

 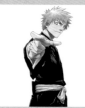

'04 WJ 7/8 DOUBLE ISSUE COVER   **'04 WJ ISSUE 33 COVER**

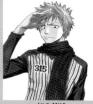 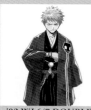

'03 WJ ISSUE 5 COVER   **'03 WJ 6/7 DOUBLE ISSUE COVER**

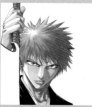 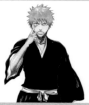

'04 WJ ISSUE 20 COVER   **'05 WJ 21/22 DOUBLE ISSUE COVER**

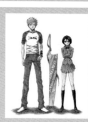

'04 WJ ISSUE 26
A title page I drew right in the middle of the Soul Society story arc, when I was feeling like I needed to draw Ichigo in street clothes and Rukia in her uniform!

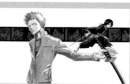

'01 WJ 36/37 DOUBLE ISSUE COVER
This brings back a lot of memories. Chapter 1 title page. I put a color tone over the characters in the back after they were colored in. The second character from the right is Shinji Hirako. There's actually another girl to Orihime's left, but she never ended up making an appearance. She was supposed to be Ichigo's classmate. Her face has been passed on to another character. Ichigo's watch was the watch I was wearing at the time.

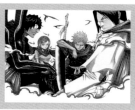

'03 WJ ISSUE 9
One scarf for everybody!! I drew this thinking I want sunglasses like the ones Chad's wearing.

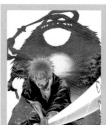

'04 ORIGINAL ANIME DVD JACKET [COVER]
The DVD jacket when "memories in the rain" (Grand Fisher episode) from '04's Anime Tour was animated. The Grand Fisher story arc wasn't too popular when it was being published, so they didn't give me too many color pages, and I had a lot of fun drawing this one.

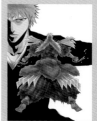

'05 ORIGINAL ANIME DVD JACKET
And this one's the DVD jacket for the following year's Anime Tour. I designed the enemy character myself, but it wasn't a character I created, so I couldn't quite grasp his image, and I made him turn around. But it still left an impression on me.

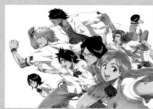

'04 WJ ISSUE 44
A title page I love!! I love everybody in it. Ichigo's watch was based on Naoto Fukazawa's "W11K." The lightning wristband Tatsuki likes to wear in the comics is the same honey color as Ichigo's hair.

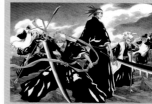

ZŌKAN JUMP HEROES POSTER
I like it because Hitsugaya, who's smaller, and Ikkaku, with his unique weapon, accent it cleanly.

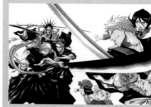

'04 WJ ISSUE 44 COVER, ISSUE 45 COVER
A connected cover when I did two consecutive front covers and color pages for the magazine. I came up with the concept of Ichigo vs. Ichigo myself. It was fun drawing it.

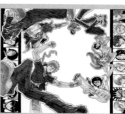

'03 WJ ISSUE 39
This is another title page I like. I like Rukia's one-piece dress. I think this is the only place you'll see Byakuya looking like this. Oh, and now that I've taken a closer look, I'm surprised the color of Mayuri's ears (?) is different.

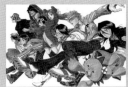

'02 WJ ISSUE 29
A title page with lots of energy I like. I like Mizuiro's hoodie and Ichigo's shoes in this one.

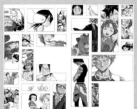

'02 WJ ISSUE 39
And this one's the one-year anniversary DVD's title page. It's simple at first glance, but it took a lot of time. I want Ichigo's goggles and Rukia's headphones. I like designing things that I want but can't find anywhere. Drawing it makes me feel like I found it. I like feeling that small sense of satisfaction.

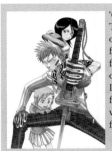

'01 WJ ISSUE 49 COVER
The first cover and opening color spread for the magazine I did for Chapter 8, the first one since Chapter 1. I had in mind to use flashy colors, which is why Ichigo's wearing a flashy outfit.

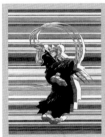

'03 CATCH PHRASE GP POSTER
The first poster I did for the Catch Phrase GP. I drew this wanting to hand-draw multi-color stripes. It took forever to do. It was fun, but I never wanna do it again.

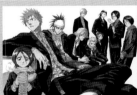

'02 WJ ISSUE 51 POSTER
A spread for the 2nd Popularity Vote. Ichigo's outfit was based on some wallpaper I saw somewhere. I like Kisuke's tie in this one. Hanataro's scarf and gloves are cute too. But man, what is Renji wearing? Is that all right?

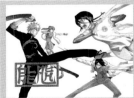

'05 WJ ISSUE 15
The first one of the Foreign Country Series. I like the hand-drawn logo. The Kanji-type logo at the bottom left is actually "BLEACH" designed in a Kanji style. The only person around me who got it without any hints was my third editor Mr. Onofusa's wife.

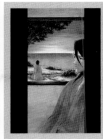

'05 WJ ISSUE 25
An illustration of Byakuya gazing at Hisana from his room. Outside the window is Byakuya's garden. A river runs through it. I had fun drawing the setting sun.

'04 WJ ISSUE 45
Rukia in the second frame is cute.

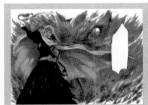

'04 WJ ISSUE 45
The first time in my life I drew flames in color. Flames are fun.

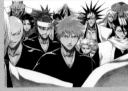

'05 WJ ISSUE 17 INSERT SUPPLEMENT COVER
When I see this illustration I remember how shocked I was when I realized the image was reversed when it was used for an ad inside the train. But then I decided to be positive and think that my skills had improved, since it still looked all right even though it was reversed.

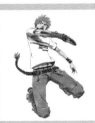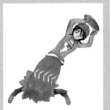
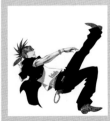

'05 WJ ISSUE 23 COVER
Characters wearing T-shirts I designed for Jump Shop. I remember coming up with design after design for these T-shirts, but kept hearing they were technically difficult to manufacture. In the end they used designs I came up with in a few hours. The cell phone on Ichigo's waist is a cell I love too much and still use to this day.

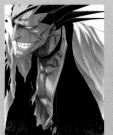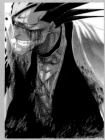

JC VOLUME 13 COVER / ILLUSTRATION
Volume 13 cover of Kenpachi that's famous among the fans. I first had him covered in blood, but they yelled at me saying "It's gonna be stacked in the bookstores!! Change it, idiot!!" So I reluctantly drew another one. Looking at it now, I think "Yeah, if a kid sees this they might get grossed out," but when you're drawing it, those sensibilities go numb *(laugh)*.

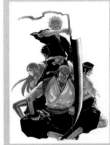

'03 WJ ISSUE 39 COVER
Designers give us a rough idea of what *Jump* covers should be, and we artists brush it up and make it look cool, but I didn't have much time for this particular one, so I drew it just like they asked me to. I have some regrets about this one to tell you the truth. I ordinarily wouldn't make Ichigo pose like this.

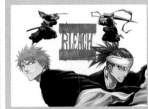

'04 WJ ISSUE 30
I like Ichigo and Renji jumping in the background. I wish I could use the computer to draw simple color illustrations like this one.

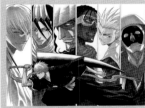

'04 WJ 6/7 DOUBLE ISSUE
Each captain has a different color shadow. I had a hard time finding the right color to bring out Kaname's skin tone. Mayuri hasn't even fought Ichigo, but he sure shows up in color a lot.

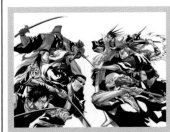

'04 WJ ISSUE 33
A title page I like. It's from around the time (volume 17) I was planning on Ichigo not appearing for an entire volume. That's why Ichigo's not in it even though it's an opening color spread.

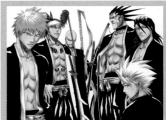

'05 WJ ISSUE 40
Title page with all-out muscles. Reeks of men. It was fun differentiating everybody's muscular structure. I wanted to draw Byakuya, Ikkaku, and Tôshirô's too, but it ended up like this for composition reasons. Too bad.

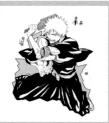

'05 WJ NEW YEAR'S CARD ILLUSTRATION
Every year the editorial office chooses one artist to draw a New Year's card for them to send out. This was when *Bleach* was chosen for 2005. Only people in the business have seen this, so I thought I'd include it.

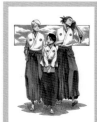

'04 WJ ISSUE 20 INSERT SUPPLEMENT FLAP
Title page for *Jump* in *Jump*'s "Prelude for the Straying Stars." I like drawing Soul Reapers in their school days. I wish I could draw some more of them. But thinking back now, doing 19 pages plus an extra 31 pages of a one-shot story for simultaneous publication is crazy.

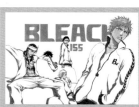

'04 WJ ISSUE 49
A title page I like for all kinds of reasons. Like the white tracksuits, the logo in the back, Uryû's slicked-back hair, Renji with his scorpion-like hair. The chevron (the design on the sleeves) was a softened version of Hummel's Hummel Angle. I chose these characters based on who might look good in this outfit.

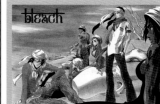

'05 WJ 21/22 DOUBLE ISSUE POSTER
The second one of the Foreign Country Series. It was just so much fun to draw fantastical clothes and accessories. I like the Indian-style logo too.

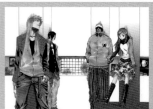

'04 WJ ISSUE 10
An illustration of everybody wearing the same color hoodie!! I like the calm feel of it. I like Uryû's shirt too. Orihime's skirt was based on L'EST ROSE.

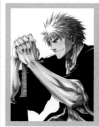

'04 CATCH PHRASE GP POSTER
A poster from the second Catch Phrase GP. By the way, it won. The phrase "Kenzan!!" that's used in all sorts of Bleach related things was thought up by the person who won.

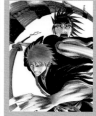

'05 VJ MAY ISSUE POSTER
Cover for *V Jump*. I like it cuz I drew it without thinking too much, yet both of them look good.

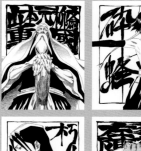 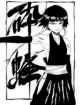 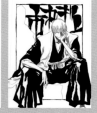 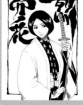 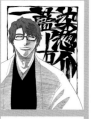
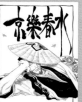 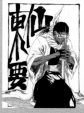 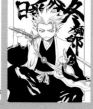
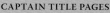
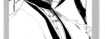

CAPTAIN TITLE PAGES
Writing the calligraphy in the background is fun every time. I didn't study calligraphy or anything. I dunno (*laugh*), I like writing with brushes. I didn't have one for Komamura so I drew one up.

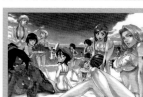

'05 WJ ISSUE 40
My first ever drawing of a beach and bathing suits. It was super fun!! Bathing suits are so nice. It was fun coming up with bathing suits that would look good for each character. Nemu's is so small, so you might not be able to tell, but I thought up the most perverted bathing suit a grown woman can wear then turned it into a school-issued bathing suit. The bottom for Kûkaku's is just a loincloth. The number one highlight is Soi Fon, who was forced by Yoruichi to hold the sliced watermelon and is holding them up with what little bosom she has. Oh, and Nanao drooping her head over her bikini top being washed away and Nemu holding it up proudly.

THE ART OF BLEACH
All Colour But The Black
CREATED BY TITE KUBO

TRANSLATION **Joe Yamazaki**
DESIGN **Courtney Utt**
EDITOR **Pancha Diaz**

Editor in Chief, Books **Alvin Lu**
Editor in Chief, Magazines **Marc Weidenbaum**
VP of Publishing Licensing **Rika Inouye**
VP of Sales **Gonzalo Ferreyra**
Sr. VP of Marketing **Liza Coppola**
Publisher **Hyoe Narita**

Printed in Singapore

Published by VIZ Media, LLC
295 Bay Street
San Francisco, CA 94133

The Art of SHONEN JUMP Edition
10 9 8 7 6 5 4 3 2 1
First printing, October 2008

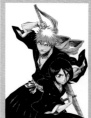

'06 WJ ISSUE 46 COVER

'05 AKAMARU JUMP SUMMER COVER
An *Akamaru Jump* cover my first editor asked me to do and I reluctantly did. But once I started, I was strangely into it. It shows in their faces. Both of them look like they're having fun.